Flat Belly Diet!

150 ALL-NEW MUFA RECIPES

FAMILY COOKBOOK

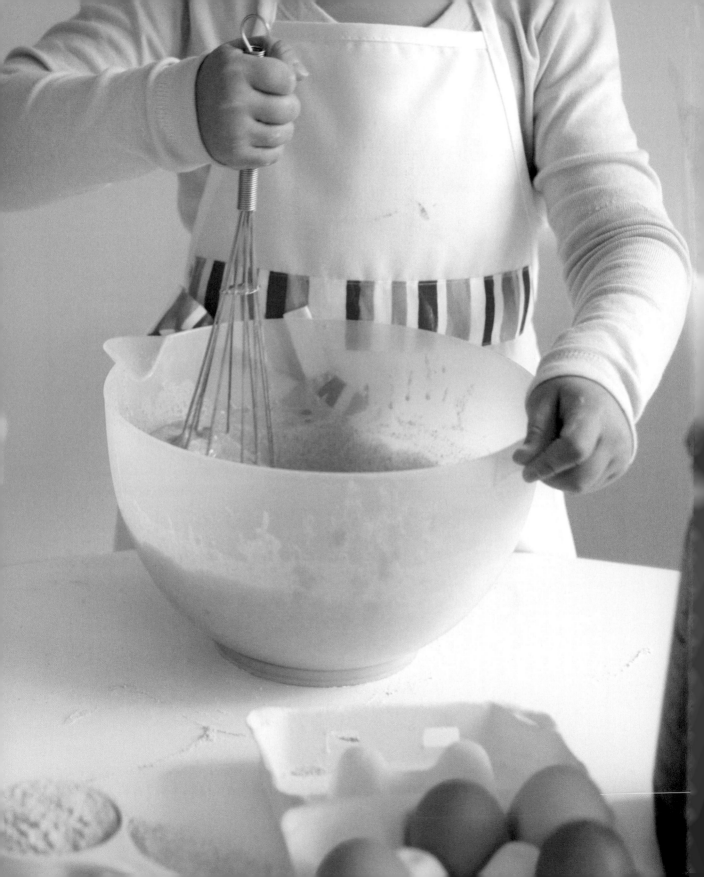

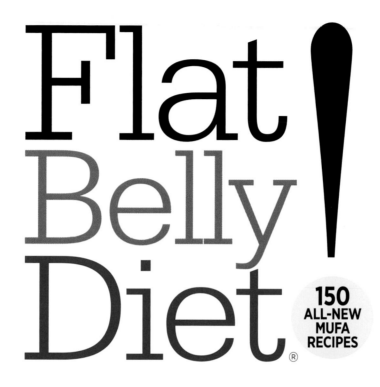

Flat Belly Diet!

150 ALL-NEW MUFA RECIPES

FAMILY COOKBOOK

By Liz Vaccariello

Editor-in-Chief

with Sally Kuzemchak, MS, RD

RODALE

© 2010 by Rodale Inc.

Rodale books may be purchased for business or promotional use or for special sales.
For information, please write to:
Special Markets Department, Rodale Inc., 733 Third Avenue, New York, NY 10017

Prevention is a registered trademark of Rodale Inc.
Flat Belly Diet is a registered trademark of Rodale Inc.

Printed in the United States of America
Rodale Inc. makes every effort to use acid-free ♾, recycled paper ♲.

Photographs © Con Poulos; prop stylist, Pam Morris; food stylist, Vivian Lui; fashion stylist, Elsa Isaac
Cover photo: Spaghetti and Meatballs (recipe page 164)
Book design by Chalkley Calderwood

Library of Congress Cataloging-in-Publication Data

Flat Belly Diet! family cookbook / by Liz Vaccariello, editor-in-chief ; with Sally Kuzemchak.
    p.   cm.
  Includes index.
  ISBN-13 978-1-60529-459-9 hardcover
  ISBN-10 1-60529-459-4 hardcover
  1. Reducing diets—Recipes. 2. Abdomen. I. Vaccariello, Liz. II. Kuzemchak, Sally.
  RM222.2.F5353 2010
  641.5'635—dc22   2009053328

Distributed to the trade by Macmillan

2 4 6 8 10 9 7 5 3 1 hardcover

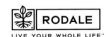

We inspire and enable people to improve their lives and the world around them
For more of our products visit rodalestore.com or call 800-848-4735

FOR KINNEY AND PEEP

Contents

Acknowledgments viii

CHAPTER
1
EAT FOR A
FLAT BELLY—AND
A HEALTHY FAMILY!
x

CHAPTER
2
WHAT YOU EAT
VS. WHAT YOUR
FAMILY EATS
20

CHAPTER
3
FLAT BELLIES
START IN THE
KITCHEN
40

CHAPTER
4
THE BEST
BREAKFASTS
56

CHAPTER
5
BETTER BAG
LUNCHES
80

CHAPTER
6
GRILL MASTERS'
FAVORITES
104

CHAPTER
7
STOVETOP
STANDARDS
134

CHAPTER
8
COMFORTING
CASSEROLES, STEWS,
AND MORE
170

CHAPTER
9
AMAZING SIDES
AND SALADS
200

CHAPTER
10
SNACKS FOR
EVERYONE
230

CHAPTER
11
DELICIOUS DESSERTS
254

APPENDIX A:
Your MUFA
Serving Chart 282

APPENDIX B:
Family Snack Pack
Guide 284

APPENDIX C:
14-Day Meal Plan 288

Endnotes 295

Index 299

Conversion Chart 309

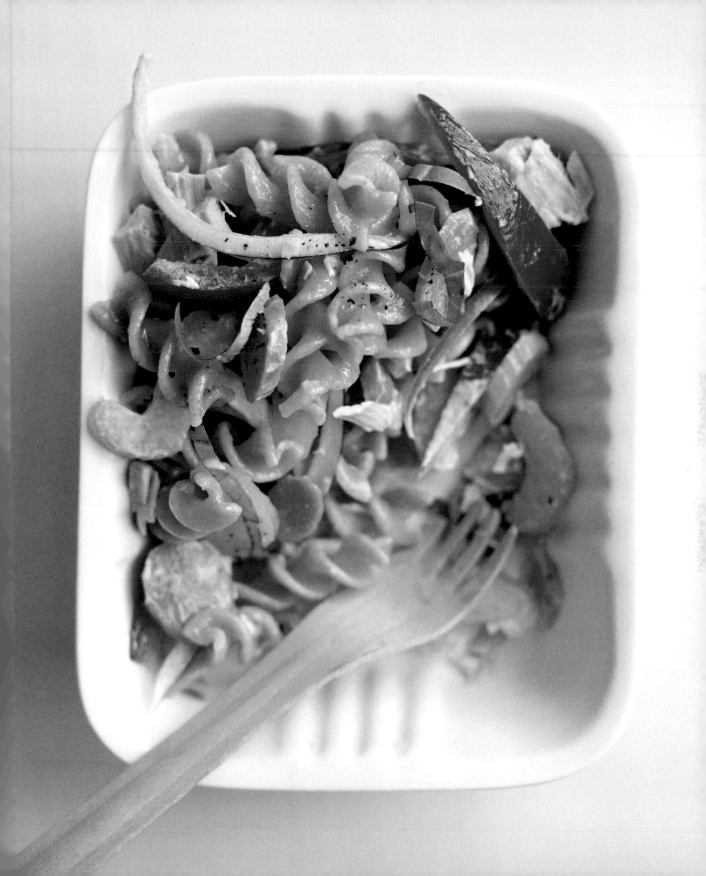

Acknowledgments

An often-quoted African proverb says that it takes a village to raise a child. As you now hold in your hands the sixth book we've produced in the *Flat Belly Diet!* series, we can assure you the same can be said for bringing books into this world, too.

In fact, it's difficult to acknowledge all of the people who helped make this book come to life, but I'd like to start with the people who made sure it would be beautiful and easy to use: Jill Armus, *Prevention*'s gifted creative director; Helen Cannavale, photo director, who assembled the amazing talents of Con Poulos, photographer; Pam Morris, prop stylist; Vivian Lui, food stylist; and Elsa Isaac, fashion stylist. Once again, you've given us something that makes us proud. Great job, everyone!

Very special thanks to Gregg Michaelson, Karen Rinaldi, Beth Lamb, Bill Stump, and Marlea Clark. To Robin Shallow, who never met an idea she didn't improve, and to Bethridge Toovell and Lauren Paul, who are tireless in their enthusiasm, support, and belief in this plan. Thanks also to Susan Graves, Courtenay Smith, and Polly Chevalier for their wise counsel and endless, sunny support. My gratitude to original *Flat Belly Diet!* coauthor Cynthia Sass, MPH, RD, and former brand editor Leah McLaughlin, who were critical to developing the original plan upon which this is all based.

Thanks are also due to the diligence of the behind-the-scenes book crew led by Andrea Au Levitt, Carol Angstadt, Chris Krogermeier, Hope Clarke, Brooke Myers, and Elizabeth Krenos—your teamwork provided the glue that kept this project, as well as several others, moving forward and on track. Thank you!

We were grateful to have recipe developers Shea Zukowski, David Bonom, and Sharon Sanders craft more great-tasting dishes for this collection. We knew they would showcase all the best ways to work with MUFAs, and they didn't miss a step. Shea also did double duty as line editor and project manager extraordinaire. And for ensuring the utmost reliability in all our Rodale recipes, thanks to our vigilant test kitchen director, JoAnn Brader, and her assistant, Stacie Petrovich. We're also glad to have had veteran copy editor Kate Slate join the crew on this round with her fresh eyes and sensible suggestions.

My gratitude to the Rodale family and their special mission, that of inspiring people to live their whole lives. And my most heartfelt thanks, of course, to CEO Maria Rodale, a leader and a friend.

Finally, Sally and I would like to thank our families, especially our children (Olivia and Sophia Vaccariello and Henry and Sam Husenits) for being an endless source of inspiration and insight into children's eating habits (and to Lori, Joni, Katharine, and Liz, who enabled us to work in peace!). And most importantly, huge thank-yous go out to our husbands, Steve Vaccariello and Joel Husenits, for so much encouragement and support through all the drafts, tastings, and late nights.

EAT FOR A Flat Belly— AND A HEALTHY FAMILY!

IF ALL THE OTHER DIETS AND THOUSANDS OF CRUNCHES YOU'VE DONE haven't made a difference to your midsection, you might be surprised by this promise: You can target belly fat by eating rich, delicious foods every day that will also leave you full, energized, and excited about food. It's true! Thanks to groundbreaking science and the tenets of the healthiest diet in the world (the Mediterranean diet), *Prevention* was able to develop the Flat Belly Diet, a remarkably

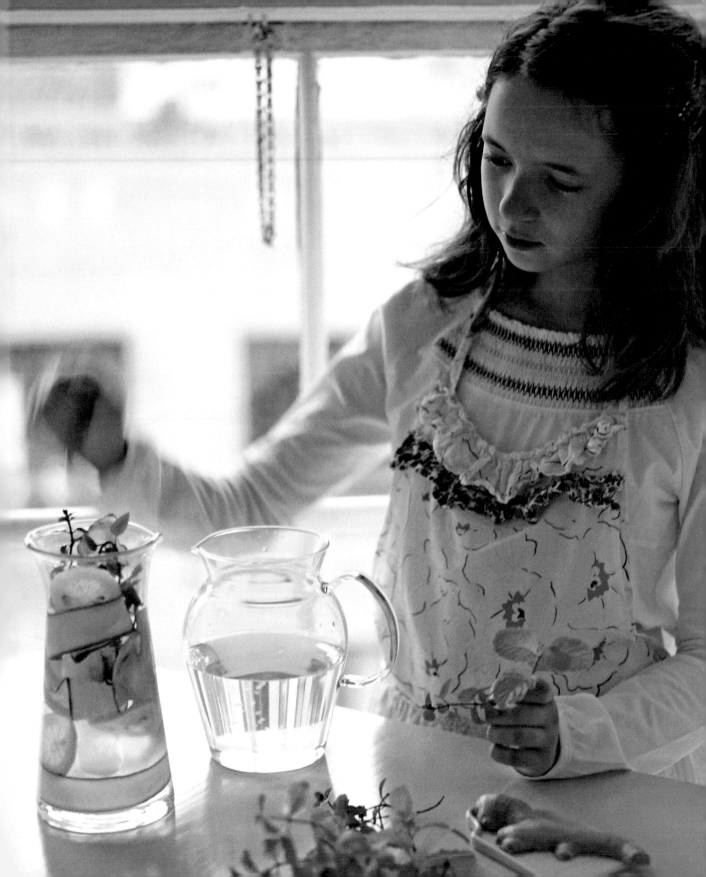

satisfying eating plan that targets belly fat and has helped thousands of people lose weight and keep it off.

Yes, I know it may sound incredible, but believe me, I know how exasperating belly fat can be. In countless letters and e-mails, I've had people all over the world describe the strenuous workout plans and crazy diets they've tried to target their trouble spots. I've been there, too. Before the Flat Belly Diet, I had tried just about everything to shrink my postbaby belly (a belly that expanded to hold twin babies, no less!). But much to my chagrin, I discovered exactly what you did: It. Just. Wouldn't. Budge. What an amazing breakthrough when we developed the diet and saw firsthand how well it worked for people. Some people in our initial test panel lost as much as 15 pounds in 32 days! And their health markers improved as well.

To help confirm what we were seeing, I asked Dr. David Katz, director of the Prevention Research Center at Yale University School of Medicine, to evaluate the diet even further. His team assessed 11 overweight women with excess belly fat, ranging in age from 35 to 65, before and after they followed the Flat Belly Diet meal plan for 4 weeks (they skipped the Four-Day Anti-Bloat Jumpstart).

His findings after only 4 weeks were truly impressive. While the women lost an average of roughly 8.5 pounds and took an average of more than 1.5 inches off their waistlines, Dr. Katz also saw a significant decrease in overall abdominal fat (including fat in the liver), which was measured before and after with MRI scans of the subjects' bellies. He also measured blood pressure, cholesterol levels, insulin sensitivity, and inflammation—and in all areas he saw lower numbers, the type of changes typically associated with a reduced risk of heart disease, cancer, and stroke. We were thrilled!

Scientific backup is important, but in reality we knew this diet worked simply by the outpouring of letters we'd received telling us so. And since our first book was published, we've listened carefully to what our readers said they wanted. We developed an online community Web site at www.flatbellydiet.com and adapted the diet for many different audiences, creating *Flat Belly Diet! Diabetes* and even *Flat Belly Diet! for Men,* for guys who want to get into the kitchen and discover the Flat Belly Diet for themselves. The truth is that the Flat Belly Diet provides an extraordinarily healthy way of eating for most people.

In fact, knowing the food on this diet has such wide appeal, I realized that there's really no reason anyone who is trying to lose weight *and* cook for her family should need to refer to separate cookbooks every night. After all, families are one of the greatest support networks that anyone who is trying to lose weight can have. Why not tap into that power by enjoying the same meals together? And the benefits certainly wouldn't have to stop there. For parents who are concerned about the dangers of childhood obesity, overhauling the family's eating style is obviously a good place to start. After all, when families share meals, lifelong patterns are developed—good habits that can serve them well into adulthood take root. That's why we decided to create this latest collection.

Even if you're the only one in your house looking to lose weight, the food on this family-friendly plan will prove appealing and satisfying for everyone else, too. You'll find dozens of ways to make nutritious meals and snacks that are delicious to family members of all ages—and while you're shedding inches and pounds, you can also feel good knowing that they're reaping the benefits these healthier, more wholesome foods can offer, including a lower risk of obesity and chronic disease and a longer, healthier life.

But what about that word *diet*?

Trust me, I'd never suggest putting your family on a diet—not in the traditional sense of the word. Many of our readers have told me over the years that they've tried so many diets, they associate the word *diet* with trying to resist favorite foods, with hunger pangs and feelings of failure. And you probably already know that kids should never *diet*. As their bodies grow and mature, children need healthy foods to fuel that development. It's also the best time for them to form a positive relationship with eating, not feel the pressure to lose weight or categorize food as "good" or "bad."

So it's officially time to rethink the word *diet*, for your sake and your family's. From this point on, regard *diet* as it was originally meant—a way of eating, the habits and routines that make you look and feel your best. In this case, you'll be trading dangerous saturated and trans fats for health-boosting monounsaturated fats and centering your meals around vegetables, fruits, whole grains, and lean proteins. (Sounds a lot better than nibbling celery all day, doesn't it?)

But before we get to the specifics of the Flat Belly way of eating, let's take another look at all the reasons we should get serious about losing weight around our middles.

WHY BELLY FAT MATTERS

Here's the plain and simple truth we need to take to heart: Not only does our vanity suffer when our bellies pooch over our waistbands, but that dreaded "muffin top" is also a serious health hazard. "Apples" who carry weight around the waist (as opposed to "pears" whose fat migrates to their hips and thighs) face unique risks. Think about it: Most of your internal organs are housed in your middle, so if you store lots of body fat there, those organs are literally encased in fat, which is a metabolically active substance that produces hormones and other substances that interact with the organs next to it. That means they have to work harder to perform all their vital functions. Over time, that can lead to long-term damage and trigger type 2 diabetes and heart disease. In fact, experts now believe that waist circumference is a better indicator of cardiovascular disease risk than measures such as body mass index (BMI).

Clearly, belly fat matters. Yet, if you're a parent, it probably won't surprise you to know that it's not just your own belly fat you need to worry about. Today's kids are bigger around the middle than they ever have been before—and their weight is at an all-time high. The latest National Health and Nutrition Examination Survey reveals that mean waist circumference has increased dramatically for boys and girls of all ages and ethnicities. Among the alarming findings: Compared with kids 10 years ago, boys ages 6 to 11 are a full inch bigger around the middle, and teenage girls carry an extra 2.5 inches of fat on their bellies. Belly fat is also

A Tale of TWO BELLY FATS

You may think of belly fat as the stuff you can see in the mirror and pinch with your fingers. That's called subcutaneous fat, meaning the fat just below the skin. Having a lot of this visible kind of fat can be hard on your heart and your health. But there's another kind of fat you can't see—and it poses serious risks for adults and children, too. Visceral fat, which begins forming during early childhood, lies deep inside your body and wraps around the internal organs. Research tells us that the more of this deep fat you have, the higher your risk of high blood pressure, diabetes, heart disease, even breast cancer and dementia. Visceral fat cells have also been found to increase inflammation, which is linked to nearly every single chronic disease.

associated with dangerous risk factors in even very young kids. A study in the journal *Obesity* found that waist circumference was significantly associated with higher total cholesterol and LDL ("bad") cholesterol levels, lower HDL ("good") cholesterol levels, and higher blood pressure in children as young as 3 years old.[1]

In the last decade, the rate of obesity among preschoolers and teens has also doubled, and it's tripled for children ages 6 to 11, according to the Institute of Medicine. Though there are new signs that rates have held steady for the past few years (instead of continuing to inch up), there's no question it's still a problem. Being overweight or obese may be tough on kids' self-esteem and confidence, but it's even worse on their health. Experts warn that the consequences of childhood obesity may actually shorten life expectancy for the next generation, since those extra pounds mean more chronic health conditions later. Here's some proof.

Diabetes

Once known as adult-onset diabetes, type 2 diabetes may now account for nearly half of all new cases among kids, studies show, and obesity is a major reason. The earlier kids develop diabetes, the higher the risk that they'll develop complications (such as kidney failure or blindness) at a young age.

Hypertension

The current prevalence of high blood pressure among school-age children is 4.5 percent, more than four times what was previously thought, according to a study from the University of Texas Health Science Center. And that figure jumps to more than 10 percent for obese kids.[2] Having high blood pressure in childhood may increase the risk of developing coronary artery disease as an adult.

Metabolic Syndrome

A cluster of health problems (including insulin resistance and high triglycerides) that dramatically increases the risk for cardiovascular disease and diabetes, metabolic syndrome (or syndrome X) affects nearly 40 percent of moderately obese kids and half of all severely obese kids. According to a recent scientific statement from the American Heart Association, metabolic syndrome has a profound impact on children's risk of future cardiovascular disease.

THE FACTS ON FAT

We know that men, women, and kids of every age are at risk of accumulating too much fat around the middle—but what does that mean for the fat on your plate? Well, talk about misunderstood. If you've been serious about your health for the last 15 years or so, you've probably noticed that the pendulum has swung wildly on this issue. For a long time, the conventional wisdom was that fat made you fat, and cutting it out would make you skinny. Remember all those boxes of fat-free cookies that flew off the shelves? Well, we all know how that story ended: People didn't get thin, and many actually gained weight because they went way overboard on calories from so many starchy, fat-free foods. Yet the high-protein diets that came along next were hardly any better. They gave the green light to all types of fat, even the kind in greasy bacon that's notorious for clogging up arteries and raising the risk of heart disease. Dieters did lose weight on those regimens—then quickly piled it all back on when the steak-and-eggs routine proved impossible to maintain in the long term.

Luckily, some of the latest weight-loss research has settled on a middle ground and proves what many of us have suspected all along: Fat is a crucial component of a healthy diet—and a surprisingly vital piece to any weight-loss plan. At the most fundamental level, fat allows your body to perform basic, life-sustaining

Baby FAT

An enormous amount of brain development occurs in the first 2 years of life—and fat plays a starring role. It's a key ingredient in the membranes of brain cells and in the insulated coating around neurons that allows transmissions to zip quickly along. That's why low-fat diets aren't recommended for babies or young toddlers and why parents have long been told to stick with full-fat milk, yogurt, and cheese for kids ages 2 years and younger. But in response to climbing rates of childhood obesity, those recommendations have recently been tweaked: The American Academy of Pediatrics now says that reduced-fat (2%) milk is preferable for kids between the ages of 12 months and 2 years who are at risk of overweight or obesity or who have a family history of obesity, high cholesterol, or cardiovascular disease. If you have a very little one in the family, talk to your pediatrician about what's best.

functions maintain, such as its temperature, cushioning and protecting your organs, making hormones or cell membranes, and absorbing fat-soluble vitamins (A, D, E, and K) from the foods you eat. Fat also imparts that all-important feeling of fullness—something that's missing from so many diets!—which wards off strong cravings and makes it easier to eat less. And of course, research has discovered that certain kinds of fat can even target the most stubborn and dangerous type of fat we carry on our bodies (a lot more on that in a minute!).

But it's easier to put the right mix of good fats on your plate—and in your family's meals—when you understand a few fat fundamentals. Here's what you need to know.

Trim These Fats

When you think about fat in food, you probably picture the thick marbling around a T-bone steak or the lard that your grandmother used to cook, well, just about everything! Those are saturated fats, the type that are mostly solid at room temperature and found in animal foods like butter, full-fat milk, and meat. (The exceptions are tropical oils like palm and coconut oil, which are high in "sat fat," too.) Trans fat is solid as well, but it's engineered to be that way through a hydrogenation process that makes it shelf stable and ideal for packaged cookies and other snack foods. Though trans fats also appear naturally in some foods, many experts consider the man-made trans fats to be the most dangerous type of fat in our diets.

But let's get back to that glob of lard: Picture it traveling through the delicate latticework of arteries around your heart. Scary thought, right? Saturated

Trans Fat TRICK

Trans fats have taken a real beating lately (with good reason, of course!). A lot of manufacturers are reducing or even eliminating trans fats from their products, but you still need to read the fine print. Check the Nutrition Facts label for zero grams of trans fats, and then skim the ingredients list: If you spot the word *hydrogenated* anywhere on the list, put the product back on the shelf. Manufacturers can claim "no trans fats" if there is less than 0.5 gram of trans fats per serving. Those little half grams can easily add up, especially if you eat two or three times the serving listed or have several trans fat–containing foods in 1 day.

fat doesn't exactly slip right through your blood vessels. Instead, it triggers the sticky buildup of LDL cholesterol along your artery walls, making it tougher for blood to push its way through. Over time, that added strain on your system sets the stage for cardiovascular disease. Trans fat also boosts the levels of LDL cholesterol. And to add insult to injury, trans fat lowers your levels of HDL cholesterol—that's the good kind that pulls bad cholesterol from your arteries and transports it to your liver for removal. Results from the Nurses' Health Study at the Harvard School of Public Health show that women who ate the highest amount of trans fat had more signs of inflammation and blood vessel damage (both harbingers of heart disease) than those who ate the lowest amount.[3]

Now that trans fat is listed on the Nutrition Facts panel of packaged foods, you can easily eliminate it from your grocery cart (see "Trans Fat Trick," page 7). You can't completely eradicate saturated fat from your diet, since it's even found in small amounts in healthy foods like nuts. But consistently replacing some saturated fat with healthier kinds—such as sautéing vegetables in olive oil (a monounsaturated fat) instead of butter or grilling a piece of salmon instead of a fatty burger for dinner—has been shown in research to help lower that dangerous LDL cholesterol. It's critical that children limit these bad fats, too: Experts now believe that arteries can actually begin the process of thickening and clogging during early childhood and that kids with high cholesterol are likely to have high cholesterol as adults.

GOOD FATS AT WORK

A dose of healthy fats every day does more than protect your heart—it also helps you reap the benefits of all the other good-for-you foods you choose to eat. That's because the fats actually help your body pull out and use vitamins and compounds that are "fat-soluble" (meaning they require some fat in order to be absorbed by the body). In a study from Iowa State University, people who ate salads with full-fat dressing soaked up more of the vegetables' carotenoids (the pigments that give color to veggies and are converted into vitamins in the body) than they did when they dressed their greens with reduced-fat dressing. Those using fat-free dressing absorbed only trace amounts of those same nutrients.

Get More Good Fats

But enough of the villains—bring on our heroes: Monounsaturated fats (aka MUFAs, pronounced MOO-fahs) and polyunsaturated fats are liquid at room temperature—like the cooking oils stashed in your pantry or the natural oils found in nuts or fatty fish like salmon—and pass easily through your blood vessels. When eaten instead of saturated fats, they can actually help lower your LDL cholesterol. In more news from the Nurses' Health Study, replacing just 5 percent of the calories from saturated fat with unsaturated fats such as MUFAs can reduce the risk of coronary disease in women by 42 percent. You've also probably heard of omega-3 fatty acids and their myriad health benefits, including protection against heart disease, depression, and even some cancers. Omega-3s are a particular type of polyunsaturated fat. Fatty fish such as salmon, mackerel, and albacore tuna are high in the omega-3s docosahexaenoic acid and eicosapentaenoic acid (aka DHA and EPA). Flaxseed, walnuts, and canola oil are rich in another omega-3 called alpha-linolenic acid, or ALA.

Why MUFAs Matter

Both polyunsaturated fatty acids and MUFAs do good things in your body, but the case for MUFAs in particular began to gain ground with the Mediterranean diet. That's the pattern of eating observed in cultures located around the Mediterranean Sea and named by researchers and epidemiologists. At the center of this diet: whole grains, seafood, and fresh fruit and vegetables, plus big helpings of MUFA-rich foods like nuts, olives, and olive oil. When researchers noticed that people in these cultures had significantly lower rates of disease and lived longer, healthier lives, the pieces began to fall in place.

Without a doubt, olive oil became the breakout star of the Mediterranean diet, and research findings poured out about its powers. In a population study of more than 20,000 Europeans published in the *American Journal of Clinical Nutrition*, higher intakes of olive oil were associated with both lower systolic (the top number) and diastolic (the bottom number) blood pressure—not surprising when you consider how monounsaturated fats move through the bloodstream more easily.[4] Likewise, in a small study published in the *Archives of Internal Medicine*, people with hypertension who ate MUFA-rich diets including olive oil showed such dramatic reductions in blood pressure that 35 percent no longer required medication to treat it.[5] Olive oil–rich diets have also been linked to significant drops in LDL cholesterol and triglycerides (another harmful fat found in the blood). And a report in *Clinical Cardiology* offered this exciting revelation: Exclusively using olive oil in cooking could cut your risk of cardiovascular disease by almost 50 percent.[6]

The impressive number of studies demonstrating olive oil's benefits prompted the FDA to approve a qualified health claim in 2004 that you may see on bottles of olive oil and some products containing it. It states that when consumed in place of saturated fats, 2 tablespoons of olive oil a day may reduce your risk of coronary heart disease. The kicker: The claim points directly to the healthy fats like MUFAs in olive oil as the reason for this special protection. However, while the heart disease connection was readily apparent, it would take more research before we would start to see the connection between these powerful MUFAs as a tool for weight loss.

MUFAS' GREATEST HITS

While olive oil may be the highest-profile MUFA, this healthful fat is found in many other foods, such as almonds, avocados, and dark chocolate—the same kinds of foods you may have banned in the past when trying to lose weight. But it's clear from mounting evidence that these foods shouldn't be relegated to the "occasional treat" category. Quite the opposite, in fact: Including MUFA-rich foods in your diet every day will usher in a slew of health perks for your entire family—and not just protection against heart disease. Here's a sampling of what else might be possible with the power of MUFAs.

Better Blood Sugar Control

For people with diabetes, controlling blood sugar (the amount of glucose circulating in the blood) is central to preventing long-term complications. But cardiovascular disease is actually the main cause of death for those with diabetes, in part because people with insulin resistance tend to have higher levels of triglycerides and LDL cholesterol. According to an analysis of studies conducted at the University of Texas Southwestern Medical Center, a diet high in

MUFAs improves blood glucose control and cholesterol levels (including a slight increase in healthful HDL) in adults with type 2 diabetes.[7] A small study published in *Diabetes Research and Clinical Practice* found that teenagers who increased their intake of MUFAs saw improvements in their hemoglobin A1c (a long-term marker of blood sugar control), plus lower LDL and total cholesterol levels, after just 3 months.[8]

Healthier Cholesterol Levels

Cardiovascular disease remains the leading cause of death in the United States, and reduced triglyceride levels and a better cholesterol profile (lower LDL and higher HDL) can lower the odds of getting it. A study of adults from Pennsylvania State University showed that a diet high in MUFAs could slash LDL levels by 14 percent in only 1 month.[9] In a study of 6-year-olds published in the *European Journal of Pediatrics*, those with the highest intake of MUFAs had higher HDL and lower LDL cholesterol and apolipoprotein B (a protein that delivers cholesterol to the cells) than kids with the lowest intake.[10] Another study from New Zealand found that when college students replaced saturated fats with monounsaturated (such as canola oil for butter), their total cholesterol levels dropped by 12 percent—and LDL by 15 percent—in under 3 weeks.[11]

WHERE THE FATS ARE

All types of oils have both unsaturated and saturated fats—it's the ratio of those fats that makes them healthy (or not). Check out the chart below to see how common oils stack up.

Oil	% Saturated	% MUFA	% Polyunsaturated
Canola	7	61	32
Flaxseed	9	16	75
Corn	13	29	58
Olive	15	75	10
Peanut	19	48	33
Palm	51	39	10
Coconut	91	7	2

Metabolic Syndrome: WHO IS AT RISK?

GROWN-UPS

According to the American Heart Association, metabolic syndrome in adults is clinically defined as having three or more of the following risk factors.

1 **Elevated waist circumference:**
   Men: 40" (102 cm) or greater
   Women: 35" (88 cm) or greater

2 **Elevated triglycerides:**
   150 mg/dL or greater

3 **Reduced HDL cholesterol:**
   Men: Less than 40 mg/dL
   Women: Less than 50 mg/dL

4 **Elevated blood pressure:**
   130/85 mm Hg or greater

5 **Elevated fasting glucose:**
   110 mg/dL or greater

KIDS

Though there's not an official clinical definition of metabolic syndrome in children, these risk factors have been used in research to identify at-risk kids.

1 **Elevated triglycerides:**
   97 mg/dL or greater

2 **Reduced HDL cholesterol:**
   Less than 50 mg/dL (less than 45 mg/dL for boys ages 15–19)

3 **Elevated fasting glucose:**
   110 mg/dL or greater

4 **Elevated waist circumference:**
   Greater than 75th percentile for age and gender

5 **Elevated blood pressure:**
   Greater than 90th percentile for age, gender, and height

Reduced Risk of Metabolic Syndrome

Having metabolic syndrome—and more than one-third of American adults currently do—means you're in serious danger of developing cardiovascular disease or type 2 diabetes. And according to a research review from the University of Alabama at Birmingham, the roots of this syndrome seem to take hold during childhood. Though it's characterized by a group of symptoms including high triglycerides and high blood pressure, the hallmarks of metabolic syndrome are abdominal obesity (the dreaded belly fat) and insulin resistance. In a 2004 review published in *Clinical Nutrition*, researchers concluded that saturated fat makes insulin resistance worse, while polyunsaturated fats and MUFAs actually improve it.[12] Another study in the *American Heart Journal* found that people were less likely to develop metabolic syndrome if they ate a diet rich in MUFAs.[13]

Improved Brain Function

Though the exact mechanism isn't understood, unsaturated fats like MUFAs may be protective against Alzheimer's disease, according to researchers from the Rush Institute for Healthy Aging in Chicago. When they followed more than 800 people ages 65 and older, they discovered that those with the highest intake of saturated fats had 2.2 times the risk of those who ate the least amount—while those who ate more unsaturated fats had a lower risk.[14] The same is seen in animal studies: Diets rich in MUFAs and polyunsaturated fatty acids improve both learning and memory, while saturated fats appear to impair them.

BEATING BELLY FAT

At the heart of our Flat Belly Diet plan are these superstar MUFAs. I know it may sound counterintuitive that you need fat to shed fat, but that's just what the science shows us. And it's not just any fat that carries these benefits: It's MUFAs. Not only have MUFAs been linked to the vast array of health benefits you've just learned about, but they've also been singled out as particularly effective at fighting overweight and obesity. What first caught our eye here at *Prevention* was a small study published in the journal *Diabetes Care*, which dropped this bombshell: While diets rich in carbs or saturated fats lead to fat deposits around the middle, a high-MUFA diet with the same number of calories actually prevents the accumulation of visceral belly fat.[15]

KIDS NEED MORE MUFAS When the National Cholesterol Education Program established its fat-intake recommendations for kids and adults, they settled on the same guidelines for both: less than 10 percent of calories from saturated fats, up to 10 percent of calories from polyunsaturated fats, and 10 to 15 percent of calories from MUFAs. But according to a study from Johns Hopkins Bayview Medical Center of more than 400 kids in grades two through five, half of them overshoot the targets for total fat and saturated fat, and half of them don't meet the recommended intake of MUFAs.[16]

When we dug into the research, we uncovered even more striking evidence: In a 2-year study of obese adults published in the *New England Journal of Medicine*, those who followed a low-fat diet lost 6 pounds, while those on the MUFA-rich Mediterranean diet dropped nearly 10.[17] The same kinds of results were seen again in a study published in the *International Journal of Obesity*: People on a diet moderate in fat and high in MUFAs lost more weight than those on a low-fat diet. Even more important, they were twice as likely as the low-fat dieters to stick with the eating pattern 18 months later.[18] A new study of nearly 500,000 Europeans published in the *Journal of Nutrition* finds that the closer people adhere to the traditional MUFA-rich Mediterranean diet, the smaller their waistlines tend to be.[19] Though no one's sure exactly why the body responds so well to MUFAs, it's clear that these amazing fats are a unique (and delicious) weapon against weight.

THE FLAT BELLY DIET PROMISE

What can you expect when you embark on the Flat Belly Diet? Well, obviously, a flatter belly! But lost pounds and inches are only meaningful if you can keep them off for good—and you'll find that this practical, realistic approach is one you can follow every day. I also know you need a lot of flexibility when you're at the center of a busy family, and the Flat Belly Diet delivers. After all, your diet should help you meet your challenges, not create new ones. Here's what else you'll get.

Newfound energy: So many diets leave you feeling drained, but the Flat Belly Diet is designed to energize you. You'll eat a full 1,600 calories a day, an amount that will allow you to lose weight but won't slow you down. It also requires that you eat regularly, which is one of the best ways to fight the fatigue that comes from having low blood sugar.

Satisfaction: The foods that fill your plate on the Flat Belly Diet are some of the same ones you've probably only dreamed about on lower-calorie plans, like peanut butter sandwiches and pesto pizza. Since these foods are rich in healthy fat, they're naturally satisfying—but because you'll be eating just the right portions of these foods at just the right times, you'll be able to savor them and still drop weight.

Choices: If you've been bored with the limited options or mind-numbing repetition of other diet plans, you'll love the way the Flat Belly Diet works. By following the basic guidelines, you can construct your own meals and snacks and swap recipes in and out as your cravings (or your schedule) change. But since some of you have told me that you thrive on structured menus, we've also included 2 weeks' worth of meal plans in the back of this book.

Smiling faces at the dinner table: Every recipe in this book was developed with families in mind. We knew this plan would only work for you if the meals tasted good to everyone and that including quick-assembly meals was a must as well. (Some don't even require any cooking—how much better does it get?) Using our recipes and tips, you can make the meals work with your calorie target and satisfy the bigger (or smaller) appetites of other family members at the same time.

Stealth HEALTH, **Family Style**

Even though you'll lose weight on the Flat Belly Diet without setting foot in a gym, you'll drop pounds faster and experience even more energy if you include some kind of activity on most days. But daily exercise is essential for everyone in your family, especially older adults who need to maintain flexibility and muscle mass and kids who are building bone (and have energy to burn!). You can all get a good workout that doesn't feel like work when you disguise it as family fun. Here are some ideas.

Opt for active outings. Instead of heading to the movies with giant buckets of popcorn, suggest excursions that get you moving, such as going ice-skating or even miniature golfing. Keep a soccer ball in the trunk of your car for impromptu games.

Take family game night outdoors. Play tag, hide-and-seek, or even a round of croquet. Whatever you're doing, you'll be moving your body a lot more than you would by sitting around the kitchen table.

Move more on vacation. Block out time to be active, such as renting bikes, hiking through a forest preserve, or taking a canoe or kayak excursion.

Organize a family Olympics. The events can be as traditional (or not!) as you'd like. Along with running and jumping contests, consider hopscotch, Frisbee, or four-square competitions.

THE GOLDEN RULES

To achieve lasting success and experience all of the wonderful benefits I've talked about—a smaller waist, more energy, reduced risk of disease—just abide by three simple Flat Belly Diet rules.

One: Eat a MUFA at Every Meal

Don't have a meal (or snack) without one serving of a MUFA food group: nuts and seeds, oils, olives, avocados, or dark chocolate. But remember that to get all the perks of these fats, they need to be eaten in combination with other healthy foods, like olive oil drizzled on a fresh green salad or peanut butter spread over warm toast. So while eating a handful of nuts can be a nutritious snack on its own, you'll want to pair it with other foods (such as canned pineapple and a cup of cottage cheese) to make it a Flat Belly Diet snack. And speaking of nuts, because they're so portable, it's smart to carry a zip-top bag of them as an easy way to get your MUFAs when you're on the road.

Two: Stick to 400 Calories per Meal

I'd love to tell you that you can gobble up bars of dark chocolate to your heart's content, but facts are facts: To drop pounds, you must put a reasonable limit on calories. Luckily, I'm not talking about a grapefruit-and-celery starvation diet. The Flat Belly Diet plan provides 1,600 calories a day, an

NEED A JUMP START?

The original Flat Belly Diet includes the Four-Day Anti-Bloat Jumpstart, a plan that quickly shrinks your middle so you start the program brimming with confidence (but inches smaller!). It temporarily removes all the foods, beverages, and behaviors that trigger gas, bloating, and belly pooch and readies your body and mind for the next phase of the Flat Belly Diet.

I haven't included the Jumpstart Plan in this book because it's lower in calories and not appropriate for all family members—especially kids. But if you'd like to get a head start yourself, you can find the plan in our *Flat Belly Diet!, Flat Belly Diet! Cookbook,* or *Flat Belly Diet! Pocket Guide*. You can also go to Flatbellydiet.com to join Flat Belly Diet online.

amount that's just right for the average 40-plus-year-old woman (for the calorie needs of children and men, see Chapter 2). It's an amount that allows you to reach your ideal body weight (and stay there) while eating foods you love and not feeling deprived. You'll spread those calories across three meals and one snack, which keeps your blood sugar stable and controls your hunger all day. Just don't be tempted to try to speed weight loss by going any lower: Eating too few calories can whittle away your muscle mass and bone density and even suppress your immune system.

Three: Never Go More Than 4 Hours without Eating

If you've ever skipped meals and gone hungry in the hopes of losing weight, you'll be thrilled to know that eating frequently just works better—and feels better, too. When you eat smaller meals regularly and dependably, you'll feel fuller and experience fewer cravings because your blood sugar levels stay stable throughout the day. (If I mapped out your blood sugar on this plan, it would look like rolling hills, not sharp peaks and dips.) Steady blood sugar also prevents the fluctuations in insulin levels that tell your body: "Store more fat!" If you've ever felt sluggish and irritable on other weight-loss plans, prepare yourself to feel a lot more energy—and none of the dreaded dieter's crabbiness.

Sassy Water

As part of the Four-Day Anti-Bloat Jumpstart, I recommend drinking a full batch of Sassy Water daily to stay hydrated and calm your digestive tract. Since Sassy Water is a yummy way for the whole family to get the fluids they need, I'm including the recipe here. It's a fun spin on plain water, but feel free to leave ingredients out, use more or less of others, or add fresh mint to the mix. And remember to make a new batch daily using fresh ingredients. Cheers!

2 liters water (about 8½ cups)
1 teaspoon grated ginger (use fresh ginger, not dried or powdered)
1 medium cucumber (peeled and thinly sliced)
1 medium lemon (thinly sliced)
12 small spearmint leaves

Combine all ingredients in a large pitcher and allow the flavors to blend overnight.

BUILD YOUR FLAT BELLY DIET MEALS

New to the Flat Belly Diet? Consider following the 14-day meal plan provided in the appendix on page 288 to get the hang of the rules and rhythm of the diet. (You're also free to swap meals in and out, depending on your preferences, since they're all 400 calories each.) Or go ahead and build your own Flat Belly meals using your favorite foods. Just pick your MUFA from the appendix on page 282, and use this simple road map.

IF YOUR MUFA IS NUTS, SEEDS, OR OIL, ADD:

○ 3 ounces lean protein

○ 2 cups raw or steamed vegetables

○ ½ cup cooked whole grain (such as brown or wild rice) or 1 whole grain bread serving (such as half of a whole wheat pita) or 1 cup fruit

Sample meal: 2 cups mesclun greens topped with 3 ounces water-packed tuna, 2 tablespoons walnuts, and 1 sliced pear

BABY BUMPS AND BREASTFEEDING

If you're pregnant or breastfeeding, it's smart to include plenty of healthful fats, including the MUFA all-stars we talk about here—like nuts, avocados, and even dark chocolate. These foods are rich in nutrients that you and your baby need, such as protein, fiber, vitamins, and the omega-3 fatty acids that are linked to better brain development in utero. But this isn't a time to be dieting. During pregnancy, you require an extra 300 calories a day in the second and third trimesters—and during lactation, an additional 500 calories per day (that's on top of the calories needed to maintain your weight). If you're experiencing a normal pregnancy, it's perfectly safe and healthy to follow the broad principles of the Flat Belly Diet, such as replacing bad fats with good ones, limiting sodium, and eating at regular intervals. Just don't get hung up on counting calories, and don't limit portions if you're still hungry.

IF YOUR MUFA IS AVOCADO OR OLIVES, ADD:

○ 3 ounces lean protein or 2 ounces lean protein plus 1 dairy (such as 1-ounce slice of reduced-fat cheese or ¼ cup shredded or crumbled cheese)

○ 2 cups raw or steamed vegetables

○ 1 cup starchy vegetables (beans, corn, peas, potatoes) or 1 cup cooked whole grain (such as brown or wild rice) or 2 whole grain bread servings (such as a full whole wheat pita, wrap, or English muffin)

Sample meal: 1 whole wheat pita filled with 2 ounces grilled chicken, ½ cup shredded reduced-fat mozzarella cheese, and ¼ cup sliced avocado, plus 2 cups salad greens tossed with 1 tablespoon balsamic vinegar

IF YOUR MUFA IS DARK CHOCOLATE, ADD:

○ 1 cup fruit

○ 1 cup dairy (such as fat-free milk or yogurt or low-fat cottage cheese) or whole grain (such as ½ cup oatmeal or 1 whole grain waffle)

Sample meal: 1 whole grain waffle topped with ¼ cup chocolate chips and 1 cup sliced strawberries

2

What You Eat
VS. WHAT YOUR
Family Eats

IF YOU'VE EVER TRIED TO LOSE WEIGHT AND COOK FOR OTHER PEOPLE
at the same time, you know that cutting calories and keeping everyone else well fed
and happy is easier said than done. Maybe you've tried the "night of a thousand
dinners" approach: You nibble a salad, your husband cooks a burger, your daughter
eats chicken nuggets, and your son noshes on a slice of pizza. Or maybe you've
heard complaints from your kids and spouse about the bland-tasting "diet" food
you're serving lately. Even worse, you may have suffered through cooking a delicious dinner for everyone, only to sit down to a prepackaged meal or diet shake
for yourself. These approaches usually work for a little while, but they all end up
fizzling out because they take an "us versus them" approach that's just too time-
consuming, too monotonous, or too impractical to maintain.

Thankfully, families of all shapes and sizes can enjoy the same flavorful, satisfying foods on this plan. Many of them are already kid-friendly staples (hello,

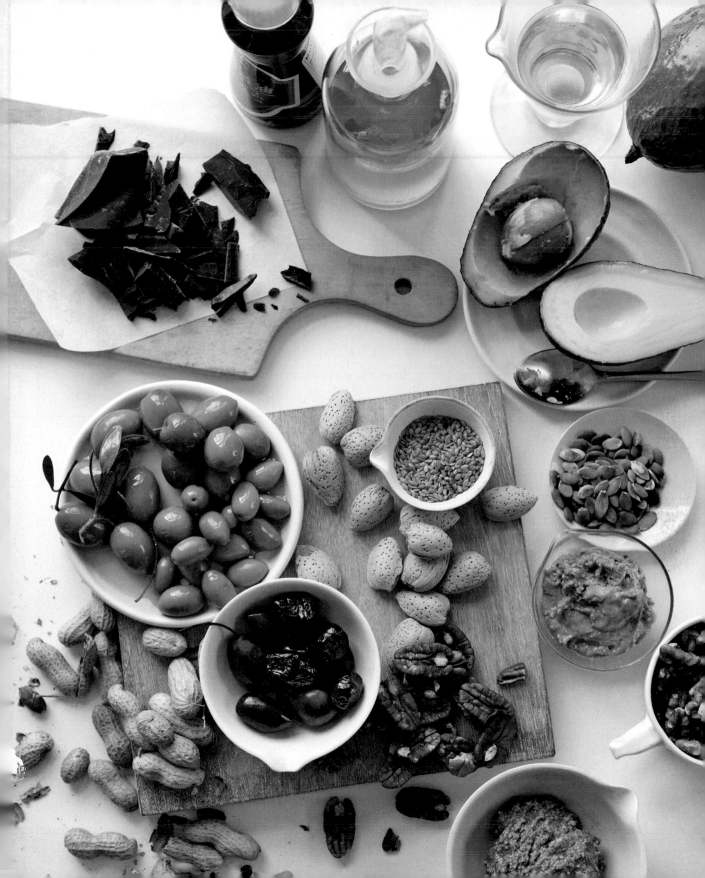

peanut butter and chocolate!). We also knew that including recipes for time-honored family dishes like tuna-noodle casserole and spaghetti and meatballs was a must, and we gave weeknight standbys like burgers and meat loaf a Flat Belly Diet makeover, too. Everyone in your family is sure to find favorites—and we'll show you plenty of ways to make the meals appealing for even the youngest (or pickiest) of eaters. Plus, we'll teach you how to tweak portions up or down for each person at your table and how to keep your calories in check even when a hungry crowd drops by for an impromptu cookout (more on all that later). But first, let's take a closer look at the logic behind this new way to eat.

THE FLAT BELLY DIET FAMILY PHILOSOPHY

t's simple: You don't have to sacrifice your own health and weight goals just because you have a family to feed. You'll reach those goals more quickly if the food truly works with the way you live (I call that being life-proof). Luckily, the Flat Belly Diet is also family-proof. Whether you're packing up lunch boxes or cooking for three generations at one table, we've got ideas for foods they'll love—and you won't have to fall off the wagon to keep them content.

If you're the one in charge of shopping for food and getting it on the table every night, this instantly makes your job a whole lot easier. And eating the same foods, together as a family, is actually good for everyone. Here's why.

You feel closer. After everyone's jam-packed days, mealtime is finally a moment to exhale. In fact, it may be the only time all day when everyone is in the same room together! It's a prime opportunity to share accomplishments, stories, and news of the day. In a survey published in the *Journal of the American Dietetic Association,* parents said that having conversations about the day was the number one reason they enjoyed family mealtime, followed closely by being together, having time to connect, and feeling an increased sense of family.[1] Mealtime brings you physically closer as you gather around the table, but also emotionally closer as you communicate with each other face-to-face—not via text messages, voice mail, or quick snatches of conversation as you dash out the door. (Just remember to turn off the TV and ignore the ringing phone while you're eating!)

Kids eat better. When families share meals together, children tend to develop healthier eating patterns and take in higher levels of key nutrients. In research

23

What You Eat vs. What Your Family Eats

from the Nurses' Health Study, boys and girls who ate dinner with their families every day got nearly one extra serving of fruits and vegetables per day, ate fewer fried foods, and drank less soda than kids who ate with their families less frequently or not at all.[2] In fact, the more often kids ate with their families, the higher their intake of fiber, calcium, iron, folate, and other vitamins and the lower their intake of saturated and trans fats.

It boosts well-being. Time and again, research has shown that regular family mealtimes are protective for kids' mental and physical wellness. In a University of Minnesota study, frequent family mealtimes were linked to lower rates of tobacco and alcohol use, fewer symptoms of depression, and higher grade point averages among adolescents.[3] Another study at the same institution found that girls whose families regularly ate meals together were less likely to engage in disordered eating behaviors. Researchers speculate that family rituals like mealtime help kids by reducing the stress in their daily lives. You've probably found that sitting down with your loved ones every night (or as often as you can) lightens your stress load, too.

Finding FAMILY MEALTIME

Making family mealtime a group priority can be tough. As much as you want to make family dinners sacred, that together time often gets squeezed out by other pressing obligations—like soccer practice, play rehearsal, and work deadlines. In a survey of parents published in the *Journal of Nutrition Education and Behavior*, a full one-third said their lives were simply too hectic for everyone to eat together.[4]

If you can't schedule activities and duties around the dinner hour, do your best to carve out special time: Pick just 1 or 2 nights a week at first and commit to eating as a family. Put it on your calendar (in ink!), just as you would a doctor's appointment or work meeting. Or designate another meal as your family mealtime—like Sunday brunch or weekday breakfast, even if you're just sitting down to bowls of cereal.

If all else fails and you're on taxi duty for your kids all evening, pull together some of the Quick-Fix Pantry Rescues to pack into a cooler (instead of zipping through the drive-thru). You and your kids can nibble them in the car—or have them at a pre- or postgame tailgate—and you'll breathe a little easier knowing you're sticking to the Flat Belly Diet and everyone's getting a healthy meal.

You transform into a supermodel. Sorry, not that kind of supermodel—the kind that shows your kids (whether they're toddlers or teenagers) the healthiest way to eat. Over the years, research has found parents are powerful influences on their children's eating habits. According to a research review conducted at Baylor College of Medicine, moms and dads strongly sway kids' food preferences and eating patterns.[5] Among the findings: Kids tend to like the same kinds of foods—and take in roughly the same number of fruits and vegetables every day—as their parents do. They're also more likely to try a new food if they see their mother eating it first. In fact, moms exert a unique influence on their children, even before birth: Some studies have found that the foods women eat during pregnancy tend to be the same types of flavors their babies end up preferring themselves. For very young kids, you may be the only guide they have for what healthy eating looks like. And older kids watch and learn from you more than you think!

FLAT BELLY PRINCIPLES FOR EVERYONE

Okay, so you're sold on eating together as a family—and, as we discussed in Chapter 1, you're thrilled to know that the same foods that melt belly fat, boost energy, and slash your risk for disease can work for your whole family. Of course, while some people in your household probably shouldn't even be thinking "belly fat" (like your teenage son, who plays three sports and eats food faster than you can unpack it from the grocery bag), it's good to know that many of the principles behind the Flat Belly Diet work for the whole family, too. In fact, they're perfect for any good-for-you eating plan. They include:

Focus on your food. Encourage everyone at the table to eat slowly, and set a leisurely pace for mealtime. You'll likely savor your food and pay attention to flavors more, and everyone will have time to tune in to those all-important fullness signals. In one study from the University of Rhode Island, women who were told to eat slowly and put down their forks between bites took in about 67 fewer calories at mealtime, yet they reported being more satisfied than those who ate faster.[6] Make it a policy to sit down at the table for meals (and snacks too, if you can swing it). Research has found that food eaten on the fly—like the stuff you scarf down while standing at the counter or passing through the kitchen—doesn't register with your brain as well because you're distracted, so you're hungrier sooner.

25

What You Eat vs. What Your Family Eats

Choose whole foods. I'm all too familiar with the realities of time-crunched family life. So packaged foods are definitely part of this plan, and in the original *Flat Belly Diet!* book we included a large list of suggested meal replacement bars, frozen meals, and fast-food options. But I encourage you to build your snacks and meals around mostly whole, unprocessed foods when you can—and we've made that especially quick and painless in the Quick-Fix Pantry Rescues sections. Sure, everyone needs a time-saving frozen dinner or energy-bar breakfast from time to time. But so many of today's processed foods have four kinds of added sugar and mile-long ingredient lists. You don't need all the extra calories, bad fats, sweeteners, and sodium that are typically crammed into packaged foods—and neither does the rest of your family.

ZONED OUT

According to the Kaiser Family Foundation, kids ages 8 to 18 spend 7.5 hours a day in front of the television, the computer, and video games or music devices—that's more than they spend on any other activity (except sleeping).[7] But more surprisingly, a recent study from Ball State University's Center for Media Design found that adults ages 45 to 54 actually log in the most media time of all—more than 9.5 hours a day of mostly TV![8] Considering that this sedentary "screen time" has been linked to a higher risk of overweight and obesity among kids, it makes sense for everyone to dial it down. Here's how.

Decide on a daily allowance as a family, and be consistent with following and enforcing it. The American Academy of Pediatrics recommends no more than 2 hours a day of screen time for kids older than 2 (children younger than 2 shouldn't watch at all).

Be economical with your TV time. Only tune in to your favorite programs, and don't use the television as "background noise."

Keep TVs, computers, and gaming systems in common areas and out of everyone's bedrooms. Ban TV (and text messaging) from mealtime.

Use a DVR to record shows, and skip through all the junk-food commercials. You'll save time, and researchers think ads for tempting foods may spark overeating.

Give younger children coupons or tokens for screen time (they can trade in any unused ones for special time with you), and set a kitchen timer to limit your older kids.

YOUR FAMILY'S CALORIE NEEDS[9]

This is how many calories kids should consume if they are getting:

	LESS THAN **30** MINUTES OF MODERATE PHYSICAL ACTIVITY PER DAY	AT LEAST **30** MINUTES OF MODERATE PHYSICAL ACTIVITY PER DAY	AT LEAST **60** MINUTES OF MODERATE PHYSICAL ACTIVITY PER DAY
KIDS 2–3	1,000	1,000	1,400
KIDS 4–8	1,300	1,400	1,800
GIRLS 9–13	1,600	1,600	2,200
BOYS 9–13	1,800	1,800	2,600
GIRLS 14–18	1,800	2,000	2,400
BOYS 14–18	2,200	2,400	3,200

Eat small amounts often. On the Flat Belly Diet, you'll be eating every 4 hours to prevent the dips in blood sugar that leave you tired, cranky, and hungry. In fact, you're actually required to eat every 4 hours! As anyone who has dealt with a hungry child knows, this approach is especially helpful for small children who don't have a lot of room in their bellies for big servings of food and for older adults who may get overwhelmed by large portions.

Keep moving. Exercise isn't a nonnegotiable on this plan, but it will help you lose weight more quickly and enhance your health even further. Proof positive: Our test panelists who exercised every day lost an average of 70 percent more body weight and 25 percent more inches on the Flat Belly Diet than the nonexercisers—and they also lost it faster. Children of all ages need physical activity, too, to build bones, strengthen muscles, develop coordination, and stave off obesity. Plus, getting kids into the habit of being active *now* ups their chances of being active adults later. So instead of always retreating to the basement for solo treadmill time, try activities you can do as a family, like walking some local trails, playing a game of backyard kickball, or hitting the public pool together.

MEETING THEIR NEEDS

27

What You Eat vs. What Your Family Eats

n Chapter 1, you learned that the Flat Belly Diet is based on a 1,600-calorie daily allowance, which is just right for an average 40-plus-year-old woman who wants to achieve and maintain an ideal body weight (and doesn't want to subsist on rice cakes or spend all day at the gym). But what about the rest of your household? As you just read, "dieting" isn't smart for any child (unless prescribed by your health care provider). Not only can it sabotage normal growth and development, but it can also set the stage for future hang-ups about food and weight. (And if you have an aging family member living with you, remember that most elderly adults don't require calorie restriction, either.) You shouldn't track the calories in your child's meals and snacks as you do for yourself, but see the chart on the opposite page for a general guide of your child's needs. As you can see, most kids require more—and sometimes much more—than you do.

You can help everyone in your household achieve good nutrition by keeping in mind some of the major goals (and challenges) at each age and stage.

Toddlers and preschoolers: Because they're so eager to learn—and imitate all the "grown-up" things you do—it's also a crucial stage for modeling positive eating habits. According to the Centers for Disease Control and Prevention, the risk for obesity doubled over the last 3 decades for children as young as 2 to 5 years old, so it's never too early to establish healthy routines that they can keep for life.[10]

Offer your young child a large variety of foods every day—but keep an eye on serving sizes, since even small kids need to learn what a normal portion looks like. Though every child is different, a good general rule for kids under the age of 6 is to serve 1 tablespoon of every food for each year in age (for example, 3 tablespoons of corn for a 3-year-old). Aim for at least three different food groups at each meal—such as grains, meat and protein, and vegetables. And don't be surprised if your preschooler wolfs down lunch one day but barely touches her PB&J the next. Appetites fluctuate wildly at this time—and young children are naturally good at regulating how much food they need—so as long as your child is growing well, there's usually nothing to worry about.

Young schoolchildren: Your child's at school all day, so a filling breakfast is key. According to a research review from the University of Florida, kids who eat breakfast have an easier time concentrating and do better on memory and problem-solving tasks, and young breakfast eaters are also less likely to become overweight or obese.[11]

And though it's a meal enjoyed away from home, school lunchtime is another area where you can make a difference. If your child buys lunch, sit down together at the beginning of the week and pick the healthiest possible options from the menu. (You can always tuck a piece of fruit or a small plastic bag of raw veggies in a schoolbag as an extra side dish.) If you're packing a lunch, fill the lunch box with small portions of nutritious foods that your child has helped choose. Kids are less likely to trade foods if together you've mapped out the kinds of items they like—or, even better, if they've helped to prepare the lunch (see Chapter 3 for ways kids can assist in the kitchen).

Tweens and teens: Thanks to major growth spurts that usually occur at this time, you'll notice that your child may be asking for seconds (or thirds) at dinnertime—that is, when you actually get to see her. When kids hit the tween and teen years, their schedules start filling up fast with clubs, sports, and socializing. With your child on the go, you suddenly have less control over what she's eating and drinking, and she's much more likely to grab a candy bar with friends than sit down for a healthy snack.

Not surprisingly, one study found that while 59 percent of young kids said they ate dinner with their families five or more times a week, only 40 percent of older teens said the same. Those older kids also reported more scheduling conflicts with family mealtimes,[12] so make some rules about which nights you expect to enjoy a family dinner together; that way, everyone can work toward a common goal.

And when you do pin your child down for a meal at home, pour a big glass of milk: Though childhood is a critical time for bone building, calcium intake dramatically drops during the tween/teen stage as kids (especially girls) swap milk for soda and sweet drinks. In fact, government food surveys reveal that girls ages 14 to 18 get only 60 percent of the calcium they need every day.

Men: Your husband already has a leg up on healthy eating—simply by being

29

What You Eat vs. What Your Family Eats

married to you. According to research from the Harvard School of Public Health, married men eat more vegetables and fewer fried foods and drink less alcohol than those who are divorced or widowed.[13]

If you're the nutritional gatekeeper of the house—in charge of the food that's stocked in the pantry and served for dinner every night—it may not come as a surprise to you that your husband feeds off (literally!) your healthy habits.

So if your spouse is looking to lose weight, you'll be glad to hear he can follow the Flat Belly Diet plan along with you. But because men are typically larger and require more food, he'll need more calories. Most men can drop pounds and still feel energized when consuming between 2,000 and 2,200 calories per day. That means he should have at least one extra 400-calorie meal or snack every day. If he's interested, he can find more details in the *Flat Belly Diet! for Men*. And if his belly is already flat, he'll still benefit from the good fats, lean protein, and antioxidant-packed vegetables on this plan—he can just enjoy larger portions of them.

speed EATING 101

It's easier for kids to slow down (and eat healthier foods) at the dinner table—but definitely not at the school cafeteria. The average lunch period lasts roughly 25 minutes for elementary schools but runs as short as 20 minutes by high school (that includes time spent in line waiting for food or milk). Even worse, some schools let students duck out of lunch early to hit the playground. That means kids are either plowing through lunch without giving thought to hunger or fullness—or running out of time and tossing most of it away. If you pack your child's lunch, include small portions of nutrient-dense foods (like peanut butter on whole grain crackers or a small thermos of turkey chili) and healthy sides that are quick to eat, like peeled orange slices and a homemade bran muffin. Avoid packing sweets, which will probably get eaten first! If your child buys lunch, ask if there's enough time to finish, and look at the menu together to find the healthiest choices. If your child's lunch period seems particularly puny, talk to the principal about your concerns. According to research published in the *Journal of Child Nutrition & Management*, the amount of food kids threw away at lunchtime dropped from 43 percent to 27 percent when they were given 10 more minutes to eat.[14]

Seniors: The basic nutritional needs of your mother or father aren't dramatically different from yours, but aging adults bring a few unique issues to the table. First, calorie needs drop because of less physical activity. But between digestive complaints, medications, and emotional changes like depression or loneliness, their appetites may also take a nosedive. If that's the case, eating smaller portions throughout the day can help meet their calorie needs (timing that fits perfectly with the Flat Belly Diet). Since the senses of taste and smell weaken with age, too, intensifying food's flavor with extra seasonings may encourage older adults to eat. (Just don't compensate with extra salt, since people of all ages get too much sodium already.) Be sure your family member also includes protein in meals and snacks. Though protein is essential for maintaining muscle mass, many older adults don't get enough because protein-rich foods tend to be harder to chew and more expensive to buy. Another key nutrient is vitamin D, which helps reduce the risk of fractures. However, as the body ages, its ability to produce vitamin D diminishes, so the Dietary Guidelines for Americans advises older adults to get extra D from supplements or foods (salmon and fortified milk, orange juice, or cereal are rich sources).

M.I.A. NUTRITION

Kids today are more at risk for becoming overweight or obese than anytime in history. But though their plates may be full, their diets are still lacking when it comes to a few significant nutrients. According to the latest Dietary Guidelines for Americans, children and adolescents are missing out on magnesium, calcium, potassium, fiber, and vitamin E. Luckily, many of the foods you enjoy on the Flat Belly Diet—including the belly-fat-melting MUFAs—also happen to be prime sources of some of those nutrients. Here's how to pick up the slack.

Magnesium

▶ **Why they need it:** It's a player in hundreds of biochemical reactions in the body and an important component of bones.

▶ **Where to find it:** Brazil nuts, bran cereal, quinoa, spinach, black beans, white or navy beans, peanuts

▶ **Featured recipe:** 5-Bean Salad (page 205)

Calcium

▶ **Why they need it:** Childhood is the most important time for forming strong bones, and calcium is critical in that process. At least 40 percent of the body's bone mass is built during the teen years.

▶ **Where to find it:** Yogurt, milk, cheese, fortified soy milk, fortified juice, fortified cereal, tofu, spinach, white beans

▶ **Featured recipe:** Crunchy Crust Mac and Cheese (page 179)

Potassium

▶ **Why they need it:** This electrolyte helps muscles contract and serves an important role in staving off hypertension—sodium doesn't have as much of an effect on blood pressure when you get enough potassium.

▶ **Where to find it:** Sweet potatoes, tomato sauce, yogurt, edamame, bananas, cod, dried apricots, cantaloupe, honeydew, orange juice

▶ **Featured recipe:** Sweet Potato Salad (page 94)

Fiber

▶ **Why they need it:** Fiber makes meals and snacks more filling and helps keep kids' digestive systems running smoothly. Fiber-rich foods also contain more antioxidant vitamins and phytonutrients and have possible cholesterol-lowering properties, too.

▶ **Where to find it:** Beans, lentils, chickpeas, whole grain cereal, apples and pears (with skin), berries, almonds, whole wheat pasta, broccoli

▶ **Featured recipe:** Almond, Oat, and Dried Cranberry-Cherry Granola (page 62)

Vitamin E

▶ **Why they need it:** This antioxidant vitamin helps protect cells against damage and may help lower the risk of heart disease, stroke, and cancer.

▶ **Where to find it:** Olive oil, canola oil, sunflower seeds, almonds, fortified cereal, peanut butter, pine nuts, wheat germ, avocado

▶ **Featured recipe:** Pan-Roasted Sunflower Seeds with Dill (page 234)

31

What You Eat vs. What Your Family Eats

HOW TO AVOID FAMILY FOOD FIGHTS

Most kids—and even many adults—are finicky about food in some way. Maybe your third-grader won't touch a green vegetable or your father-in-law can't stand even the sight of fish. As frustrating as this can be, it's truly better to be patient than to push it.

You may have grown up with a firm "clean your plate!" policy, but experts today agree that this timeworn tenet isn't healthy or productive and won't make anyone a better eater. In fact, a study at Cornell University found that preschool children who were forced to finish their meals at home ate 41 percent more during snack time at daycare, possibly because having no control over how much they eat interferes with their ability to self-regulate.[15] Respecting other people's food preferences (even little people) is central to fostering positive attitudes toward eating—not to mention keeping mealtime civil!

That said, it's still important to (gently) encourage your picky eater to try new foods and flavors. After all, eating a larger variety of foods ups the odds of hitting more important nutrients every day. So here are some strategies to try.

Start small. Don't expect a picky eater to dive into a heaping portion of an unfamiliar food, but it's reasonable to request that she try a tiny amount before passing judgment. One effective tactic is to establish this family rule: Everyone must take at least one small bite of a new food before saying "no, thank you." Or, if your child will eat just one or two bites of meat—but is scared off by a whole slice—put just those two pieces on her plate for starters. Ten years ago, Sally, my coauthor, started giving her veggie-phobic husband three lettuce leaves in a small dish, smothered in vinaigrette, along with dinner. Today, he's eating huge green salads nightly and even ordering them at restaurants (while she beams with pride).

Stay the course. Research from the UK found that it can take up to 10 exposures before a school-age child will try a new vegetable[16]—and it may take years of watching you eat asparagus before your teen (or your aforementioned veggie-phobic husband!) will try a spear himself. Even if your finicky eater has rejected foods before, continue to put them on the table—and try a couple of new spins. For example, if frozen green beans are too mushy, steamed fresh ones (drizzled with raspberry salad dressing) could be a big hit. Avocado slices may get an "eww," but guacamole and baked chips are gobbled up. Bone-in chicken breasts?

33

What You Eat vs. What Your Family Eats

No way. Chicken tenders they can pick up and dunk into sauce? More, please. And as crazy as it sounds, shape can make a difference: Some kids turn their noses up at carrot coins but happily devour carrot sticks.

Make it appealing. With just a little effort, you can make new foods seem downright delicious (and completely nonthreatening) to picky eaters. Serve a small portion with a yummy dip or alongside his current favorites. If your child's never tried pesto, stir some into a bowl of fun-shaped pasta like corkscrews or wagon wheels. For a fish-fearing family member, start with a mild whitefish like tilapia instead of stronger-flavored salmon, and pair it with a side dish she already loves.

Consider giving your dish a fun name. In research from Cornell, kids ate nearly twice as many carrots when they were labeled "X-Ray Vision Carrots" than they did when they were simply called "Carrots"—plus, they continued to eat more of the veggies the following days, even when there were no fun monikers. The researchers also found the same with grown-ups: When a meal was given a descriptive, yummy-sounding name, adults rated it tastier than those with boring-sounding labels.[17] So when your family asks what's for dinner, get creative with your answer and they might just eat more. (You'll find more ideas for making food family-friendly in Chapter 3.)

Get sneaky. Yes, it's important for your child to learn to love the natural flavors and textures of foods like fruits and vegetables. After all, the foods kids grow up eating are more likely to be the ones they'll choose as adults. But when all else fails, employing some stealth-health strategies will deliver the important nutrients your picky eaters need—and they'll be none the wiser. Grated carrots and zucchini can go undercover in spaghetti sauces and meatballs. Purees of sweet potatoes hide well in muffin and pancake batter. You'll also find this strategy in some of our recipes, such as Dark Chocolate Zucchini Bread (page 269) and Stovetop Meat Loaf with Mushroom Gravy (page 166). In research from Pennsylvania State University, kids who ate pasta with pureed broccoli and cauliflower snuck into the sauce ate just as much as kids who had regular sauce—and ate fewer total calories overall (adding veggies boosts the nutrient content but lowers the overall calorie density).[18]

Tread lightly. Battling over broccoli won't make your picky eater dig in—he's more likely to dig in his heels instead. Avoid criticizing your child over food choices. Food is one major area where kids can (and will!) assert their control.

HOW TO PREVENT EMOTIONAL EATING

I f you've ever treated yourself to an extra piece of chocolate cake after a work promotion or crunched your way through a bag of salt-and-vinegar potato chips when you're angry with your spouse, you know how difficult it is to escape emotional eating. Almost everyone has used food as comfort—not just nourishment—in times of sadness, stress, anxiety, and even joy.

To get a handle on your pattern of emotional eating, you need to first learn how to distinguish real hunger from emotional hunger. The real deal feels like stomach-growling, anything-will-do emptiness. But when a strong emotion collides with a strong craving, it's likely all in your head (not in your belly). Finding ways to process your feelings that don't involve food, like venting to a friend or taking a stress-relieving run, can help steer you away from the snack cabinet and ease your emotional burden.

But kids aren't immune to emotional eating, either. In fact, some of the coping mechanisms that you may have surrounding food probably have their roots in childhood. Did your parents take you out for dessert when you made the swim team? Was cheese pizza your go-to stress snack during college study sessions?

PUTTING YOURSELF FIRST

Do your spouse and kids get top billing in your life? When was the last time you put a task for yourself at the beginning of your to-do list? Many women are so focused on the needs of their families that they forget all about themselves—and may even feel guilty when they do cash in me-time for a trip to the mall or a movie with friends. But if you want to permanently change your weight—and therefore your health and your life—you need to get greedier with your time and energy. We're not suggesting you ditch your responsibilities and spend all your time at the spa (though that does sound awfully nice). We simply mean that changing your health habits requires that you reserve special time for yourself every day: to write in a food journal, attend a morning yoga class at the gym, or prepare healthy snacks. When you give yourself permission to take that time, you'll feel energized and self-confident. And ultimately, that makes you a better parent and a better spouse.

Strong connections like these between food and emotions can develop very early on—and it can take a long time to undo those links.

Thankfully, there are a number of ways you can help your child avoid having so many issues with emotional eating later in life. Here are some helpful tips.

Don't use food as a reward. You don't want your child to associate food with being "good." Find alternative ways to show your pride (like stickers for little kids or an upgrade in allowance for older ones), and consider celebrating special milestones with experiential rewards (like a family bowling trip or movie night when everyone pulls straight A's).

Stay positive about food. Maybe you remember having to sit at the table until you choked down your overcooked lima beans (or being punished for trying to feed them to the dog!). Or perhaps you were an overweight child and can painfully recall your parents withholding dessert.

For most people, those are the types of situations that create negative associations around food and eating—and are exactly the types of memories you don't want for your own children. Instead, focus on the message that food is important fuel for the body, that the healthy foods that keep our bodies running like well-oiled machines should come first (but that sensible portions of dessert and other treats can have a place, too). If you stock a kitchen full of healthy, appealing foods and model good eating habits yourself, you'll reinforce those positive messages every day.

Keep mealtime pleasant. Family meals should be a source of comfort for everyone, not a time for quarrels or stressful conversation. Though you may be tempted to discuss difficult issues at the dinner table (you are, after all, sitting down together in one place!), find another time for that.

In one survey of parents, arguments at the dinner table were actually associated with a higher overall fat consumption, perhaps because families ate fatty foods to cope with the stress of disagreements. And always make a point to keep the TV set off during family dinners. Not only does television put a serious damper on togetherness, it's also been linked in studies to a lower intake of fruits and veggies and a higher intake of fat in both kids and adults.

WEIGHTY ISSUES

All children have growth spurts that can trigger sudden weight gain, and lots of kids pack on pounds when puberty starts. But the current rates of childhood obesity are frightening: Nearly one in five kids is obese, and being heavy during childhood can have lasting effects. One study published in the *New England Journal of Medicine* found that 64 percent of kids who are obese at ages 10 to 14 are obese at age 25.[19] So it's natural to be worried about your child's health if she's carrying extra weight. If you're concerned, follow this advice.

DO:

Talk to your child's pediatrician (privately) to get her opinions and insight. She can tell you if the weight gain is normal—and if not, the best course of action to take.

Give lots of praise and encouragement to bolster your child's self-esteem. She may be feeling self-conscious and even have suffered some teasing at school. Let her know that she is special and loved.

Eat dinner together as a family, and plan active family outings whenever you can.

Make healthy foods accessible, like placing low-fat yogurt cups, cut-up vegetables, and washed fruit on a low shelf in the refrigerator. Keep junk food to a minimum (and out of sight).

DON'T:

Criticize your child about her weight or point out slimmer kids her age.

Single her out from the rest of the family with separate food or exercise policies. Instead, make any new health-boosting initiative—like fewer fast-food meals or more after-dinner walks—a family affair.

Talk about "dieting" or your own hang-ups about your weight. In a study from Pennsylvania State University, 5-year-old girls whose mothers dieted were more likely to be aware of dieting and weight-loss strategies themselves. Other research found that teen girls whose moms had weight worries developed their own body-image anxieties. Be sure your daughter (or son) knows that you're following this plan to get healthier and feel better.

Put your child on any kind of weight-loss diet unless your health care provider recommends it. When you restrict her intake, you risk depriving her of important nutrients she needs now.

HOW TO LOSE WEIGHT WHEN YOUR FAMILY DOESN'T NEED TO

We wrote this book to help you incorporate the Flat Belly Diet into your family life because you're much more likely to meet your goals if the meals and snacks you make for yourself can be shared with your whole family. But even though everyone can enjoy the same kinds of foods, you must be especially mindful about your portions of those foods. To shed belly fat—the stubborn and irritating fat that's so difficult to disguise and so dangerous to your health—sticking to the three core rules of the Flat Belly Diet is absolutely essential. Trust me, there will be times you'll be put to the test, like when your husband brings home an extra-cheese pizza or your carefully scheduled day goes haywire. But follow these five pointers, and you're more likely to stay on track no matter what.

Measure up. After a few mornings of carefully measuring out 2 tablespoons of peanut butter for your toast, you may be tempted to start winging it. Resist the urge to guesstimate portions, especially those of high-calorie MUFAs like nuts, oils, and avocado. Even though these foods are brimming with the power to help you lose inches, they're also calorie dense: They pack a lot of calories in a very small space. Just an extra drizzle of oil here or a few more walnut halves there can add up to a very real roadblock to weight loss. The portions of MUFAs on this plan were carefully and precisely calculated—and you'll need to follow them to a T to reap the rewards.

Here's another surprising way those measuring spoons will serve you well: They nix the chance that you'll be too skimpy with your MUFA servings. Downsizing your MUFAs might seem like a speedier route to a flat belly, but you truly need that full ¼ cup of dark chocolate chips or 1 tablespoon of pesto sauce to experience the unique health benefits—and, just as important, the feelings of fullness and satisfaction they impart that will keep hunger away.

So now is the time to head to the local discount store and stock up on extra measuring cups and spoons so you'll always have a clean set on hand (and buy some for work if you frequently dine at your desk).

Enlist your family's help. To be successful, your home environment must support your weight-loss goals, and you may need your family's help to make that happen. Ask your husband to keep his stash of sweets in a high cabinet out of your reach (or better yet, at his office). If your mother-in-law loves to whip up

Keeping an Eye Out for EATING Disorders

Most people (even children) take a stab at losing weight from time to time, but some take it to unhealthy extremes. According to the National Eating Disorders Association, more than half of teenage girls—and almost a third of teenage boys—use some kind of unhealthy behavior to control weight, such as skipping meals, smoking cigarettes, vomiting, or taking laxatives. Girls are especially vulnerable during the teenage years: Forty percent of newly identified cases of anorexia occur in girls ages 15 to 19. Listed below are some of the red-flag signs of disordered eating.[20] If you spot any of these, talk to your family member or health care provider right away, since eating disorders are most treatable when caught early.

○ Being highly critical of herself; complaining frequently about being "fat"

○ Avoiding family mealtime and/or developing strange eating habits, such as cutting food into tiny pieces

○ Exercising excessively or obsessively

○ Not menstruating (or menstruation becoming irregular)

○ Intensely fearing certain foods or the idea of gaining weight

○ Appearing listless or depressed

○ Spending more time than normal in the bathroom

home-baked goodies, tell her how much you and the kids would enjoy a batch of Crunchy Peanut Butter Cookies (page 259) or Pecan Bars (page 265). Don't be afraid to spell out your needs. Chances are when your family sees how important this is to you, they'll pitch in and help.

Keep junk food out of the house. How many times have you brought home cookies and chips "for the kids"—but ended up digging into them yourself? The truth is, children get junk food in plenty of other places, from treats at school to snacks at friends' houses. So why keep a stockpile of it in your own home, especially if you can't resist the siren call of their favorite candy tucked away in the cupboard?

If you want to give the kids a treat, take a special outing to the ice-cream shop for cones. Remember that an occasional planned splurge like this won't derail your efforts as long as you're prudent about choices and portions (like sticking to a child-size scoop of sorbet instead of gelato) and balance it out with some extra physical activity (like a run the next morning). That's far better than the constant temptation of a half-gallon carton stashed in your freezer.

Plan ahead. I know that you don't have a lot of extra time, especially if you're shuttling kids around to activities or caring for an aging family member. Planning is fundamental to any weight-loss plan, but I promise it won't put a strain on your schedule. In fact, we designed the Flat Belly Diet so that you can get a lot done in just a little time. For example:

- **In 5 minutes you can . . .** assemble a couple of Snack Packs from the list on page 284 so eating is a no-brainer on an especially frenzied day.
- **In 10 minutes you can . . .** map out the next day's meals and snacks so you're guaranteed to stick with the plan.
- **In 60 minutes you can . . .** hit the grocery store and stock enough food for a week's worth of delicious meals—without having to dash back to the market midweek or, even worse, grab takeout on your way home from work. (You can log on to Flatbellydiet.com to get customized shopping lists each week based on the recipes you select.)

Put it in writing. I strongly encourage you to keep a food journal throughout this process (especially early on, when you're still getting the hang of the food plan). A large body of research has shown that people who keep one have better overall success at losing weight and maintaining that loss. A food journal works wonders on weight loss in a few ways: It makes you more mindful of food choices (why bother sneaking that handful of cheese curls if you have to write it down?). And if your weight loss seems to have stalled, it can uncover hidden sources of calories, like those spontaneous glasses of Chardonnay during dinner.

It's also a permanent record of your accomplishments. When you're craving a motivation boost, flip back over the days to see all the healthy, positive choices you've made, and you'll be instantly empowered to recommit to your goals. If you take a moment to jot down your thoughts and feelings, in addition to your meals and snacks, you'll also get a sense of how your emotions affect your food choices and where your stumbling blocks might be (late-night stress eating, anyone?).

We've created a *Flat Belly Diet! Journal* to make it easier for you to track your meals and MUFAs, but your food journal doesn't have to be fancy or official-looking. And even if you have time to track only a couple of days each week, you'll still reap the benefits of this simple but powerful tool.

39

What You Eat vs. What Your Family Eats

3

Flat Bellies START in the Kitchen

~~~~~~

NOW THAT YOU'RE ARMED WITH THE TOOLS AND KNOW-HOW FOR shedding your belly fat for good—and feeding your family a healthier, more nourishing diet in the process—it's time to put this plan into action. To harness the fat-melting power of MUFAs and drop pounds and inches all over, head straight for your own kitchen. When you know how to whip up delicious, satisfying, fat-burning meals and snacks, losing weight is so much easier (and so much yummier)—and you're set up for lasting success.

What's so special about doing it yourself? Preparing your own food means you're in control of what you eat every day. The more you're in control, the better your chances of sticking to the basic rules of this plan—the same rules that will lead to weight loss and a lower risk of chronic disease throughout your life. For instance,

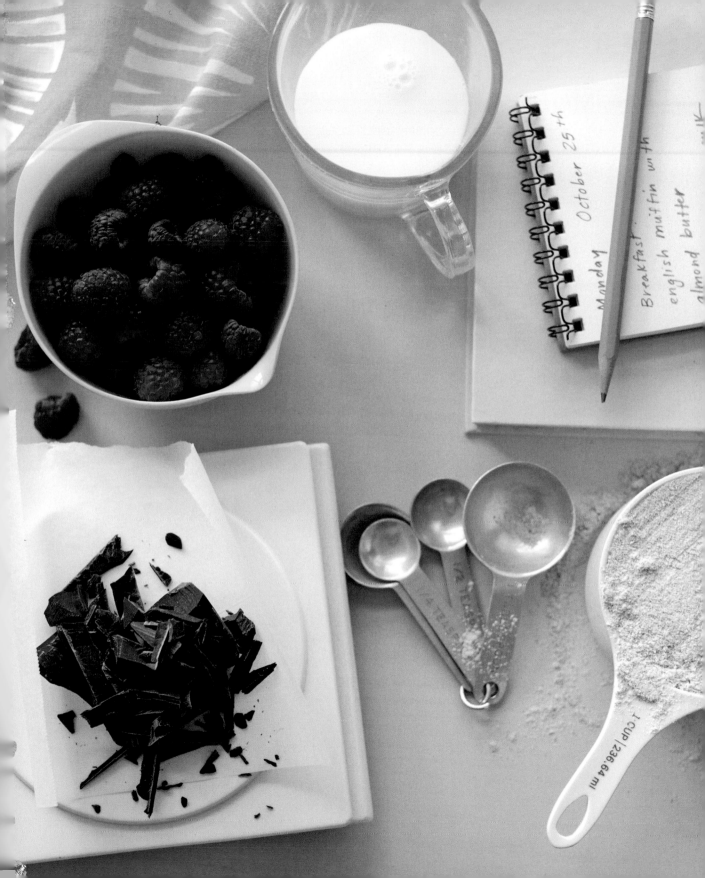

Monday   October 25th

Breakfast:
english muffin with
almond butter
milk

MUFAs Save You MONEY

Everyone knows that making meals at home is cheaper than ordering out. But simply following the Flat Belly Diet will stretch your food dollar, too. You'll spend less by eating smaller quantities of nutrient-dense foods, like a small handful of peanuts or a single square of high-quality chocolate. And since some MUFAs on this plan are rich in protein too (such as nut butters, seeds, and edamame), you'll be buying less meat every week—one of the biggest-ticket items in the grocery store.

it takes less than a minute to measure out pasta, tomato sauce, and olive oil for the perfect Flat Belly Diet 400-calorie plate of spaghetti that fills you up (without filling out your waist). But order the pasta at your favorite Italian spot, and all bets are off in terms of being able to choose your own ingredients. To illustrate this point, Sally, my wonderful coauthor, likes to tell clients about a friend of hers in the restaurant business who revealed the secret to a delicious marinara: a stick of butter melted right into the pot! Talk about a secret ingredient!

So it's no wonder that people who cook less and eat out more end up busting their calorie budgets. In research conducted at the University of Memphis, women who dined out more than five times a week took in nearly 300 additional calories a day—and almost 400 more milligrams of sodium—than women who ate out less often.[1] Does five times a week sound like a lot to you? When you tally up all those work lunches, take-out dinners, and pizza deliveries, you can see just how easy it is to reach that number. Those extra 300 calories a day will pad your frame with a whopping 30 pounds every year!

The same happens with kids. According to a study from the University of California, San Diego, restaurant meals eaten by children are 55 percent higher in calories and contain significantly more saturated fat than the average meals served at home.[2] Even worse, older kids and teens are more likely to get their fix at fast-food restaurants. In surveys, adolescents say they hit fast-food joints as often as twice a week—the same amount that led to a significant increase in body mass index for teen and tween girls in a study conducted at the University of Washington.[3] Other research at Louisiana State University found that kids who eat fast food take in not only more calories, fat, and sodium but also fewer fruits and vegetables and lower levels of vitamins A and C than those who don't.[4]

Believe me, I'm not suggesting that you boycott your favorite bistro or send your take-out menus through the shredder. Eating out is a fact of life for today's busy families and a much-needed break from DIY dining. But you'll lose weight more quickly—and your whole family will eat a healthier overall diet—if most of your meals come from your kitchen. In fact, in a recent survey from the Food Marketing Institute, 92 percent of adults admitted that they eat more healthfully at home than they do when dining out.[5]

And no, you won't be stuck at the stove all day! We know that families also need flexibility, which is why we included lots of dishes that can be made in 20 minutes or less. Or you can shave off time by following the "Make It Faster" tips we've included with the recipes. When time is really, really short, turn to our Quick-Fix Pantry Rescues for ASAP hunger relief.

GETTING YOUR FAMILY ON BOARD

Whether you consider yourself a top chef in the kitchen or a just-the-basics cook, you know that preparing a meal is easier with a little help. So far I've talked a lot in this book about the importance of everyone in the family eating a healthy diet and sharing those foods together and of creating a positive environment where good-for-you foods are valued. But to achieve those goals, it's important to get your family involved at the ground level.

When family members help plan and prepare meals with you, a few wonderful things happen. At the most basic level, they learn to place an importance on

UNHAPPY MEALS

Looking for a nutritious fast-food kids' meal? Good luck! According to a 2008 study published in the *American Journal of Clinical Nutrition,* only 3 percent of kids' meals at fast-food restaurants meet the federal nutrition guidelines used for school lunches. Of the more than 51,000 possible combinations of entrées, sides, and drinks, more than 65 percent were too high in fat, more than half contained too much sodium, and about three-quarters had too little iron, vitamin A, and calcium. Surprisingly, chicken-based meals were less likely to meet nutrition guidelines than those with burgers. Nearly all the meals that made the grade were deli sandwiches paired with fruit and milk.[6]

Ordering a **Flat Belly** MEAL

If you're heading out to a restaurant, feel confident that you can still have fun with your family and put together a safe, Flat Belly Diet–worthy meal from the menu. To make that easier, follow this plan.

Order a protein. One serving of protein (such as a chicken breast or piece of fish) is 3 ounces, or roughly the size of a deck of cards or a woman's palm. Be warned that you'll get twice this (maybe more) at most restaurants. So either split your meat or poultry with your spouse or ask if the restaurant has a child- or senior-size portion.

Hold the fat. Ask your server if your meat, poultry, or fish can be cooked without added fat. Order salads and veggies plain, and request olive oil and balsamic vinegar on the side.

Pick your carb. Choose either a roll from the bread basket or a whole grain side dish (such as brown rice) or cup of fruit. Most restaurant rolls tip the scales, and you'll want to stick to the equivalent of one standard slice of bread—so tear large rolls in half, then place the bread basket out of reach. If you're opting for a side of grains, eyeball your ½-cup serving (about the size of a tennis ball) and push away the rest with your fork. One cup of fruit is about the size of a baseball.

Add a MUFA. Bring along a plastic bag containing 2 tablespoons of nuts or seeds to add to your salad, steamed veggies, or fish. Or ask your waiter to bring you some olive oil—just remember to pack a tablespoon for accurate measuring!

cooking. Developing a taste for home-cooked meals means they'll simply prefer the flavors of whole, largely unprocessed foods over packaged and fast foods that are brimming with things like sodium and preservatives. If they consistently choose those healthier foods, they're more likely to stay at a healthy weight and live a longer life. In helping to prepare meals, they'll also make important connections about nutrition as they watch how food groups are balanced and see what sensible portions look like—two things they definitely won't learn at the burger place!

Kitchen helpers feel a sense of ownership in the finished product—and when they're involved in the preparation of a healthy dish, they're much more likely to eat it. In a study from Columbia University in New York City, children who participated in a program that involved them in cooking vegetables and whole grains reported a higher preference for those foods and ate more of them in the school cafeteria than kids who didn't cook.[7] Researchers from the University of Minnesota found that middle- and high-schoolers who regularly helped with dinner prep at home took in less fat and more fruits, vegetables, fiber, folate, and vitamin A than kids who didn't pitch in.[8]

And, of course, when kids are cooking in the kitchen with you, they're not playing video games or gobbling up chips in front of the television set (and neither is your spouse if he's pitching in, too!). It transforms that predinner hour into bonding time. Simply put, cooking brings your family together. And even if you can only find time for a Sunday brunch group effort, you'll still have that weekly shared experience—a time when everyone can work as a unit and have fun, then enjoy the finished product as a family.

CALLING ALL COOKS

Maybe you're thinking, *Dream on, Liz*. If your kids treat the kitchen as the place they dump their backpacks—and your husband couldn't ID a garlic press if his life depended on it—you might feel like you have your work cut out for you. But the reality is, lots of kids love to help (little kids especially yearn to do all the grown-up things they see you do). And if the kitchen is typically your domain, your spouse might simply feel out of his element there—but that doesn't mean he's not willing and able to pitch in if you give him a job to do. Here are four ways to make this happen.

Boosting CONFIDENCE-Building SKILLS

According to research, kids who learn to prepare meals report a higher "self-efficacy" (or confidence in their abilities) for cooking. Older kids gain experience that will serve them well later, when they're on their own and fending for themselves (think of all those college kids who barely know how to boil water!). And for young children, simple tasks like spreading peanut butter onto bread with a butter knife or measuring out a cup of flour will help hone their still-developing fine-motor skills.

THE NAME GAME

Want to spark motivation even more? Name a dish after your family member if he had a big hand in making it—think "Eggs à la Grandpa" or "Kate's Spicy Noodles." Then occasionally request their signature dishes (and watch the proud looks spread across their faces!).

Give them a say. Meal prep begins with meal planning, and it's important that your family has input on the menu. Look through this book together, and talk about which dishes look or sound especially good to each person. Everyone can even take turns picking a new recipe and be in charge of tracking down the ingredients in the pantry or making a list of what's needed at the market.

Assign age-appropriate jobs. Even if they're too young or inexperienced to head up dinner preparations alone, all family members can take on jobs—big and small—that will help them feel invested in the meal. For the recipes in this book, we've made it simple to dole out duties to kitchen helpers: Just look for the "Make It a Team Effort" box that accompanies some of the recipes for specific ideas on how anyone can pitch in. In the meantime, here are 20 specific tasks they can tackle in the kitchen right now—and that you can subtract from your own list!

YOUNG KIDS CAN:
o Measure dry ingredients like oatmeal
o Stir pancake or muffin batter
o Load berries into the blender
o Dry lettuce in the salad spinner
o Rinse off vegetables
o Put liners in a muffin tin
o Spread pesto onto pizza crusts
o Sprinkle nuts into cereal
o Snap the ends off green beans
o Put place mats and napkins on the table

OLDER KIDS CAN:

o Grate cheese

o Operate a hand mixer or blender

o Measure liquid ingredients

o Whisk salad dressing together

o Drop cookie dough onto a baking sheet

o Roll chicken breasts or fish fillets in breading

o Crack eggs

o Cut herbs with kitchen scissors

o Put garlic cloves through a press

o Pour drinks and arrange silverware on the table

Grow a garden. There's nothing that piques an interest in cooking like growing your own fresh ingredients. Picking that first ripe red pepper or strawberry instills pride, satisfaction, and motivation to turn the harvest into a meal, no matter what your age. And if you've ever tasted a fruit or vegetable straight from the stem, you also know how much tastier fresh produce really is. Many studies have shown that when kids grow a garden, they're actually more willing to taste the fruits (and veggies) of their labors. One recent study from St. Louis University found that children who grew up eating homegrown fruits and vegetables were twice as likely to get five servings a day—and they reported liking the taste of fruits and veggies much more than kids who didn't eat fresh produce.[9] The same goes for adults: In research from Michigan State University, men and women who participated in a community garden ate fruits and vegetables 1.4 times more per day and were 3.5 times more likely to eat produce nearly every day than nongardeners.[10] Even if you have space for only a container of tomato plants on a balcony or small pots of herbs on your windowsill, your family will still reap the benefits. Look through this book to find recipes that feature the crops you've grown.

Offer gratitude and praise. Be sure your family members know that you appreciate their assistance—and that you enjoy spending time with them in the kitchen. Make a big deal about it at the dinner table when they've lent a hand. Both kids and adults thrive on positive reinforcement, so if you want their help again, take care to tell them just how truly helpful they are.

KEEP A **KID-SAFE** KITCHEN

It's fun and rewarding to have your children prepare meals with you, but remember to review these commonsense safety precautions before you start cooking.

○ Pull out plastic measuring cups and bowls for little ones to use instead of breakable glass ones.

○ Keep blenders and food processors unplugged if your young child is helping you put ingredients into them.

○ Turn all pot handles toward the back of the stove so young kids can't reach them or accidentally knock pots off the stovetop.

○ Always supervise older children who are using knives, and remind them to always point the blade away from themselves. Younger kids should use plastic knives when cutting or spreading.

○ If you have an electric stove, warn kids that the stovetop may still be hot even if the burner is off.

○ Make sure kids understand the basics of food safety—such as using separate cutting boards for meats and veggies and always washing their hands before and after handling food.

MAKING MUFAS FAMILY-FRIENDLY

The MUFAs that will melt away belly fat and slash your risk for disease are naturally delicious. (What's not to love about a handful of buttery cashews or a piece of rich dark chocolate?) And we've designed the recipes in this book to appeal to kids and grown-ups alike. But I know all too well that it can take a little extra effort for some family members to dive into their meals. If you're going to spend time making a dish, you want to make sure it's not only something that's nutritious for everyone, but also something everyone will actually eat.

First, ditch the notion that you dine on "grown-up" food while your children nosh on "kid food." You can start with the same basic ingredients and, with just a few tweaks here and there, make meals and snacks even more family-friendly. Here are some ideas to get you started.

Divide and conquer. Different family members may be fussy about the ingredients in their meal. You know the routine: Your husband doesn't like onions, your son wants extra cheese, and your daughter won't touch anything green.

When you're assembling food for these kinds of eaters, deconstruct the meal and allow everyone to "build" theirs instead. Some meals naturally lend themselves to this concept. Give everyone individual whole wheat pizza shells or whole grain tortillas, and arrange bowls of toppings or fillings to make a pizza or burrito "bar." Do the same with breakfast: Everyone gets a bowl of plain cooked oats and chooses from spices, dried fruits, and nuts and seeds for toppings. When family members are in charge of making their own meals, they feel more in control (and therefore more likely to dig in!).

Take a walk on the mild side. Kids taste foods in different ways than adults do. They typically prefer mild or sweet flavors—and they're usually not as accepting of the spicy or even slightly bitter flavor of some grown-up favorites. When possible, avoid spicing their portion of food too much. Then either allow them to add some spice once they've tasted it or season it with something you already know they love, like a little garlic or a sprinkle of grated Parmesan. And if your

Shopping WITH KIDS

If you're the designated food shopper in your household, you're probably used to speeding through the aisles on autopilot. But when your kids tag along, you can teach them valuable lessons about nutrition while you get your groceries. Here's how to make the trip worthwhile.

Draw up a shopping list of healthy choices together (such as bananas, yogurt, and brown rice) before you go.

Talk about the different colors and varieties of produce; while you're walking the aisles, allow kids to pick a special fruit or vegetable that looks particularly good to them.

Name different food groups as you're placing foods in the cart, and explain how they help the body in different ways, such as "Dairy builds strong bones" or "Grains boost your energy level."

Point out different foods and talk about balancing ones that help the body grow (like beans) with those that are "sometimes" treats (like chips).

Give your child practice making her own good choices. Ask her to choose between two kinds of whole grain crackers or select fun-shaped pasta.

Look at food labels with older kids, comparing grams of sugar in cereals or sizing up the fat in different kinds of ice cream. Point out sneaky labeling tricks, such as "fruit punch" packing mostly sugar.

child (or spouse!) is likely to reject a food because he "doesn't like the little green things," do the same for toppings like scallions and chopped basil.

Up the fun quotient. You know the old saying about real estate: "location, location, location"? When it comes to kids and food, think "presentation, presentation, presentation." For many kids, the way food looks is just as vital as—and sometimes even more vital than—how it tastes. That said, I know you don't have a ton of extra time to make sailboats out of squash or spell out your child's name with raisins. But in very little time and with very simple tools, you can turn something basic into something special. Use a cookie cutter to make tuna-salad-sandwich stars and hearts, skewer fruit chunks onto a kebab stick, or squeeze a mustard smiley face on a sandwich. Another surefire trick: Make one of our breakfast recipes for dinner. Kids get a kick out of unexpected twists, and you'll still be feeding everyone a healthy meal (and sticking to the Flat Belly Diet plan for yourself).

Add a dip. It's a universal truth: Kids love to dunk their food. So instead of serving a sauce on top of their main course, simply pour it into a small dish and serve it on the side as a dip. Many of the recipes in this book, like Fish Nuggets with Tartar Sauce (page 177) or Shrimp and Broccoli with Peanut BBQ Sauce (page 144), include a pretty tasty dunking dip served on the side. When all else fails, remember that 1 tablespoon of ketchup has just 15 calories and 167 milligrams of sodium—and if it makes their scrambled eggs or chicken disappear, it's well worth it.

Keep the quality. Nobody likes mushy, lifeless vegetables. Raw ones are a much easier sell, especially if they're arranged on a tray as an "appetizer" for hungry family members before dinner's ready. And when you're cooking veggies, take care to use a technique that either preserves some of the vegetable's natural crunch (like steaming or blanching) or enhances sweetness or crispiness (like roasting).

Lose the utensils. I'm not asking that you forgo proper table manners, but turning a knife-and-fork dinner into something handheld may actually encourage your child to gobble it up. That's one reason foods like burritos, tacos, pizza, and burgers are so popular with kids. But these hands-on meals don't have to be unhealthy: Scrambled eggs and Canadian bacon are just as good for you when they're rolled into a tortilla and eaten at the bus stop instead of at the breakfast table. And you'll find MUFA-friendly makeovers in this book for no-fork-required favorites like Easy Barbecue Pita Pizzas (page 241), Grilled Shrimp Rolls (page 115), and Caramelized Onion and Swiss Burgers (page 128).

GET COOKING: MUFAS 101

Ready to dive in? It's time to get familiar with the stars of this plan—the MUFAs. Here's a primer on everything you need to know about buying, storing, and cooking with your new favorite fats.

Oils

▶ **Buy them:** Look for oils that are expeller-pressed, a chemical-free extraction process that lets the oil keep its natural color, aroma, and nutrients. Delicate oils like flaxseed should be cold-pressed, which means they're pressed in temperatures below 120° F. Only buy an amount you'll use in about 2 months. Any longer and the oil will deteriorate and become stale and bitter-tasting.

▶ **Store them:** Most oils should be kept in a cool, dark place (the back of your pantry is ideal). A few exceptions are flaxseed and walnut oils, which break down more quickly in warm temperatures and do best in the refrigerator.

▶ **Use them:** Drizzle oil on salads, veggies, and grilled meats and fish or into marinades and dressings. Pick up an oil "mister" at a kitchen gadget store, which allows you to spray a fine mist of oil on foods.

▶ **Serving:** 1 tablespoon

Olives and Tapenade

▶ **Buy them:** You'll find a great selection of olives at many grocery store deli counters or olive bars, as well as jarred on the shelf. Pick up jarred tapenade that lists olives as the main ingredient and contains about 40 calories per tablespoon.

▶ **Store them:** Keep olives and tapenade in their original jars or in airtight containers in the refrigerator.

▶ **Use them:** Yummy by themselves as a snack or appetizer, olives can also be tossed into salads or included in meat dishes and pasta sauce. Tapenade serves as a creative fill-in for traditional condiments on sandwiches or sauces. Though olives and tapenade are rich in healthy fats, they also tend to be salty—so limit

Bagged LUNCH Alternatives

There are few lunchtime staples as dependably delicious as a PB&J. But if your child's school district has banned peanuts from the lunchroom out of a concern for food allergies, you'll be happy to hear that other butters go just as well between two slices of whole wheat. Two tablespoons of almond butter or sunflower butter each equal one MUFA serving, and both pack even more vitamin E and fiber per serving than peanut butter. (Just check the policy at your child's school to see if other nuts and seeds are allowed.)

olive dishes to no more than once a day to keep your sodium intake in check.

▶ **Serving:** 10 olives or 2 tablespoons tapenade

Nuts, Nut Butters, and Seeds

▶ **Buy them:** Select nuts that are labeled plain and/or raw. Avoid oil-roasted or salted varieties, which add extra fat and calories as well as sodium (dry-roasted without salt are fine). Shelled nuts shouldn't be dark, mottled, or shriveled. When buying nuts in their shells from a bulk bin, avoid any that rattle (that means they're old and dry) or have a lot of cracks or holes in the shells. Bypass additive-packed nut butters and look for brands labeled "all-natural" instead. Your pick should contain only small amounts of salt, oil, or sugar (which can be listed as molasses or evaporated cane juice). Steer clear of seeds that are discolored or shriveled or smell rancid or musty.

▶ **Store them:** Stash nuts and seeds in airtight containers and keep them in a cool, dry place like your pantry. Raw, unshelled nuts will last 6 to 12 months; shelled nuts keep 3 to 4 months. You can also freeze shelled nuts for up to a year. Natural nut butters have a layer of oil resting on top, and trying to mix it in is a sloppy task. So store the jar upside down to incorporate the oil back into the nut butter, and keep opened jars in the refrigerator. If you find it hard to spread, remove the lid and warm the jar in the microwave for 10 seconds or spoon your serving into a glass dish and heat.

▶ **Use them:** Sprinkle nuts and seeds onto salads and cooked veggies or into pasta, yogurt, cereal, or pancake or muffin batter. Chop or grind them up for a crunchy breading for fish or chicken. Or toss them with dried fruit in a zip-top bag for an easy, portable snack. Bond with your kids over straight-from-the-jar spoonfuls of nut butter. Swirl it into oatmeal, blend it into smoothies, or spread it onto waffles, apple slices, or whole grain crackers.

▶ **Serving:** 2 tablespoons

Avocados

▶ **Buy them:** Select fruits that are quite firm or give just slightly when gently pressed. Bypass avocados that are bruised, cracked, or indented. Scan ingredient lists on guacamole. Avocado should be listed first.

▶ **Store them:** You can ripen a very hard avocado on the counter for 24 to 48 hours; putting it in a paper bag will shorten ripening by a day. Keep ripe avocados in the refrigerator and use within 1 to 2 days.

▶ **Use them:** With a sharp knife, slice the avocado lengthwise all around the pit. Then gently turn the two halves in opposite directions to separate. Discard the pit and either peel away the skin or scoop the fruit out with a spoon. Avocados can be mashed for dips or spreads or sliced and chopped for sandwiches and salads.

▶ **Serving:** One-fourth of an avocado (about $1/4$ cup)

Dark Chocolate

▶ **Buy it:** Check labels for the words *semisweet*, *bittersweet*, or *extra bittersweet*. Choose chocolate that contains at least 60 percent cacao. Stock up on chips, bars, and chunks.

Darkness and LIGHT

When it comes to your health, dark chocolate trumps milk chocolate because it contains more natural flavonoids, compounds in the cocoa bean that act as antioxidants in the body to block cell damage. But because it packs less sugar, dark chocolate is not as sweet as milk chocolate.

So if your kids prefer the flavor of their favorite milk chocolate bar, that's okay. Just don't give up entirely. Dark chocolate that has a lower percentage of cacao (60 percent versus a more intense 85 percent) will taste less bitter, so it might just be a good compromise.

▶ **Store it:** Keep unopened chocolate in a cool, dry place (not above 75°F or you risk a soft, gooey mess). Opened chocolate should be stored in an airtight container or bag in the refrigerator or freezer. Stored chocolate may develop a slight white coating, which is perfectly safe to eat.

▶ **Use it:** Savor it straight up, melted onto fresh fruit, baked into muffins or quick bread, grated into oatmeal or yogurt . . . we're sure you and your kids will think of something!

▶ **Serving:** 1 ounce or ¼ cup chips

FOOD-PREP BASICS

Technique: Roasting

▶ **Claim to fame:** Transforms plain vegetables into a golden, crispy side dish that rivals french fries.

▶ **How:** Toss vegetables (I especially love cauliflower and asparagus) with canola oil, sprinkle with salt and pepper, and spread on a rimmed baking sheet or broiler pan. Bake at 400°F for 30 to 45 minutes, or until browned and crispy around the edges.

Technique: Grilling

▶ **Claim to fame:** Quickly cooks meat, fish, tofu, and poultry without adding a lot of fat or creating dirty pans

▶ **How:** Preheat gas grills for 10 to 15 minutes and charcoal grills for 20 to

The 5/20 RULE

When you don't have time to crunch the numbers on a food package's Nutrition Facts panel, use this quick-and-dirty way to quickly tell if a product is worth your time: Check out the "% Daily Value" numbers. If you spot 5 percent or less, the food is low in that nutrient—which is great for nutrients you want less of (like cholesterol, saturated fat, and sodium) but not for those you want more of (like fiber and calcium). If it's 20 percent or more, it's high (ideal for fiber, vitamins, and minerals but not so good for saturated fat, sodium, and sugar).

30 minutes (the coals should be mostly gray). Add your food and drizzle with marinade a few times during cooking. Use a meat thermometer to check temperature, and remove from the grill when it's within 10 degrees of doneness—it will continue to cook when it's off.

Technique: Stir-Frying

▶ **Claim to fame:** Creates one-dish, one-pot dinners that cook in record time (with little fat) and are loaded with healthy veggies that keep their crunch

▶ **How:** Cut vegetables and a protein (such as meat, poultry, or tofu) into small pieces. Heat a wok or skillet and add 1 to 2 teaspoons of oil. Add the protein and stir constantly until cooked through. Toss in vegetables, spices, and sauce and stir until the vegetables are crisp-tender and everything is well mixed.

Technique: Poaching

▶ **Claim to fame:** Infuses fish like salmon, sea bass, cod, and halibut with low-fat flavor

▶ **How:** Place fillets in a skillet with just enough liquid to cover them. (Make a simple poaching liquid by adding chopped veggies like carrot and celery, lemon juice, salt, and herbs to water.) Heat until slightly simmering and cook for 20 to 30 minutes, or until the fish flakes easily with a fork and is opaque all the way through.

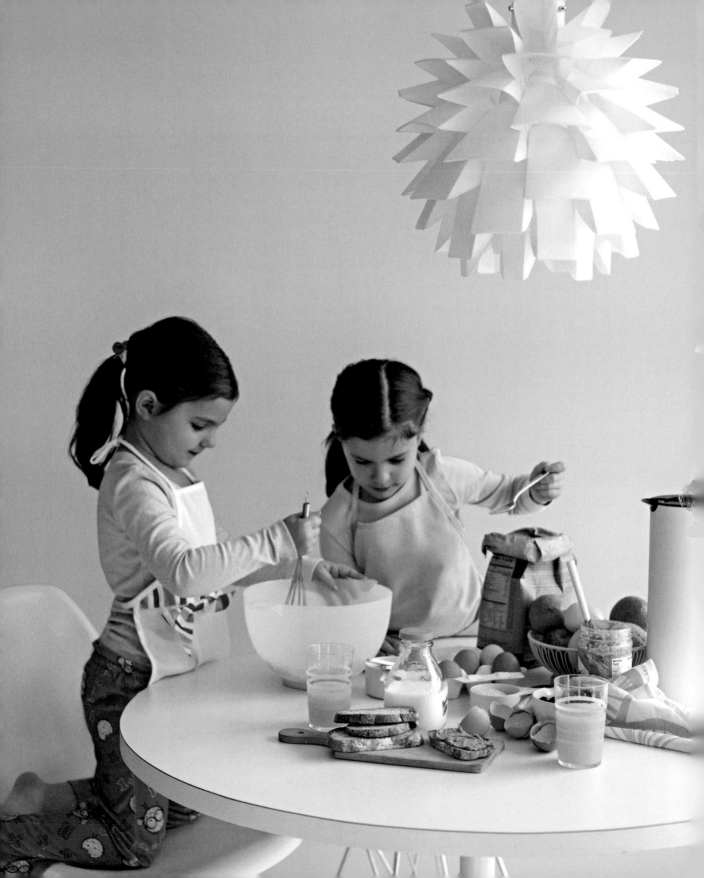

The Best

BREAKFASTS

- Pomegranate-Strawberry Smoothie
- Apricot-Peach Smoothie
- Maple-Pecan Oatmeal
- Almond, Oat, and Dried Cranberry-Cherry Granola
- Scrambled Egg "Pizza"
- Italian-Style Eggs
- Pan-Fried Cheddar Polenta
- Vegetable Frittata

- Pesto Pinwheels
- Chocolate-Stuffed French Toast
- Walnut-Pear Pancake with Maple Syrup
- Berry Good Peanut Butter Scones
- Lemon-Blueberry Buttermilk Muffins
- Banana Split Muffins
- Maple-Pecan Cinnamon Rolls

Pomegranate-Strawberry Smoothie

1 SERVING / 264 CALORIES / MUFA: FLAXSEED OIL

Brimming with good-for-you antioxidants, this breakfast beverage also travels well. Pour your smoothie in a thermos and take it with you for a midmorning or afternoon snack. Shake well to recombine before drinking.

5 MINUTES

⅓ cup pomegranate juice
2 teaspoons honey
¾ cup frozen unsweetened strawberries
2 tablespoons fat-free plain yogurt
1 tablespoon flaxseed oil
4 ice cubes

Nutrition per serving

- 264 calories
- 4 g protein
- 34 g carbohydrates
- 14 g fat
- 1.5 g saturated fat
- 0 mg cholesterol
- 25 mg sodium
- 3 g fiber

1. Combine the pomegranate juice and honey in a small cup. Whisk to dissolve the honey completely.

2. Combine the strawberries, yogurt, oil, ice cubes, and pomegranate mixture in a blender. Process for 1 to 2 minutes, or until thick and smooth. Pour into a glass.

MAKE IT A TEAM EFFORT Kids will like the added fruit flavors of smoothies made with fruit-juice cubes. Buy a plastic ice-cube tray to make cubes from the juice in which pineapple, pears, and other fruits are canned. Place a fine strainer over a measuring cup with a pouring spout. Dump the fruit into the strainer. Have the kids pour the juice into the ice-cube tray. Place in the freezer until solid. Remove the cubes from the tray, and have the kids pack them into zip-top plastic bags that they have labeled for longer storage.

MAKE IT A FLAT BELLY DIET MEAL: Serve with 8 whole wheat crackers (70) and 1 piece reduced-fat mozzarella string cheese (70). **Total meal: 404 calories**

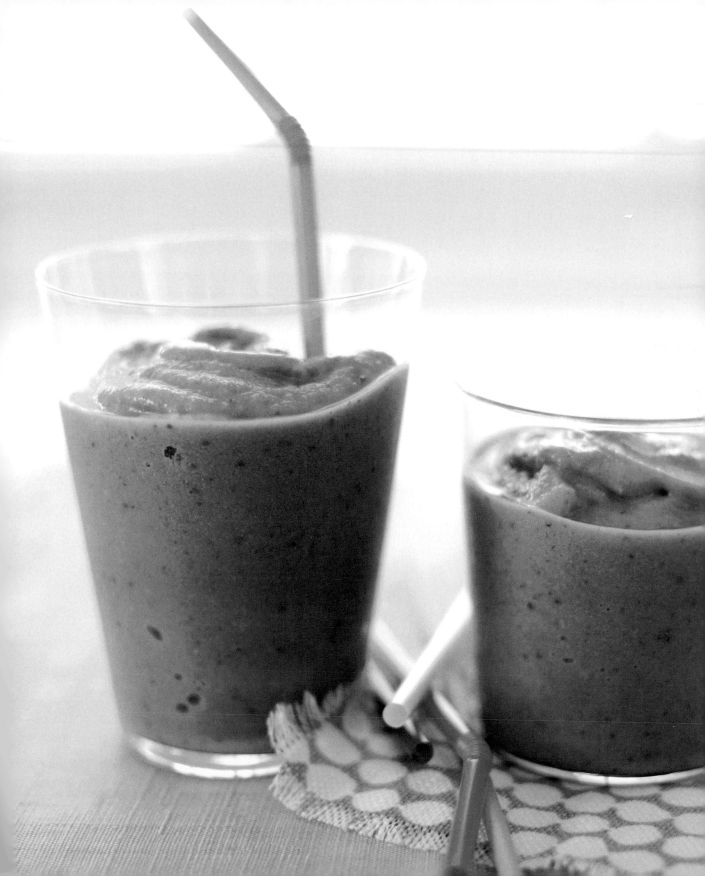

Apricot-Peach Smoothie

1 SERVING / 293 CALORIES / MUFA: WALNUT OIL

Local peaches always seem to be the sweetest. Buy plenty when they are in season and store them, peeled and sliced, in the freezer.

5
MINUTES

½ cup apricot nectar
2 teaspoons honey
⅛ teaspoon ground cinnamon
1 cup frozen unsweetened
   peaches, coarsely chopped
1 tablespoon walnut oil
4 ice cubes

Nutrition per serving
○ 293 calories
○ 2 g protein
○ 44 g carbohydrates
○ 14 g fat
○ 1 g saturated fat
○ 0 mg cholesterol
○ 5 mg sodium
○ 2 g fiber

1. Combine the apricot nectar, honey, and cinnamon in a small cup. Whisk to dissolve the honey completely.

2. Combine the apricot mixture, peaches, oil, and ice cubes in a blender. Process for 1 to 2 minutes, or until thick and smooth. Pour into a glass.

MAKE IT A FLAT BELLY DIET MEAL: Serve with 1 hard-cooked egg (78) and 1 clementine (35).
Total meal: 406 calories

Maple-Pecan Oatmeal

4 SERVINGS (½ CUP EACH) / 274 CALORIES / MUFA: PECANS

Rolled oats are, as the name implies, a flattened version of whole grain oats. The thinner the oat, the faster it cooks, making this breakfast a perfect and easy option for a cold morning.

10 MINUTES

½ cup pecans
1¾ cups 1% milk
1 cup old-fashioned rolled oats
¼ cup maple syrup
1 teaspoon vanilla extract
¼ teaspoon salt
⅛ teaspoon ground cinnamon

Nutrition per serving
○ 274 calories
○ 8 g protein
○ 34 g carbohydrates
○ 12 g fat
○ 1.5 g saturated fat
○ 5 mg cholesterol
○ 190 mg sodium
○ 3 g fiber

1. Place the pecans in a medium skillet and cook over medium-high heat, shaking the pan often, for 3 to 5 minutes, or until lightly toasted. Transfer to a cutting board to cool, then coarsely chop.

2. Combine the milk, oats, maple syrup, vanilla extract, salt, and cinnamon in a medium saucepan. Bring to a simmer over medium heat and cook, stirring occasionally, for 5 minutes, or until the oatmeal is tender. Stir ¼ cup of the pecans into the oatmeal. Serve sprinkled with the remaining ¼ cup pecans.

MAKE IT A FLAT BELLY DIET MEAL: Serve with 1 sliced banana (105). Total meal: 379 calories

Almond, Oat, and Dried Cranberry-Cherry Granola

12 SERVINGS (½ CUP EACH) / 293 CALORIES / MUFA: ALMONDS

Once you have the master recipe down pat, feel free to substitute other types of nuts and dried fruit to make your own special house blend. Just be sure to keep the amounts the same.

45 MINUTES

4 cups old-fashioned rolled oats

1½ cups sliced almonds

1 teaspoon ground cinnamon

¼ teaspoon ground nutmeg

¼ teaspoon salt

¾ cup honey

2 tablespoons canola oil

½ teaspoon almond extract

½ cup dried cranberries

½ cup dried tart cherries

Nutrition per serving

○ 293 calories
○ 7 g protein
○ 46 g carbohydrates
○ 10 g fat
○ 0.5 g saturated fat
○ 0 mg cholesterol
○ 50 mg sodium
○ 6 g fiber

1. Preheat the oven to 300°F. Coat a large baking sheet with cooking spray.

2. Combine the oats, almonds, cinnamon, nutmeg, and salt in a large bowl. Combine the honey, oil, and almond extract in a separate bowl. Pour the honey mixture over the oat mixture and stir well to combine. Spread evenly on the baking sheet.

3. Bake, stirring every 10 minutes, for 38 to 40 minutes, or until lightly toasted. Remove from the oven and stir in the cranberries and cherries. Cool completely and store in an airtight container.

MAKE IT A FLAT BELLY DIET MEAL: Serve with 6 ounces fat-free vanilla yogurt (130). Total meal: 423 calories

Scrambled Egg "Pizza"

4 SERVINGS / 232 CALORIES / MUFA: OLIVE OIL

Serving typical morning fare cleverly disguised as a pizza is a quick way to put a new twist on the ordinary breakfast routine.

15 MINUTES

- 4 **large eggs**
- 2 **large egg whites**
- 1/8 **teaspoon salt**
- 1/8 **teaspoon ground black pepper**
- 1 **whole wheat tortilla (8")**
- 1/4 **cup olive oil**
- 1 **tomato, chopped**
- 1/2 **teaspoon dried oregano**
- 1 **tablespoon shredded reduced-fat Italian cheese blend**

Nutrition per serving
- 232 calories
- 8 g protein
- 6 g carbohydrates
- 19 g fat
- 3.5 g saturated fat
- 210 mg cholesterol
- 230 mg sodium
- 1 g fiber

1. Beat the whole eggs, egg whites, salt, and pepper in a bowl. Set aside.

2. Brush both sides of the tortilla with some of the oil. Heat a nonstick skillet (large enough to hold the tortilla) over medium heat. Place the tortilla in the skillet and cook for about 1 minute, or until golden. Turn with tongs and cook for about 1 minute, or until crisp. Place on a cutting board or platter.

3. Return the skillet to the heat. Add two-thirds of the remaining oil. Swirl to coat the pan. Add the eggs. Stir with a silicone spatula and cook for about 2 minutes, or until set. Spoon evenly over the tortilla.

4. Return the pan to the heat. Add the remaining oil. Swirl to coat the pan. Add the tomato and oregano. Toss for 2 minutes, or until the tomato starts to get juicy. Spoon evenly over the eggs. Sprinkle with the cheese. Cut into 4 wedges with a pizza cutter and serve.

MAKE IT A TEAM EFFORT On a weekend when you have more time, have the kids add their own nutritious toppings to the pizza, like steamed broccoli florets or spinach leaves.

MAKE IT A FLAT BELLY DIET MEAL: Serve with 2 ounces Canadian bacon (104) and 1 cup cantaloupe balls (60). Total meal: 396 calories

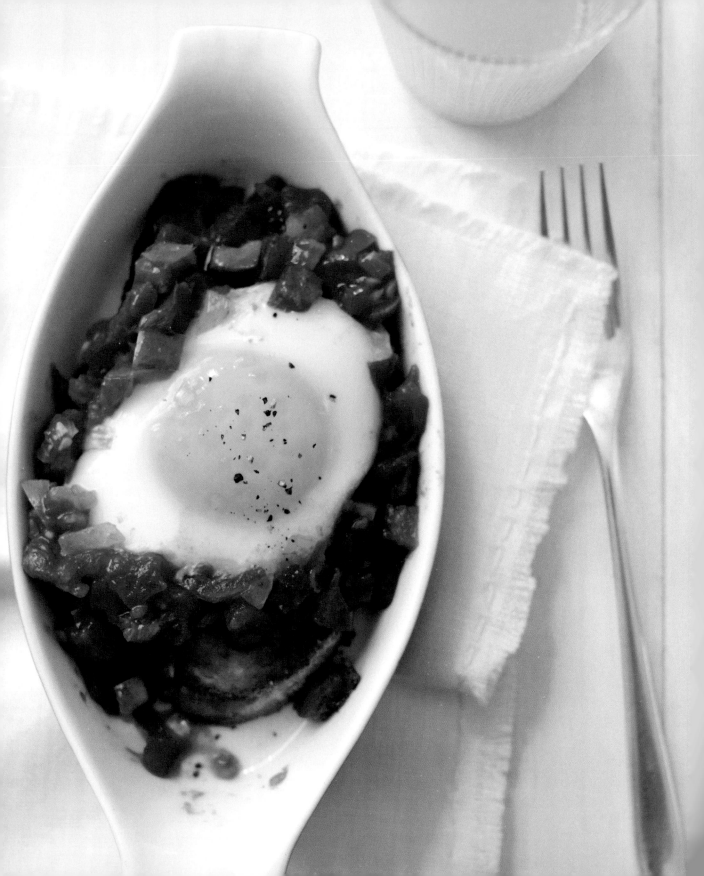

Italian-Style Eggs

4 SERVINGS / 309 CALORIES / MUFA: CANOLA OIL

If your kids prefer keeping the component parts of a meal separate, by all means serve the toast on the side. However, using the bread as a base for the sauce and eggs is a great way to enjoy every bite.

15 MINUTES

- 4 slices (½" thick) French or Italian bread (about 4 ounces)
- ¼ cup canola oil
- ¼ cup finely chopped onion
- ¼ cup finely chopped green bell pepper
- 6 plum tomatoes, chopped
- ⅛ teaspoon salt
- ⅛ teaspoon ground black pepper
- 4 large eggs

Nutrition per serving
- 309 calories
- 11 g protein
- 23 g carbohydrates
- 20 g fat
- 3 g saturated fat
- 210 mg cholesterol
- 350 mg sodium
- 2 g fiber

1. Heat a large nonstick skillet over medium-high heat. Brush 1 side of each bread slice with some of the oil. Place oil side down in the pan. Brush the tops with oil. Cook for about 2 minutes on each side, or until toasted. Place a slice of toast on each of 4 plates. Set aside.

2. Return the pan to medium heat. Add the remaining oil, the onion, and bell pepper. Cook, stirring, for 2 minutes, or until the vegetables have softened. Stir in the tomatoes, salt, and black pepper. Bring to a boil. Reduce the heat to medium-low and cook for 5 minutes, or until the tomatoes make a chunky sauce. With a large spoon, create 4 indentations in the sauce.

3. Break 2 of the eggs into 2 custard cups. Gently tip each egg into 1 of the indentations in the sauce. Repeat with the remaining 2 eggs. Cover and simmer for 6 to 8 minutes, or until the whites are completely set.

4. Use a large spoon to lift each egg and accompanying sauce onto each plate, either next to or on top of the toast. Spoon any remaining sauce evenly around the egg.

MAKE IT A FLAT BELLY DIET MEAL: Serve with ¾ cup orange juice (82). Total meal: 391 calories

Pan-Fried Cheddar Polenta

4 SERVINGS / 349 CALORIES / MUFA: CANOLA OIL

If you're in a hurry, use store-bought precooked polenta to cut your cooking time in half, and serve topped with onions and cheese.

30 MINUTES

¼ cup canola oil
1 small onion, chopped
2 garlic cloves, minced
¼ teaspoon dried thyme
3 cups water
¼ teaspoon salt
¾ cup instant polenta
1 cup (4 ounces) shredded reduced-fat sharp Cheddar cheese
1 tablespoon all-purpose flour

Nutrition per serving
○ 349 calories
○ 11 g protein
○ 28 g carbohydrates
○ 23 g fat
○ 5 g saturated fat*
○ 20 mg cholesterol
○ 660 mg sodium*
○ 2 g fiber

1. Coat an 8" x 8" baking pan with cooking spray.

2. Heat 3 tablespoons of the oil in a large nonstick skillet over medium-high heat. Add the onion, garlic, and thyme. Cook, stirring occasionally, for 3 to 4 minutes, or until slightly softened.

3. Combine the water and salt in a medium saucepan. Bring to a boil over medium-high heat and whisk in the polenta in a steady stream. Cook, stirring occasionally, for 3 to 5 minutes, or until the polenta thickens. Remove from the heat and whisk in the onion mixture and the cheese. Pour into the baking pan, smooth with a spatula, and cool completely.

4. Turn the cooled polenta out onto a cutting board. Use a sharp knife to cut the polenta into 8 rectangles. Spread the flour on a plate and lightly coat the rectangles. Wipe out the skillet and heat 2 teaspoons of the oil over medium-high heat. Add 4 polenta rectangles and cook for 3 minutes per side, or until lightly browned. Transfer to a plate to keep warm and repeat with the remaining 1 teaspoon oil and polenta.

Limit saturated fat to no more than 10 percent of total calories—about 17 grams per day for most women or 21 grams for most men—and sodium intake to no more than 2,300 milligrams.

MAKE IT A FLAT BELLY DIET MEAL: Serve with 1 cup sliced strawberries (54). Total meal: 403 calories

Vegetable Frittata

8 SERVINGS / 140 CALORIES / MUFA: TAPENADE

Because this frittata is baked instead of cooked in a skillet, it's almost effortless. It makes a wonderful dish to serve for a weekend brunch.

40 MINUTES

1 zucchini, thinly sliced

1 large or 2 medium tomatoes, thinly sliced

¼ sweet onion, thinly sliced

2 tablespoons whole wheat bread crumbs

1 teaspoon herbes de Provence

8 large eggs

4 large egg whites

¼ teaspoon salt

¼ teaspoon ground black pepper

1 cup green tapenade

1. Preheat the oven to 350°F. Coat a 13″ x 9″ baking dish with cooking spray.

2. Spread the zucchini in the baking dish. Top with the tomatoes and onion. Sprinkle evenly with the bread crumbs and herbes de Provence. Beat the whole eggs, egg whites, salt, and pepper in a bowl. Pour over the vegetables.

3. Bake for 25 to 30 minutes, or until the eggs are set and the top is golden. Remove and let sit for 5 minutes before cutting into 8 pieces. Dollop 2 tablespoons of tapenade on each serving.

MAKE IT AHEAD For quick breakfasts during the week, bake a frittata on the weekend, cool completely, and refrigerate, covered with plastic wrap. Individual servings may be reheated in the microwave or eaten at room temperature.

Nutrition per serving

○ 140 calories

○ 9 g protein

○ 5 g carbohydrates

○ 10 g fat

○ 2 g saturated fat

○ 210 mg cholesterol

○ 390 mg sodium

○ 1 g fiber

MAKE IT A FLAT BELLY DIET MEAL: Serve with 1 English muffin (135) spread with 2 teaspoons trans-free margarine (53) and 2 slices reduced-sodium turkey bacon (70). **Total meal: 398 calories**

Pesto Pinwheels

4 SERVINGS (2 SLICES EACH) / 185 CALORIES / MUFA: PESTO SAUCE

This egg roulade is as simple to prepare as a jelly roll. Kids can help by spreading the pesto-cheese mixture like frosting on a cake.

30 MINUTES

- 3 cups baby spinach
- 2 tablespoons all-purpose flour
- 4 large eggs
- 2 large egg yolks
- 1/8 teaspoon salt
- 1/8 teaspoon ground black pepper
- 1/8 teaspoon paprika
- 1/2 cup fat-free small curd cottage cheese
- 1/4 cup pesto sauce
- 8 cherry tomatoes, quartered

Nutrition per serving
- 185 calories
- 12 g protein
- 9 g carbohydrates
- 12 g fat
- 3 g saturated fat
- 320 mg cholesterol
- 350 mg sodium
- 2 g fiber

1. Wash the spinach and place in a saucepan with any water clinging to its leaves. Cover and cook, tossing, for about 3 minutes, or until wilted. Drain and rinse with cold water. Squeeze dry and set aside.

2. Preheat the oven to 350°F. Coat a glass or ceramic 13" x 9" baking dish with cooking spray. Set aside.

3. Place the flour in a mixing bowl and whisk in 1/4 cup water until smooth. Add the whole eggs, egg yolks, salt, pepper, and paprika. Beat until smooth. Pour into the baking dish. Bake for 15 minutes, or until firm. Set the egg sheet aside to cool.

4. Process the cottage cheese and reserved spinach in a food processor until smooth. Add the pesto and pulse to mix.

5. Spread the mixture over the egg sheet. Starting at 1 long side, roll the egg sheet into a tube like a jelly roll. Cut crosswise into 8 slices. Serve with the tomatoes on the side.

🕐 MAKE IT AHEAD Tuck plastic wrap over and around the sides of the unsliced egg roll. Cover tightly with foil and refrigerate for up to 3 days. Slice and let return to room temperature before serving.

MAKE IT A FLAT BELLY DIET MEAL: Serve with 1/2 cup grapes (52) and Pomegranate-Strawberry Smoothie (page 58), but omit the flaxseed oil (144). **Total meal: 381 calories**

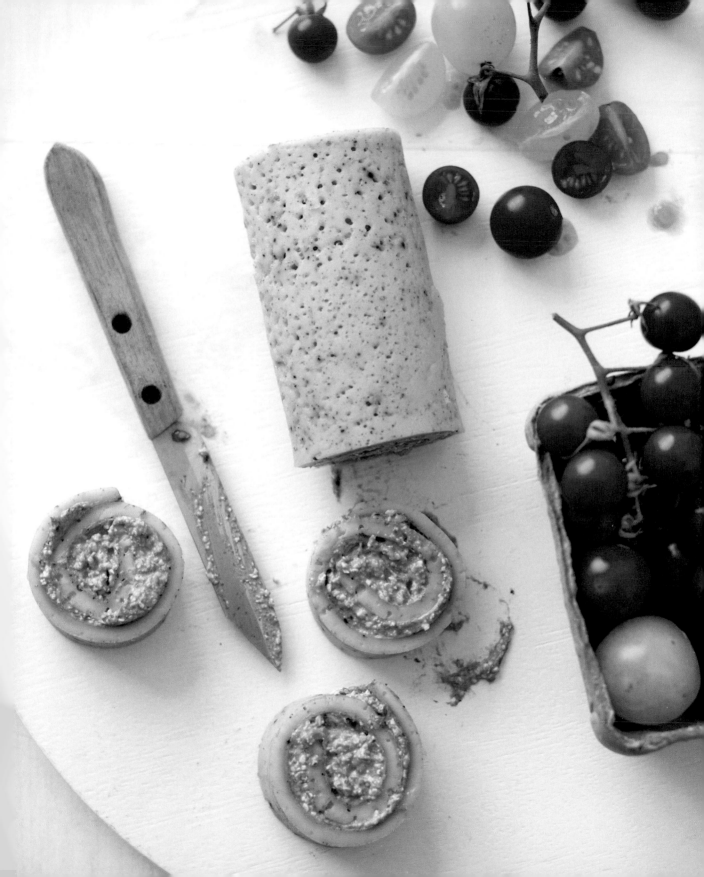

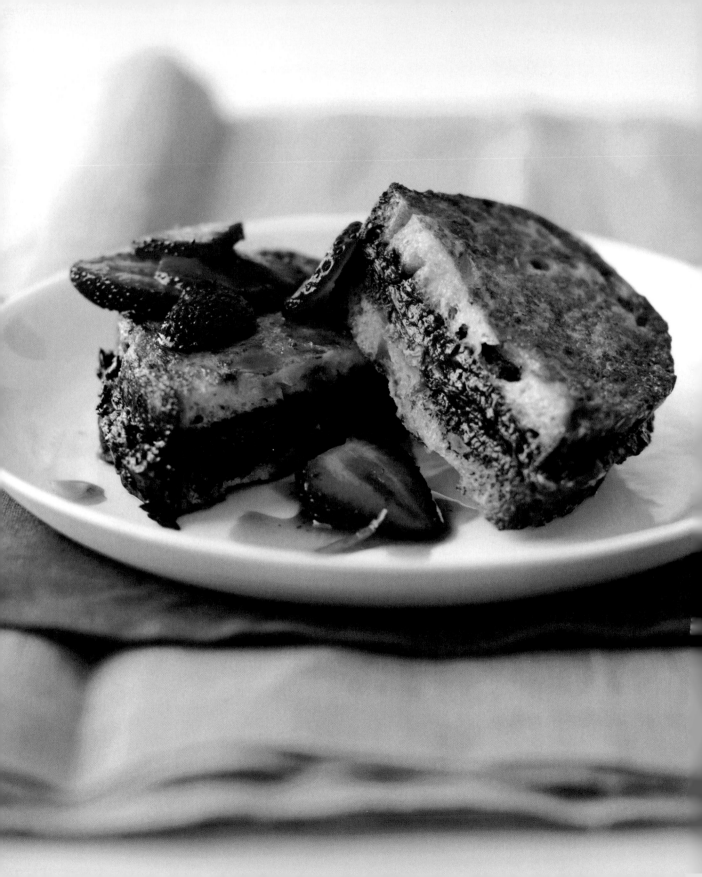

Chocolate-Stuffed French Toast

4 SERVINGS / 416 CALORIES / MUFA: CHOCOLATE

Could there be anything better than chocolate for breakfast? Look to this dish when you want a decadent start to your weekend. Neufchâtel cheese contains one-third less fat than regular cream cheese, making it a great alternative in most recipes.

25 MINUTES

4 ounces semisweet chocolate, finely chopped

3 ounces Neufchâtel cheese, at room temperature

2 cups sliced strawberries

1 tablespoon sugar

1 teaspoon grated orange zest

6 ounces Italian bread, cut on the diagonal into 8 slices (½" thick)

2 large eggs

2 large egg whites

1 teaspoon vanilla extract

1 tablespoon trans-free margarine

Nutrition per serving
- 416 calories
- 14 g protein
- 48 g carbohydrates
- 20 g fat
- 10 g saturated fat*
- 120 mg cholesterol
- 420 mg sodium
- 5 g fiber

1. Combine the chocolate and cheese in a small bowl and mix well. Combine the strawberries, sugar, and orange zest in a separate bowl.

2. Spread one-fourth of the chocolate mixture on 4 slices of the bread. Top each with a second slice and press lightly to form a sandwich.

3. Combine the whole eggs, egg whites, and vanilla extract in a medium bowl. Working one a time, dip both sides of each sandwich in the egg mixture and set on a plate.

4. Melt the margarine in a large nonstick skillet over medium heat. Wait for the foam to subside, then add the sandwiches and cook until golden and cooked through, about 4 minutes per side. Serve hot, topped with the strawberry mixture.

Limit saturated fat to no more than 10 percent of total calories—about 17 grams per day for most women or 21 grams for most men—and sodium intake to no more than 2,300 milligrams.

MAKE IT A FLAT BELLY DIET MEAL: A single serving of this recipe counts as a Flat Belly Diet Meal without any add-ons!

Walnut-Pear Pancake with Maple Syrup

6 SERVINGS / 395 CALORIES / MUFA: WALNUTS

Also known as a Dutch baby, this German-style baked pancake is a real crowd-pleaser. Once out of the oven, it deflates quickly—but it stays delicious to the last bite.

40 MINUTES

2 tablespoons trans-free margarine

2 pears, peeled, cored, and sliced

5 tablespoons sugar

1 cup all-purpose flour

¼ teaspoon ground cinnamon

¼ teaspoon salt

1 cup 1% milk

3 large eggs, lightly beaten

1½ teaspoons vanilla extract

1¼ cups walnuts, chopped

¼ cup maple syrup

Nutrition per serving
- 395 calories
- 10 g protein
- 49 g carbohydrates
- 19 g fat
- 2.5 g saturated fat
- 110 mg cholesterol
- 180 mg sodium
- 4 g fiber

1. Preheat the oven to 400°F.

2. Melt the margarine in a large ovenproof nonstick skillet over medium-high heat. Add the pears and cook, stirring occasionally, for 4 to 5 minutes, or until lightly browned and tender. Stir in 2 tablespoons of the sugar and cook for 1 minute longer. Remove from the heat.

3. Meanwhile, combine the flour, cinnamon, salt, and remaining 3 tablespoons sugar in a bowl. Stir in the milk, eggs, and vanilla extract until smooth. Fold in the walnuts.

4. Pour the batter over the pears and transfer the skillet to the oven. Bake for 22 to 24 minutes, or until the pancake is puffed and golden. Cut into 6 wedges. Drizzle with maple syrup and serve hot.

MAKE IT A FLAT BELLY DIET MEAL: A single serving of this recipe counts as a Flat Belly Diet Meal without any add-ons!

Berry Good Peanut Butter Scones

8 SERVINGS / 429 CALORIES / MUFA: PEANUT BUTTER

Because of the berry mixture they contain, these grab-and-go scones actually taste remarkably like peanut butter and jelly sandwiches—but with far less mess!

25 MINUTES

2 cups all-purpose flour
½ cup packed light brown sugar
1 teaspoon baking soda
1 teaspoon cream of tartar
¼ teaspoon salt
1 cup natural unsalted creamy peanut butter
1 package (5 ounces) mixed dried berries (about 1 cup)
¾ cup fat-free plain Greek yogurt
1 large egg

Nutrition per serving

○ 429 calories
○ 13 g protein
○ 58 g carbohydrates
○ 17 g fat
○ 2 g saturated fat
○ 25 mg cholesterol
○ 250 mg sodium
○ 4 g fiber

1. Preheat the oven to 400°F. Line a heavy baking sheet with parchment paper.

2. Combine the flour, brown sugar, baking soda, cream of tartar, and salt in a food processor. Pulse to combine.

3. Add the peanut butter by spoonfuls to the flour mixture. Pulse until the mixture is combined and looks like sand. Transfer to a mixing bowl and stir in the berries.

4. Stir the yogurt and egg together in a small bowl and add to the flour mixture. Stir with a spoon until combined. Use your hands, if necessary, to ensure that all of the flour is incorporated.

5. Transfer the dough to a lightly floured work surface and pat into a circle about 1" thick. Cut the dough into 8 equal wedges. Arrange the wedges on the baking sheet and bake for 15 minutes, or until lightly browned. Let cool slightly and serve warm.

MAKE IT A FLAT BELLY DIET MEAL: A single serving of this recipe counts as a Flat Belly Diet Meal without any add-ons!

Lemon-Blueberry Buttermilk Muffins

6 SERVINGS (2 MUFFINS EACH) / 402 CALORIES / MUFA: CANOLA OIL

Lemons and blueberries are a perfect combination—and this recipe affords you 2 muffins as a Flat Belly Diet serving! What could be better than that?

25 MINUTES

1¾ cups cake flour
⅔ cup blueberries
⅔ cup sugar
¾ cup low-fat buttermilk
6 tablespoons canola oil
2 large eggs
1 tablespoon grated lemon zest
¾ teaspoon lemon extract
1½ teaspoons baking powder
¼ teaspoon baking soda
¼ teaspoon salt

Nutrition per serving
○ 402 calories
○ 7 g protein
○ 58 g carbohydrates
○ 16 g fat
○ 2 g saturated fat
○ 70 mg cholesterol
○ 330 mg sodium
○ 1 g fiber

1. Preheat the oven to 375°F. Line a 12-cup muffin pan with paper liners. Measure out and set aside 2 tablespoons of the flour in a small bowl. Add the blueberries and toss. Set aside.

2. Combine the sugar, buttermilk, oil, eggs, and lemon zest and extract in a large bowl. Combine the remaining flour, the baking powder, baking soda, and salt in a separate bowl. Add the flour mixture to the buttermilk mixture and stir until smooth (the batter will be thin). Fold in the blueberries.

3. Fill the muffin cups two-thirds full and bake for 16 to 17 minutes, or until the tops are lightly golden and a toothpick inserted in the center comes out clean. Cool in the pan on a rack for 5 minutes. Remove the muffins from the pan and cool completely on the rack.

MAKE IT A FLAT BELLY DIET MEAL: Serve with ½ cup blackberries (31). Total meal: 433 calories

Banana Split Muffins

12 SERVINGS / 287 CALORIES / MUFA: WALNUTS

All the flavors of a banana split are loaded into these amazing muffins—chocolate, vanilla, walnuts, and (of course) banana—making them a dessert-worthy breakfast!

20 MINUTES

1½ cups walnuts, coarsely chopped

1½ cups all-purpose flour

¾ cup semisweet chocolate mini baking chips

1 tablespoon baking powder

½ teaspoon ground cinnamon

½ teaspoon salt

½ cup packed dark brown sugar

¼ cup canola oil

¼ cup fat-free plain Greek yogurt

¼ cup fat-free milk

1 large egg

1 very ripe banana, mashed (about ⅓ cup)

1 teaspoon vanilla extract

Nutrition per serving
- 287 calories
- 5 g protein
- 33 g carbohydrates
- 17 g fat
- 3 g saturated fat
- 20 mg cholesterol
- 230 mg sodium
- 2 g fiber

1. Preheat the oven to 375°F. Coat a 12-cup muffin tin with cooking spray.

2. Measure ½ cup of the walnuts into a food processor and grind to a fine meal. Place the ground walnuts, flour, chocolate chips, baking powder, cinnamon, and salt in a large bowl and stir until thoroughly combined.

3. Combine the brown sugar, oil, yogurt, milk, egg, banana, and vanilla extract in a medium bowl and stir until smooth. Add the banana mixture to the flour mixture and stir until thoroughly combined. Stir in the remaining 1 cup walnuts and mix well (the batter will be thick).

4. Fill the muffin cups three-fourths full and bake for 13 to 15 minutes, or until the tops spring back lightly when touched. Remove the muffins from the pan and let cool on a rack.

⧗ MAKE IT **FASTER** This batter is very thick, like cookie dough, so try using an ice cream scoop to fill the tins quickly and easily.

MAKE IT A FLAT BELLY DIET MEAL: Serve with 1 pear (103). Total meal: 390 calories

Maple-Pecan Cinnamon Rolls

12 SERVINGS / 366 CALORIES / MUFA: PECANS

Forget that cinnamon-roll-at-the-mall temptation! Wrap leftovers in plastic wrap and freeze in an airtight bag as individual servings. Let stand on the counter until thawed, and then pop in the microwave for 30 seconds until warmed.

2 HOURS 50 MIN

1 cup whole milk
½ cup packed light brown sugar
1 tablespoon active dry yeast
2 large eggs
¼ cup fat-free plain Greek yogurt
1 tablespoon vanilla extract
4 cups white whole wheat flour
2 tablespoons ground cinnamon
½ teaspoon salt
½ cup raisins
3 tablespoons trans-free margarine
¾ cup maple syrup
1½ cups pecans, coarsely chopped

Nutrition per serving
○ 366 calories
○ 28 g protein
○ 62 g carbohydrates
○ 11 g fat
○ 1.5 g saturated fat
○ 35 mg cholesterol
○ 125 mg sodium
○ 6 g fiber

1. Warm the milk in the microwave until the temperature reaches 100° to 110°F, 30 to 40 seconds. Stir in the brown sugar and yeast and let the mixture sit for 10 minutes, or until bubbles form. Combine the eggs, yogurt, and vanilla extract in a separate bowl.

2. Combine the flour, 1 tablespoon of the cinnamon, and the salt in a large bowl of a stand mixer with a dough hook. Slowly add the milk and yogurt mixtures while the mixer is running on low. Knead for 8 minutes, adding the raisins after about 5 minutes. Coat the bowl and dough with cooking spray. Cover and keep in a warm place until the dough is doubled in bulk (about 1 hour).

3. Meanwhile, mix the margarine and ¼ cup of the maple syrup in a small bowl and set aside. Combine 1 cup of the pecans, ¼ cup of the syrup, and the remaining 1 tablespoon cinnamon in another small bowl and set aside. Coat a 13" x 9" baking dish with cooking spray and pour the remaining ¼ cup syrup over the bottom. Cover with the remaining ½ cup pecans. Set aside.

4. Punch down the dough and transfer to a lightly floured work surface. Roll the dough into a rectangle about ½" thick. Spread the margarine mixture over the dough, leaving a 1" border around the edges. Slowly pour the pecan-syrup mixture into the center and spread over the margarine mixture.

5. Starting on a long side, carefully roll the dough into a log shape. Slice into 12 equal pieces. Arrange the pieces cut side up in the baking dish. Cover and let rise in a warm place for 45 minutes.

6. Preheat the oven to 350°F. Bake the rolls uncovered for 30 minutes, or until golden brown. Let cool slightly and serve warm.

MAKE IT A FLAT BELLY DIET MEAL: Serve with ¾ cup fat-free milk (62). Total meal: 428 calories

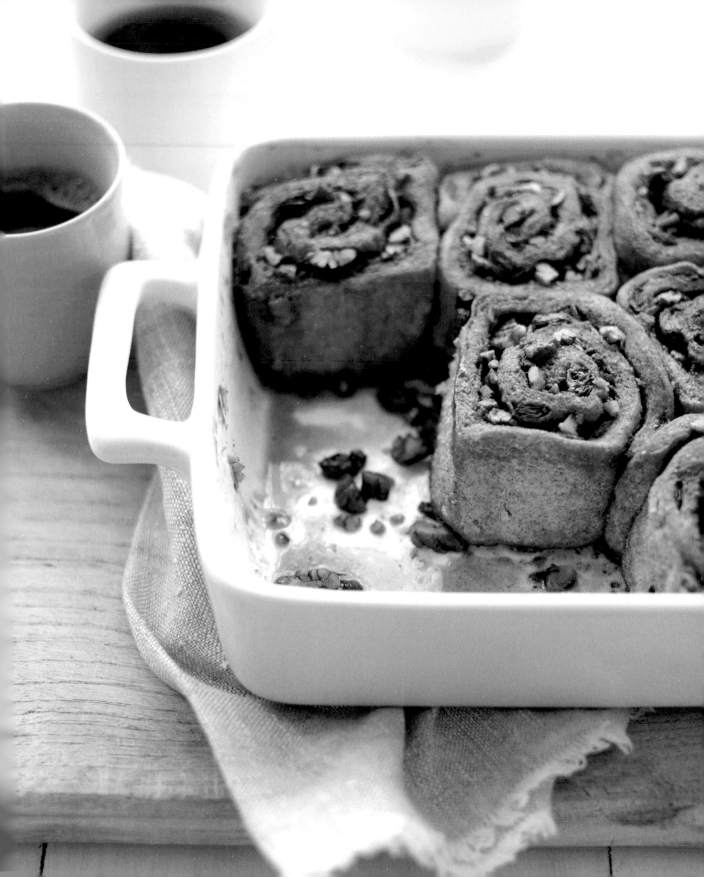

QUICK-FIX PANTRY RESCUES

Waffle Warm-Up

Spread 2 frozen whole grain waffles (140) with 2 tablespoons **peanut butter** (188) and 1 tablespoon apricot preserves (48). **Total Calories = 376**

Super-Quick Breakfast Wraps

Warm $\frac{1}{2}$ cup low-sodium canned black beans, rinsed and drained (100), in the microwave, then stir in 2 tablespoons salsa (10) and mash in $\frac{1}{4}$ cup **Hass avocado** (96). Divide ingredients between two 8" whole wheat tortillas (212) and roll up burrito-style. **Total Calories = 418**

Basic Banana Wrap

Spread 2 tablespoons **peanut butter** (188) on an 8" whole wheat tortilla (106). Top with 1 sliced banana (105) and drizzle with 1 teaspoon honey (21). Roll up burrito-style. **Total Calories = 420**

Greek Shake

Blend 6 ounces fat-free plain Greek yogurt (90), 1 tablespoon **flaxseed oil** (120), 2 tablespoons honey (128), $\frac{1}{4}$ cup fat-free milk (21), and 6 ice cubes (0) until smooth. Serve with $\frac{1}{2}$ toasted 6" whole wheat pita (60). **Total Calories = 419**

Honey-Walnut Oatmeal

Cook $\frac{1}{2}$ cup oatmeal (160) with $\frac{1}{2}$ cup evaporated fat-free milk (100) and $\frac{1}{2}$ cup water (0). Top with 2 tablespoons toasted **walnuts** (82) and 1 tablespoon honey (64). **Total Calories = 406**

Menu for a Weekend Brunch

Vegetable Frittata (page 67)

Tropical Fruit Salad (page 256)

Oven-Roasted Potatoes (below)

SERVES 8

⏲ **The night before:** Assemble Vegetable Frittata and a double batch of Tropical Fruit Salad and refrigerate until morning.

⏲ **About 90 minutes before serving:** Prepare Oven-Roasted Potatoes by coarsely chopping 2 pounds small red potatoes and toss with 2 tablespoons olive oil, 1 tablespoon chopped fresh rosemary, 1 teaspoon salt, and ½ teaspoon ground black pepper.

⏲ **About 1 hour before serving:** Preheat the oven to 350°F. Arrange the potatoes on a baking pan and bake for 45 minutes, or until browned. At the same time, put the frittata in the oven for 30 minutes, or until puffed and golden.

MAKE IT A FLAT BELLY DIET MEAL: Enjoy the frittata topped with tapenade (140), along with the fruit salad (omit the avocado) (177) and roasted potatoes (104). **Total meal = 421 calories**

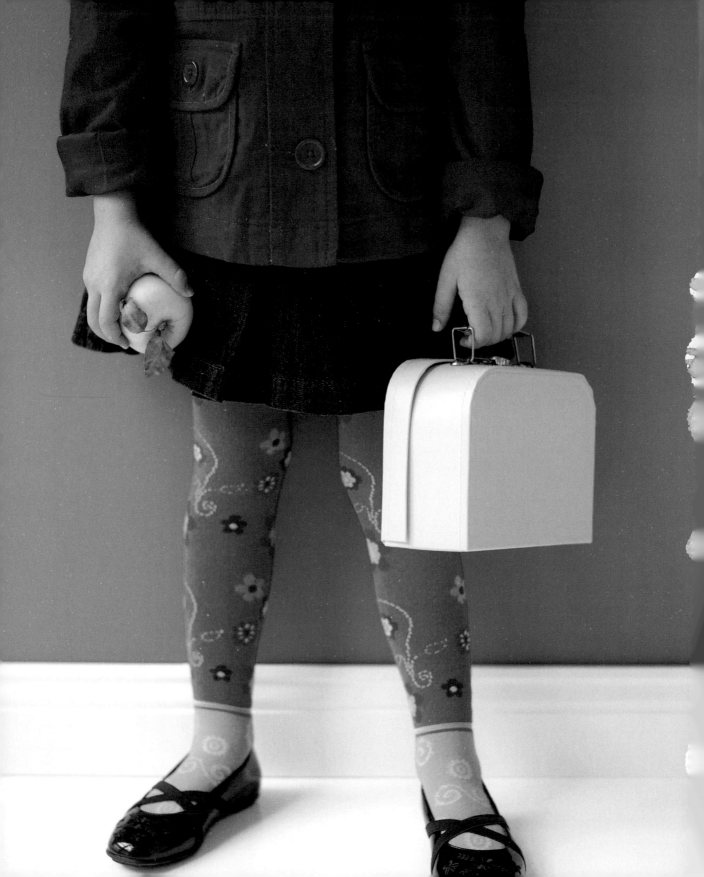

5

Better Bag LUNCHES

- ○ Peanut Butter–Strawberry Wrap
- ○ Grilled Tomato and Cheese
- ○ Chicken and Creamy Pepper Jelly Wrap
- ○ Turkey, Avocado, and Cheddar Panini
- ○ Seared Salmon BLT
- ○ Thai Butterfly Pasta Salad
- ○ Chicken Salad with Wheat Crackers
- ○ Tuna Rotini Salad Toss

- ○ Sweet Potato Salad
- ○ Penne Pasta Salad
- ○ Middle Eastern Chopped Salad
- ○ Curried Waldorf Salad
- ○ Quinoa Salad with Cherries and Pecans
- ○ Avocado-Orange Salad
- ○ Orange, Apple, and Jicama Slaw with Shrimp

Peanut Butter–Strawberry Wrap

1 SERVING / 332 CALORIES / MUFA: PEANUT BUTTER

Kids adore peanut butter and jelly sandwiches. This version ramps up the fiber while cutting down the unwanted sugar that's in the jelly.

Lay the tortilla on a work surface. Spread with the peanut butter. Cover with the strawberries. Roll into a tube. Slice on the diagonal into the desired number of pieces.

1 whole wheat tortilla (8")
2 tablespoons natural unsalted crunchy peanut butter
½ cup sliced strawberries

MAKE IT
**A TEAM
EFFORT**

Spreading peanut butter evenly can be a real challenge for young cooks. Help them out by warming the peanut butter and tortilla in the microwave for 15 seconds or so and letting them spread with the back of a spoon.

Nutrition per serving
○ 332 calories
○ 10 g protein
○ 31 g carbohydrates
○ 19 g fat
○ 2 g saturated fat
○ 0 mg cholesterol
○ 230 mg sodium
○ 7 g fiber

MAKE IT A FLAT BELLY DIET MEAL: Serve with 1 cup 1% milk (102). Total meal: 434 calories

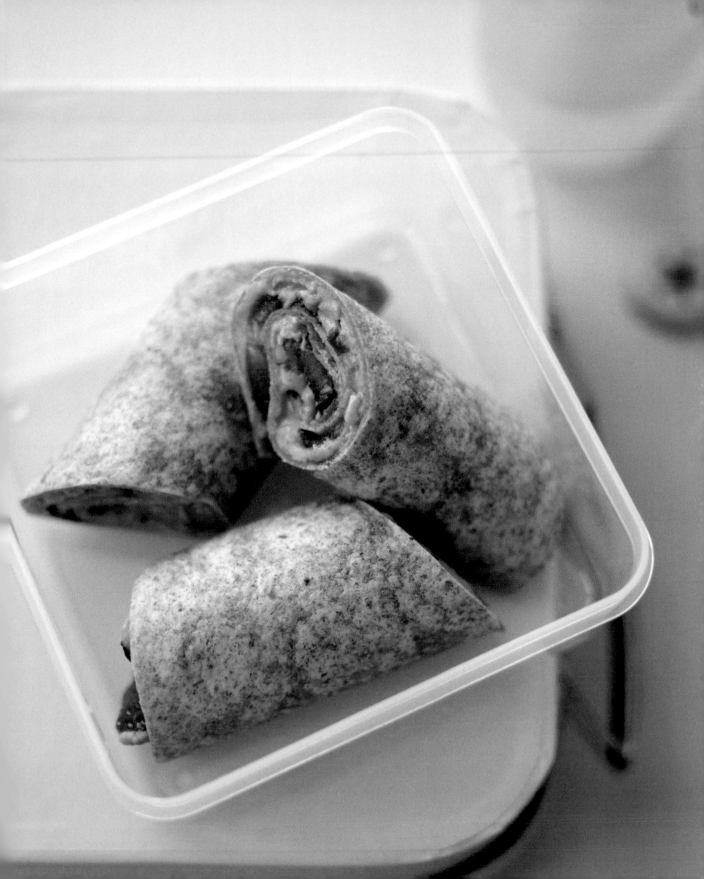

Grilled Tomato and Cheese

1 SERVING / 358 CALORIES / MUFA: CANOLA OIL

Grilled cheese with tomato soup is such a classic combination. Here the two are paired in a hearty sandwich that takes only minutes to prepare.

10 MINUTES

- 2 slices whole wheat bread
- 1 tablespoon canola oil
- 1 slice (1 ounce) reduced-fat provolone cheese
- 1 teaspoon whole grain mustard (optional)
- ¼ cup baby spinach
- 1 small tomato, thinly sliced

Nutrition per serving
- 358 calories
- 14 g protein
- 32 g carbohydrates
- 21 g fat
- 4 g saturated fat*
- 15 mg cholesterol
- 540 mg sodium
- 5 g fiber

1. Lay the bread on a work surface and brush 1 side of both slices with oil until all the oil is absorbed. Flip 1 slice oiled side down and top with the cheese, mustard (if using), spinach, and tomato. Top with the second slice of bread, oiled side up.

2. Set a cast-iron skillet over medium-high heat for 2 to 3 minutes, or until the surface is very hot. With a spatula, transfer the sandwich to the skillet. Cook for 1 minute, pressing with the spatula, until browned on the bottom. Flip and cook for 1 minute, pressing lightly with the spatula, until browned on the second side. If the cheese is not quite melted, remove the pan from the heat, cover, and let sit for 30 seconds. Halve on the diagonal.

Limit saturated fat to no more than 10 percent of total calories—about 17 grams per day for most women or 21 grams for most men—and sodium intake to no more than 2,300 milligrams.

MAKE IT A TEAM EFFORT With adult supervision, kids can learn the important life skill of stovetop cooking. A toasted sandwich makes a good entry recipe. It's easy and fast, and it rewards the young cook with warm melted cheese.

MAKE IT A FLAT BELLY DIET MEAL: Serve with 1 apple (77). Total meal: 435 calories

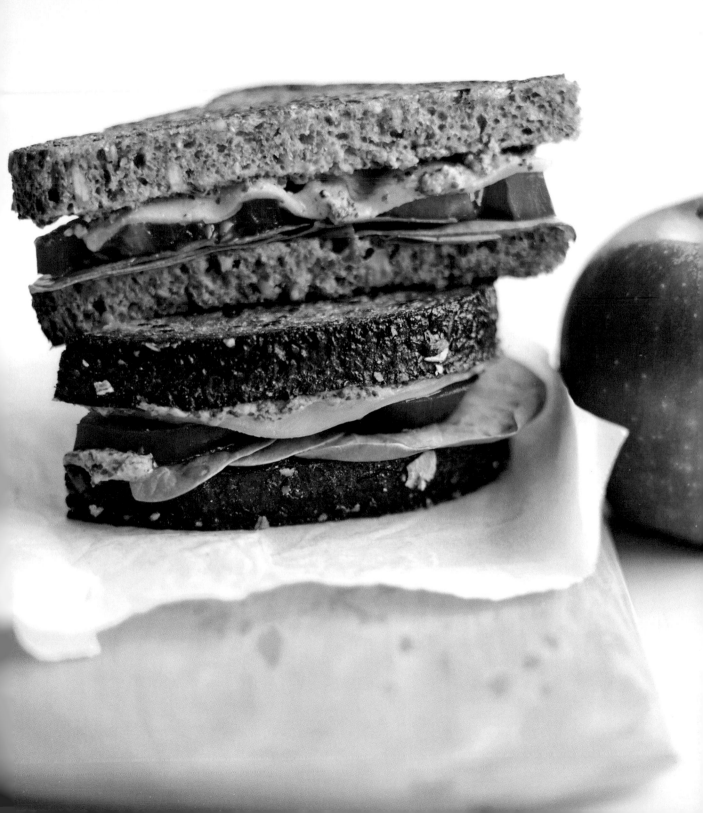

Chicken and Creamy Pepper Jelly Wrap

1 SERVING / 309 CALORIES / MUFA: CANOLA OIL MAYONNAISE

If you're so inclined, add a couple of dashes of hot pepper sauce to the mayonnaise for extra flavor flair. Jalapeño jelly is usually more sweet than spicy, so it shouldn't pose a problem for most palates.

5 MINUTES

- 1 whole wheat tortilla (8″)
- 1 tablespoon canola oil mayonnaise
- 2 teaspoons jalapeño jelly
- 2 ounces cooked boneless, skinless chicken breast, sliced
- 2 leaves red romaine, torn

Nutrition per serving
- ○ 309 calories
- ○ 14 g protein
- ○ 27 g carbohydrates
- ○ 15 g fat
- ○ 1 g saturated fat
- ○ 35 mg cholesterol
- ○ 350 mg sodium
- ○ 3 g fiber

Lay the tortilla on a work surface. Spread with the mayonnaise. Swirl the jelly into the mayonnaise. Top with the chicken and romaine. Fold up burrito-style. Cut in half.

MAKE IT AHEAD Precooked chicken breasts are a huge time saver, and poaching your own is a great way to save money, too, since raw chicken is usually cheaper. For every pound of chicken, bring 3 cups water to a simmer in a skillet. Add 1 celery rib, chopped, and 1 bay leaf and simmer for 1 minute. Add the chicken and cook uncovered for 6 minutes, or until cooked through. Remove the chicken from the poaching liquid (which can be discarded). When the chicken is cool enough to handle, prepare it as directed in the recipe.

MAKE IT A FLAT BELLY DIET MEAL: Serve with 1 cup cherry tomatoes (27) and 1 peach (59). Total meal: 395 calories

Turkey, Avocado, and Cheddar Panini

4 SERVINGS / 329 CALORIES / MUFA: AVOCADO

The classic Italian pressed sandwich is usually made with white-flour bread, such as ciabatta, but we use regular whole wheat instead for the extra fiber boost.

25 MINUTES

- 8 slices whole wheat bread
- 6 teaspoons Dijon mustard
- 6 slices reduced-fat Cheddar cheese (3 ounces)
- 1 Hass avocado, cut into 16 slices
- ½ pound sliced reduced-sodium deli turkey breast
- 1 cup arugula leaves

Nutrition per serving
- ○ 329 calories
- ○ 24 g protein
- ○ 32 g carbohydrates
- ○ 12 g fat
- ○ 4 g saturated fat*
- ○ 35 mg cholesterol
- ○ 950 mg sodium*
- ○ 7 g fiber

1. Brush 1 side of each bread slice with ¾ teaspoon mustard. Top 4 of the slices with 1 slice cheese, 4 slices avocado, 2 ounces turkey, and ¼ cup arugula. Top with ½ slice of the remaining cheese. Set remaining bread slices mustard side down over the cheese.

2. Lightly coat a large nonstick skillet with cooking spray and warm over medium heat. Add 2 sandwiches to the skillet and set a second heavy skillet on top of the sandwiches. Cook, pressing down slightly, for 2½ to 3 minutes per side, or until the bread is golden and the cheese melts. Transfer to a cutting board and cut each in half on the diagonal. Repeat with remaining 2 sandwiches, recoating the pan with spray as necessary.

* Limit saturated fat to no more than 10 percent of total calories—about 17 grams per day for most women or 21 grams for most men—and sodium intake to no more than 2,300 milligrams.

MAKE IT A FLAT BELLY DIET MEAL: Serve with 1 small, sliced red bell pepper (28) and 6 dried apricot halves (51). Total meal: 408 calories

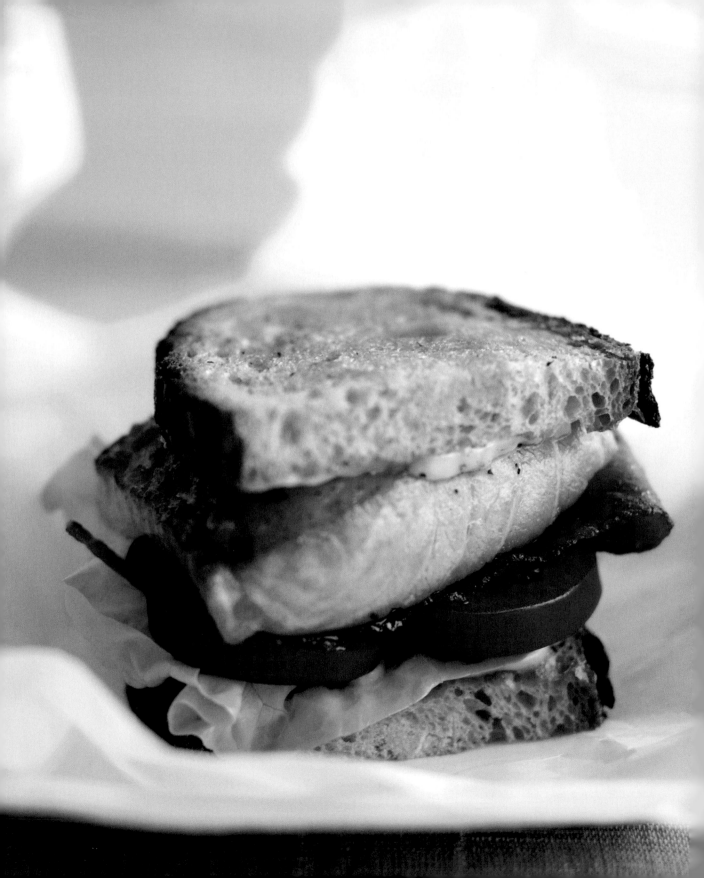

Seared Salmon BLT

4 SERVINGS / 367 CALORIES / MUFA: CANOLA OIL MAYONNAISE

Here's the secret to the best salmon: Never overcook it. Salmon is perfectly done when it becomes opaque but is still moist on the inside.

25
MINUTES

- 4 slices turkey bacon
- 4 skinless salmon fillets (3 ounces each)
- ¼ teaspoon salt
- ¼ teaspoon ground black pepper
- ¼ cup canola oil mayonnaise
- 4 slices whole wheat bread, toasted and halved
- 4 small Boston lettuce leaves
- 1 tomato, cut into 8 slices

Nutrition per serving
- 367 calories
- 23 g protein
- 15 g carbohydrates
- 23 g fat
- 2.5 g saturated fat
- 80 mg cholesterol
- 450 mg sodium
- 2 g fiber

1. Coat a medium nonstick skillet with cooking spray and heat over medium-high heat. Add the bacon and cook for 2 minutes per side, or until crisp. Transfer to a plate and set aside.

2. Return the skillet to medium-high heat. Sprinkle the salmon with the salt and pepper and add to the skillet. Cook for 4 minutes per side, or until the fish flakes easily with a fork. Transfer to a plate.

3. Spread 1½ teaspoons mayonnaise on each of the 8 bread halves. Arrange 4 bread halves on a work surface mayonnaise side up and top each with 1 lettuce leaf, 2 tomato slices, 1 slice of bacon, and 1 salmon fillet. Set the remaining bread halves mayonnaise side down over the salmon.

MAKE IT A FLAT BELLY DIET MEAL: Serve with ½ cup unsweetened applesauce (52).
Total meal: 419 calories

Thai Butterfly Pasta Salad

4 SERVINGS (1 CUP EACH) / 319 CALORIES / MUFA: TAHINI

This dish keeps well in an airtight container in the refrigerator, so you can pack several days' lunches ahead of time.

15 MINUTES

- 4 ounces multigrain farfalle (bow tie) pasta
- ½ cup frozen baby peas
- ½ cup tahini
- ¼ cup warm water
- 1 tablespoon honey
- 1 tablespoon reduced-sodium soy sauce
- ¼ teaspoon salt
- ⅛ teaspoon ground black pepper
- 1 roasted pepper, chopped (about ½ cup)

1. Bring a medium pot of water to a boil over high heat. Add the pasta and cook according to package directions. Place the peas in a colander and drain the pasta over the peas. Rinse the peas and pasta together with cold water.

2. Meanwhile, whisk the tahini, water, honey, soy sauce, salt, and black pepper in a bowl.

3. Add the roasted pepper, pasta, and peas to the dressing and toss to coat.

MAKE IT A TEAM EFFORT A good-quality kitchen scale makes an excellent investment in healthier eating because you know exactly the amount of an ingredient you need. Kids can improve their math skills at the same time by helping with the weighing.

Nutrition per serving
- ○ 319 calories
- ○ 11 g protein
- ○ 33 g carbohydrates
- ○ 17 g fat
- ○ 2 g saturated fat
- ○ 0 mg cholesterol
- ○ 500 mg sodium
- ○ 4 g fiber

MAKE IT A FLAT BELLY DIET MEAL: Serve with ½ cup canned juice-packed pineapple chunks (54).
Total meal: 373 calories

Chicken Salad with Wheat Crackers

1 SERVING / 297 CALORIES / MUFA: CANOLA OIL MAYONNAISE

If you don't have any pickle relish in the house, substitute the same amount of minced dill pickles instead. This recipe is designed to be a portable serving for one, but feel free to multiply the recipe if you like.

5 MINUTES

2 ounces precooked boneless, skinless chicken breast, finely chopped (see page 86)

1 tablespoon canola oil mayonnaise

1 teaspoon drained pickle relish

6 low-sodium whole wheat crackers

1. Combine the chicken, mayonnaise, and pickle relish in a transportable plastic container. Stir and seal. Refrigerate.

2. Serve with the crackers.

Nutrition per serving

○ 297 calories
○ 14 g protein
○ 21 g carbohydrates
○ 17 g fat
○ 1.5 g saturated fat
○ 35 mg cholesterol
○ 209 mg sodium
○ 3 g fiber

MAKE IT A FLAT BELLY DIET MEAL: Serve with 1 cup baby carrots (53) and 1 cup watermelon balls (46). Total meal: 396 calories

Tuna Rotini Salad Toss

4 SERVINGS (1½ CUPS EACH) / 404 CALORIES / MUFA: CANOLA OIL MAYONNAISE

White tuna is loaded with valuable omega-3s, a type of fat that helps reduce inflammation. But if you're concerned about mercury levels found in seafood, opt for canned salmon or light tuna (versus white tuna) in this recipe.

25 MINUTES

6 ounces multigrain rotini pasta

¼ cup canola oil mayonnaise

¼ cup chopped fresh basil

¼ teaspoon salt

¼ teaspoon ground black pepper

2 cans (5 ounces each) water-packed solid white tuna, drained

2 celery ribs, thinly sliced

1 large red bell pepper, cut into 1½"-long strips

2 carrots, thinly sliced

½ red onion, thinly sliced

1. Bring a large pot of water to a boil. Add the pasta and cook according to package directions. Drain, rinse under cold water, and drain again. Transfer to a bowl.

2. Stir in the mayonnaise, basil, salt, and black pepper. Add the tuna, celery, bell pepper, carrots, and onion and toss again.

* Limit saturated fat to no more than 10 percent of total calories—about 17 grams per day for most women or 21 grams for most men—and sodium intake to no more than 2,300 milligrams.

Nutrition per serving

○ 404 calories
○ 27 g protein
○ 41 g carbohydrates
○ 14 g fat
○ 1.5 g saturated fat
○ 40 mg cholesterol
○ 630 mg sodium*
○ 4 g fiber

MAKE IT A FLAT BELLY DIET MEAL: A single serving of this recipe counts as a Flat Belly Diet Meal without any add-ons!

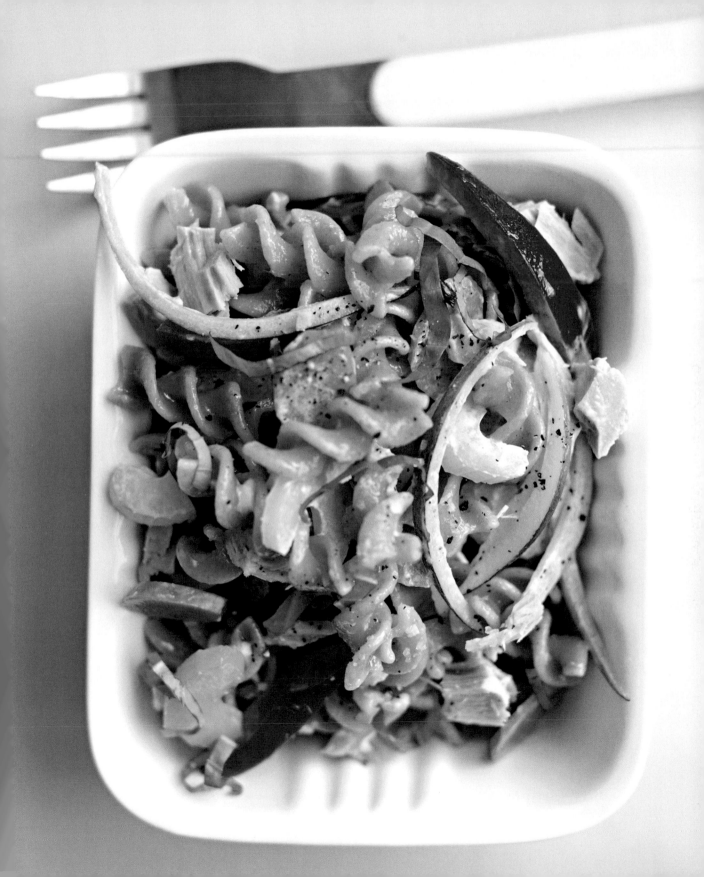

Sweet Potato Salad

4 SERVINGS (½ CUP EACH) / 190 CALORIES / MUFA: SUNFLOWER SEEDS

At your next family picnic, try switching this recipe in for your usual potato salad. Sweet potatoes are an excellent source of vitamin C and beta-carotene. For a change from spinach, try using arugula or red romaine if you like.

15 MINUTES

1 large sweet potato (about ¾ pound), peeled and cut into 1" cubes
⅓ cup fat-free plain yogurt
1 tablespoon honey
⅛ teaspoon salt
⅛ small red onion, thinly sliced
2 cups baby spinach
½ cup sunflower seeds

Nutrition per serving
○ 190 calories
○ 6 g protein
○ 25 g carbohydrates
○ 8 g fat
○ 1 g saturated fat
○ 0 mg cholesterol
○ 150 mg sodium
○ 5 g fiber

1. Place a steamer basket over boiling water and steam the sweet potato for 10 to 15 minutes, or until just tender. Place in a bowl and chill in the refrigerator.

2. Whisk the yogurt, honey, and salt together in a large bowl. Add the chilled sweet potato along with the onion, tossing to coat. Serve on a bed of spinach leaves. Sprinkle each serving with 2 tablespoons sunflower seeds.

MAKE IT A FLAT BELLY DIET MEAL: Serve with 2 ounces precooked chicken breast (81) and 1 cup green or red grapes (104). **Total meal: 375 calories**

Penne Pasta Salad

4 SERVINGS (2 CUPS EACH) / 424 CALORIES / MUFA: PESTO SAUCE

This dish is delicious served either warm or cold, although for best presentation serve right away; the broccoli will seem less vibrant if you refrigerate overnight.

25 MINUTES

- 6 ounces multigrain penne pasta
- 2 cups broccoli florets
- 12 ounces precooked skinless, boneless chicken breast, cut into 1/2" pieces (see page 86)
- 1 cup grape tomatoes, halved
- 1/4 cup pesto sauce
- 1 tablespoon extra-virgin olive oil
- 1 tablespoon fresh lemon juice
- 1/4 teaspoon salt
- 1/8 teaspoon ground black pepper

1. Bring a large pot of water to a boil. Add the pasta and cook according to package directions. Add the broccoli to the pot for the last 2 minutes of cooking. Drain the pasta and broccoli, rinse under cold water, and drain again. Transfer to a large bowl.

2. Add the chicken, tomatoes, pesto, oil, lemon juice, salt, and pepper and toss well.

Nutrition per serving
- ○ 424 calories
- ○ 36 g protein
- ○ 38 g carbohydrates
- ○ 14 g fat
- ○ 3 g saturated fat
- ○ 75 mg cholesterol
- ○ 360 mg sodium
- ○ 4 g fiber

MAKE IT A FLAT BELLY DIET MEAL: A single serving of this recipe counts as a Flat Belly Diet Meal without any add-ons!

Middle Eastern Chopped Salad

4 SERVINGS (2 CUPS EACH) / 338 CALORIES / MUFA: OLIVE OIL

Even salad skeptics will be won over by the fresh flavors in this amazing multitextured dish.

25 MINUTES

¼ cup extra-virgin olive oil
2 tablespoons red wine vinegar
1 garlic clove, minced
½ teaspoon salt
¼ teaspoon ground black pepper
3 tomatoes
1 cucumber, peeled, seeded
1 red bell pepper
1 green bell pepper
8 ounces precooked boneless, skinless chicken breast
¼ red onion, finely chopped
2 tablespoons chopped parsley
2 tablespoons crumbled feta cheese
2 whole wheat pitas (6")

1. Whisk together the oil, vinegar, garlic, salt, and black pepper in a large bowl.

2. Seed the tomatoes and coarsely chop. Chop the cucumbers, bell peppers, and chicken into similar-size pieces. Add to the oil mixture along with the red onion, parsley, and feta.

3. Divide among 4 bowls. Toast the pitas and cut each into 4 wedges. Serve 2 wedges per person.

Nutrition per serving
○ 338 calories
○ 22 g protein
○ 22 g carbohydrates
○ 18 g fat
○ 3.5 g saturated fat
○ 50 mg cholesterol
○ 510 mg sodium
○ 5 g fiber

MAKE IT A FLAT BELLY DIET MEAL: Serve with 3 tablespoons hummus (78). Total meal: 416 calories

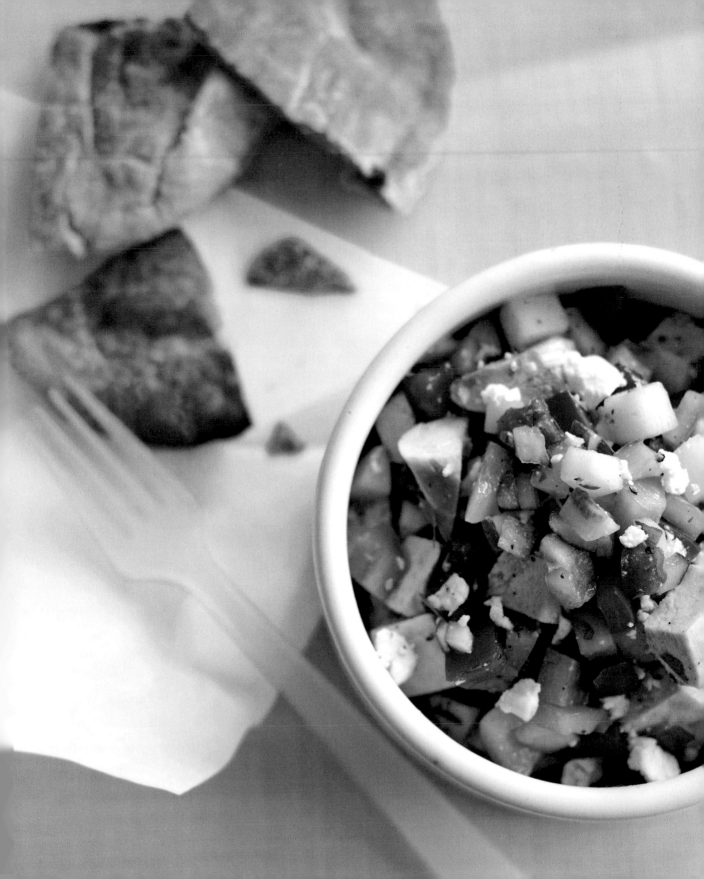

Curried Waldorf Salad

4 SERVINGS (1½ CUPS EACH) / 391 CALORIES / MUFA: WALNUTS

This salad offers the perfect opportunity to transform a few leftovers (namely, cooked chicken and brown rice) into a completely new dish.

15 MINUTES

½ cup walnuts, coarsely chopped

1 cup fat-free plain Greek yogurt

1 tablespoon mild curry powder

1 pound precooked boneless, skinless chicken breast, chopped (see page 86)

2 cups cooked brown rice

2 celery ribs, chopped

1 Granny Smith apple, chopped

¼ cup chopped red onion

6 dried apricot halves, chopped

Nutrition per serving
○ 391 calories
○ 36 g protein
○ 37 g carbohydrates
○ 11 g fat
○ 1.5 g saturated fat
○ 65 mg cholesterol
○ 130 mg sodium
○ 5 g fiber

1. Place the walnuts in a medium skillet and cook over medium-high heat, shaking the pan often, for 3 to 5 minutes, or until lightly toasted. Transfer to a plate to cool.

2. Combine the yogurt and curry powder in a large bowl. Add the walnuts, chicken, rice, celery, apple, onion, and apricots and toss to thoroughly combine. Serve at room temperature and refrigerate any unused portions.

MAKE IT A FLAT BELLY DIET MEAL: A single serving of this recipe counts as a Flat Belly Diet Meal without any add-ons!

Quinoa Salad with Cherries and Pecans

4 SERVINGS (1 CUP EACH) / 378 CALORIES / MUFA. PECANS

When we made this dish in our test kitchen, some of our tasters said they thought it was so delicious they'd eat it for breakfast!

25 MINUTES

1 cup quinoa, rinsed and drained
½ cup pecans
½ teaspoon olive oil
1 red onion, chopped
1 tablespoon honey
¼ teaspoon ground cinnamon
2 cups dark, sweet cherries, fresh or frozen
2 tablespoons chopped parsley

Nutrition per serving
○ 378 calories
○ 10 g protein
○ 57 g carbohydrates
○ 14 g fat
○ 1.5 g saturated fat
○ 65 mg cholesterol
○ 5 mg sodium
○ 7 g fiber

1. Bring 1½ cups water to a boil in a medium saucepan. Add the quinoa, cover, and reduce the heat to low. Simmer for 12 to 15 minutes, or until the water is absorbed. Uncover and allow to cool.

2. Meanwhile, place the pecans in a medium nonstick skillet and cook over medium-high heat, shaking the pan often, for 3 to 5 minutes, or until lightly toasted. Transfer to a plate to cool.

3. Heat the oil in the same skillet. Add the onion and cook for 5 to 7 minutes, or until beginning to brown. Remove from the heat and stir in the honey and cinnamon. Set aside to cool.

4. While the onion mixture and quinoa cool, pit the fresh cherries, if using, or thaw the frozen cherries in the microwave according to package directions. Coarsely chop the cherries and combine with the quinoa, pecans, and onion mixture in a large bowl. Toss well and sprinkle with the parsley.

MAKE IT A FLAT BELLY DIET MEAL: A single serving of this recipe counts as a Flat Belly Diet Meal without any add-ons!

Avocado-Orange Salad

4 SERVINGS (½ CUP SALAD AND 1 CUP GREENS EACH) / 120 CALORIES / MUFA: AVOCADO

The bright citrus flavors play nicely against the smooth, buttery texture of avocado in this easy-to-put-together salad.

15 MINUTES

1 tablespoon olive oil
1 tablespoon chopped fresh cilantro
1 teaspoon fresh lemon juice
¼ teaspoon salt
1 large navel orange
1 Hass avocado, sliced
1 slice sweet onion, chopped
4 cups mixed baby greens

1. Whisk together the oil, cilantro, lemon juice, and salt in a large bowl.

2. Cut the peel and pith off the orange. Hold the orange over the oil mixture and cut between the membranes to release the orange segments, allowing them to drop into the bowl along with their juices. Add the avocado and onion. Toss gently to combine. Serve the salad mixture on a bed of greens.

Nutrition per serving
○ 120 calories
○ 2 g protein
○ 11 g carbohydrates
○ 9 g fat
○ 1 g saturated fat
○ 0 mg cholesterol
○ 160 mg sodium
○ 5 g fiber

MAKE IT A FLAT BELLY DIET MEAL: Serve with 2 slices whole wheat bread (140), 2 ounces deli roast beef (63), and 1 ounce reduced-fat provolone cheese (58). **Total meal: 381 calories**

Orange, Apple, and Jicama Slaw with Shrimp

4 SERVINGS (2 CUPS SLAW AND 5 SHRIMP EACH) / 370 CALORIES / MUFA: PUMPKIN SEEDS

When working with jicama, make sure to wash and peel it just before using because (like potatoes and avocados) the flesh will darken when exposed to air.

20 MINUTES

3 tablespoons fresh lime juice

3 tablespoons chopped fresh cilantro

2 teaspoons sugar

½ teaspoon salt

1 jicama, peeled and cut into thin strips

1 large apple, peeled, cored, and cut into thin matchsticks

1 can (11 ounces) mandarin orange segments, drained

½ cup shelled unsalted dry-roasted pumpkin seeds

1 tablespoon olive oil

¾ pound peeled and deveined large shrimp

1. Whisk together the lime juice, cilantro, sugar, and ¼ teaspoon of the salt in a large bowl. Add the jicama, apple, orange segments, and pumpkin seeds. Toss well.

2. Heat the oil in a large nonstick skillet over medium-high heat. Sprinkle the shrimp with the remaining ¼ teaspoon salt and add to the skillet. Cook for 2½ to 3 minutes per side, or until opaque. Serve the slaw topped with the shrimp.

Nutrition per serving
- 370 calories
- 24 g protein
- 43 g carbohydrates
- 13 g fat
- 2.5 g saturated fat
- 130 mg cholesterol
- 430 mg sodium
- 12 g fiber

MAKE IT A FLAT BELLY DIET MEAL: A single serving of this recipe counts as a Flat Belly Diet Meal without any add-ons! To serve as part of another FBD Meal, omit the pumpkin seeds and shrimp (187).

QUICK-FIX PANTRY RESCUES

Salmon Surprise

Mix half of a 6-ounce pouch of pink salmon (137) with 1 tablespoon **canola oil mayonnaise** (100) and 2 tablespoons chopped roasted pepper (8). Spread on 2 rye crispbreads (62) and serve with ¼ cup raisins (123). **Total Calories = 430**

Olive Spread Wrap

Mash together 2 ounces Neufchâtel cheese (148) and 10 pitted and chopped **black olives** (50). Spread on one 8″ whole wheat tortilla (106) and fill with 2 ounces low-sodium sliced deli ham (61) and ½ cup baby spinach (5). Serve with ½ cup grapes (52). **Total Calories = 422**

Turkey on Rye

Combine 1 tablespoon **canola oil mayonnaise** (100) and 1 tablespoon horseradish (7). Spread mixture on 2 slices rye bread (165) and arrange

2 ounces reduced-sodium deli turkey (61) between them. Serve with 1 apple (77). **Total Calories = 410**

Pineapple-Edamame Salad

Combine ½ cup pineapple tidbits (59) with 1 cup **edamame** (244), 1 chopped scallion (5), 2 ounces chopped precooked chicken breast (81), and 2 cups mixed greens (18). **Total Calories = 407**

Nutty Noodles

Cook 2 ounces multigrain noodles (203) according to package directions. Meanwhile, combine 2 tablespoons **peanut butter** (188), 1 tablespoon soy sauce (0), 1 teaspoon minced garlic (15), and ¼ teaspoon crushed red-pepper flakes (0), if desired. Drain the noodles, reserving 2 tablespoons of the cooking liquid. Toss with the peanut mixture, adding the reserved liquid to coat. **Total Calories = 406**

Menu for a Hearty Picnic

Middle Eastern Chopped Salad (page 96)

Whole Wheat Pita

Hummus

Dried Apricots

SERVES 4

⊙ **The night before:** Make Middle Eastern Chopped Salad.

⊙ **The morning of the picnic:** Pack along ¾ cup hummus to go with the pita called for in the salad recipe and 2 dozen dried apricots.

MAKE IT A FLAT BELLY DIET MEAL: Enjoy the chopped salad (338) with *either* 3 tablespoons hummus (78) or 6 apricot halves (51). **Total meal = 416 calories (with hummus) or 389 calories (with apricots)**

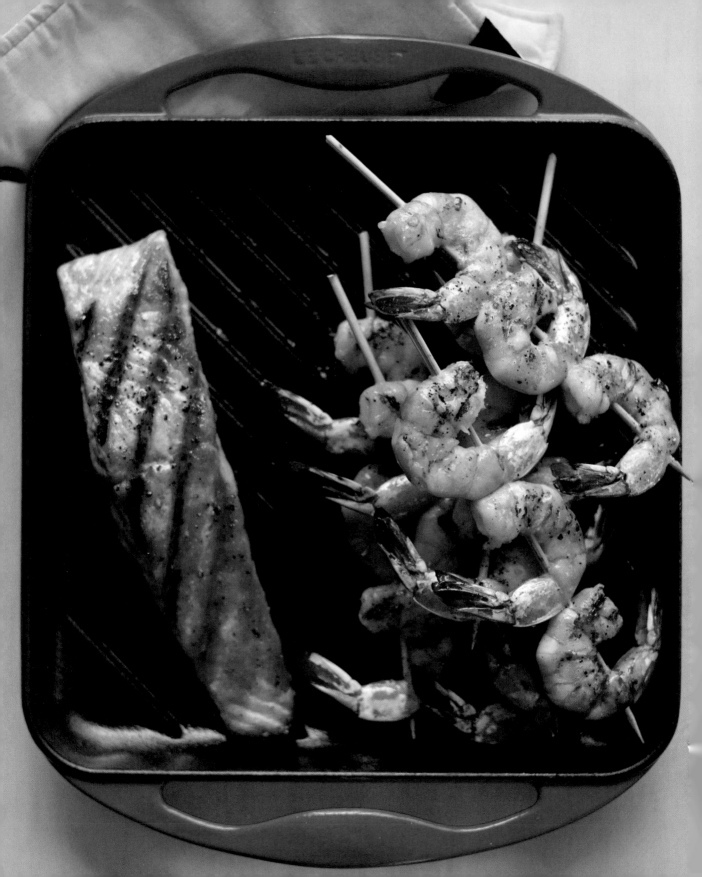

6

Grill
MASTERS' FAVORITES

- Italian Vegetable Spiedini
- Grilled Zucchini Boats
- Chili-Dusted Avocado Potatoes
- Seared Portobello "Steaks"
- Grilled Tofu Cutlets
- Lemon Shrimp with Roasted Peppers
- Grilled Shrimp and Zucchini Tostadas
- Grilled Shrimp Rolls
- Salmon with Sizzling Sesame Scallions
- Grilled Tilapia with Balsamic Vinaigrette
- Grilled Chicken Breasts with Pan-Roasted Tomatoes and Olives

- Mediterranean Chicken Kebabs with Lemon-Tahini Sauce
- Tandoori Chicken Thighs
- Barbecue Turkey Burgers with Avocado Mash
- Grilled Turkey and Bok Choy with Chile-Garlic Sauce
- Spice-Rubbed Pork Tenderloin with Avocado, Cucumber, and Onion Salad
- Caramelized Onion and Swiss Burgers
- Barbecued Pork Tenderloin
- Grilled Flank Steak with Chimichurri Sauce
- Marinated Beef Tip Roast

Italian Vegetable Spiedini

4 SERVINGS / 266 CALORIES / MUFA: OLIVE OIL

Spiedini is the Italian word for kebabs. Whatever you call them, these grilled seasoned vegetables with pasta are delightful.

25 MINUTES

- 8 very small onions
- 1 yellow summer squash (about ½ pound)
- 2 tablespoons panko bread crumbs
- 2 tablespoons grated Parmesan cheese
- ¼ teaspoon dried thyme
- ¼ teaspoon rubbed sage
- ⅛ teaspoon salt
- ⅛ teaspoon ground black pepper
- 8 cherry tomatoes
- 4 tablespoons extra-virgin olive oil
- 3 ounces multigrain rotini pasta
- 1 tablespoon minced parsley

Nutrition per serving
- 266 calories
- 7 g protein
- 27 g carbohydrates
- 15 g fat
- 2.5 g saturated fat
- 0 mg cholesterol
- 200 mg sodium
- 4 g fiber

1. Preheat the grill to medium. Bring a medium pot of water to a boil.

2. Meanwhile, wash the onions but do not peel. Trim away the root tips and cut an X in the root end with a small knife. Place in a large microwaveable zip-top storage bag. Halve the squash lengthwise. Cut each half crosswise into 8 chunks. Place in the bag with the onions. Seal about halfway. Place the bag in the microwave and arrange the vegetables in a single layer. Cook on medium power for 90 seconds, or just until heated. Remove carefully and set aside until cool enough to handle. Trim away the onion skins and discard.

3. Combine the bread crumbs, cheese, thyme, sage, salt, and pepper in a shallow glass or ceramic baking dish. Add the cooked onions and squash and the tomatoes. Drizzle with 1 tablespoon of the oil. Toss to coat the vegetables with the crumb mixture. Thread the vegetables onto 4 long metal skewers. Reserve the remaining crumb mixture.

4. Grill the skewers over direct heat, turning, for 8 minutes, or until browned on all sides. Move to indirect heat and continue cooking for 10 minutes, or until the squash is tender. Remove and gently slide the vegetables into the dish of reserved crumb mixture. Set aside.

5. Meanwhile, add the pasta to the boiling water and cook according to package directions. Drain and add to the vegetable dish with the remaining 3 tablespoons oil and the parsley. Toss and serve.

MAKE IT A FLAT BELLY DIET MEAL: Serve with 3 ounces grilled beef tenderloin (134).
Total meal: 400 calories

Grilled Zucchini Boats

4 SERVINGS / 163 CALORIES / MUFA: OLIVES

This rustic vegetable dish has only a fraction of the saturated fat of a version made with pork sausage, thanks to the Italian soy sausage in the stuffing.

55 MINUTES

2 zucchini (½ pound each), halved lengthwise

3 ounces Italian soy sausage, crumbled

½ small onion, finely chopped

8 cherry tomatoes, finely chopped

40 pitted black olives, chopped

1 egg white, beaten

4 tablespoons (1 ounce) shredded reduced-fat four-cheese Italian blend

1 tablespoon fine dried whole wheat bread crumbs

¼ teaspoon ground black pepper

1 teaspoon olive oil

Nutrition per serving
- 163 calories
- 8 g protein
- 12 g carbohydrates
- 11 g fat
- 2 g saturated fat
- 5 mg cholesterol
- 640 mg sodium*
- 5 g fiber

1. Preheat the grill to medium. Set out a 12" x 12" sheet of heavy-duty foil.

2. Meanwhile, scoop out the flesh of each zucchini with a melon baller or spoon, leaving about a ¼" shell. Finely chop the flesh and transfer to a large nonstick skillet. Add the sausage, onion, tomatoes, and olives. Cover and cook over medium-high heat, tossing occasionally, for 5 minutes, or until the vegetables release their liquid. Uncover and cook for about 3 minutes to evaporate the liquid. Spread the mixture on a rimmed baking sheet to cool.

3. Return the mixture to the pan. Add the egg white, 3 tablespoons of the cheese, the bread crumbs, and pepper, tossing to mix. Drizzle the oil on the zucchini shells and rub to coat all surfaces. Pack the stuffing mixture into the zucchini shells and press in firmly. Sprinkle with the remaining 1 tablespoon cheese. Set the zucchini on the sheet of foil.

4. Place the zucchini on the grill rack over indirect heat. Grill for about 40 minutes, or until the zucchini are cooked to desired tenderness.

* Limit saturated fat to no more than 10 percent of total calories—about 17 grams per day for most women or 21 grams for most men—and sodium intake to no more than 2,300 milligrams.

MAKE IT AHEAD The zucchini can be stuffed (make sure the stuffing mixture is completely cool) and refrigerated, covered in plastic wrap, for up to 2 days before grilling. The zucchini can also be grilled, cooled, and refrigerated in an airtight container for up to 3 days. Serve at room temperature or reheat in the microwave.

MAKE IT A FLAT BELLY DIET MEAL: Serve with ½ cup cooked carrots (27) and Golden Rice Pilaf (page 227), but omit the pistachios (184). Total meal: 374 calories

Chili-Dusted Avocado Potatoes

4 SERVINGS / 290 CALORIES / MUFA: AVOCADO

Who needs meat for dinner when this hearty vegetable grill can take center stage?

45 MINUTES

2 large russet (baking) potatoes
2 teaspoons canola oil
¾ teaspoon chili powder
⅛ teaspoon salt
4 slices low-fat turkey bacon
1 Hass avocado, cut into 16 slices
½ cup (2 ounces) shredded reduced-fat Cheddar cheese
¼ cup fat-free sour cream (optional)
Hot-pepper sauce (optional)

Nutrition per serving
○ 290 calories
○ 10 g protein
○ 37 g carbohydrates
○ 12 g fat
○ 3 g saturated fat
○ 20 mg cholesterol
○ 330 mg sodium
○ 5 g fiber

1. Preheat the grill to medium. Coat 1 side of a large sheet of heavy-duty foil with cooking spray.

2. Cut each potato lengthwise into 4 slices. Trim the rounded sides slightly so each slice sits flat. Rub evenly with the oil. Sprinkle the chili powder and salt evenly over the potatoes.

3. Grill the potatoes over direct heat for 5 minutes per side, or until browned. Place on the foil and place over indirect heat for 20 minutes, or until tender when pierced with a knife. Meanwhile, place the turkey bacon over direct heat. (If you're concerned that the bacon will fall through the grates, use a grill basket or another sheet of foil.) Grill for 1 minute per side, or until crisp. Transfer to a plate and set aside.

4. When the potatoes are tender, leave them over indirect heat and top each piece with a half slice of the bacon, 2 slices of avocado, and 1 tablespoon of the cheese. Grill for about 4 minutes to melt the cheese. Serve hot topped with sour cream and hot sauce (if desired).

MAKE IT A TEAM EFFORT
No need for you to do all the dirty work. Have the kids roll up their sleeves and get out the vegetable brush to scrub the spuds. They can also use a table knife to help you slice the avocado.

MAKE IT A FLAT BELLY DIET MEAL: Serve with 2 cups mixed greens (18) tossed with 1 tablespoon feta cheese (25), 2 tablespoons dried cranberries (49), and 1 tablespoon balsamic vinegar (14). Total meal: 396 calories

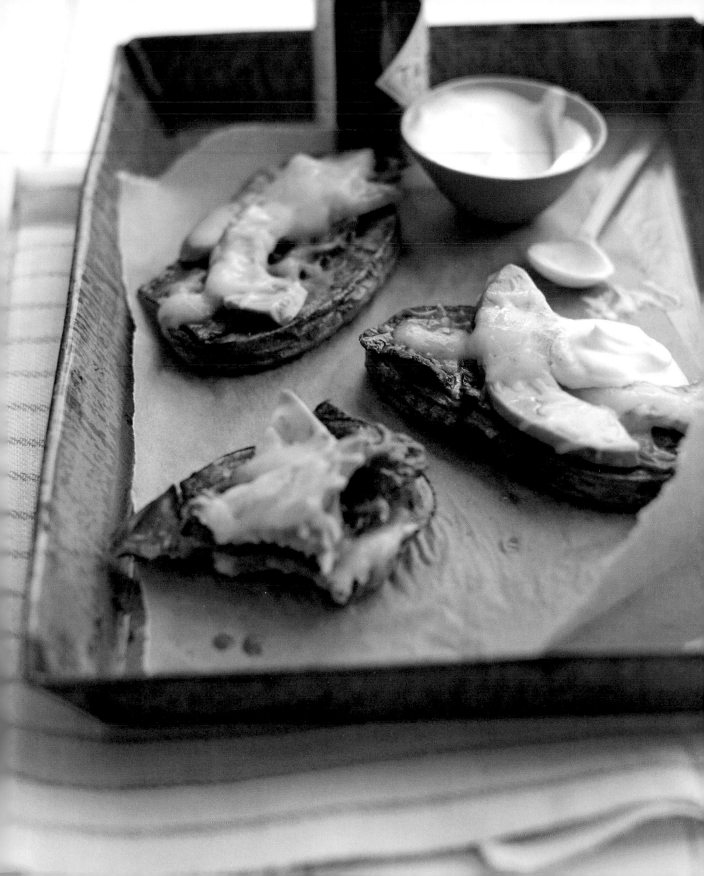

Seared Portobello "Steaks"

4 SERVINGS / 230 CALORIES / MUFA: TAHINI

Grilled portobello mushroom caps may be a trendy restaurant entrée, but they are so easy to make at home, there's no reason to go out.

20 MINUTES

2 teaspoons olive oil
1 garlic clove, minced
¾ teaspoon minced fresh rosemary
⅛ teaspoon salt
4 large portobello mushroom caps (about 4 ounces each)
½ roasted pepper, coarsely chopped (about ¼ cup)
½ cup tahini
Pinch of ground red pepper (optional)
¼ cup lukewarm water
2 teaspoons minced parsley (optional)

Nutrition per serving

○ 230 calories
○ 7 g protein
○ 12 g carbohydrates
○ 18 g fat
○ 2.5 g saturated fat
○ 0 mg cholesterol
○ 350 mg sodium
○ 3 g fiber

1. Preheat the grill to medium.

2. Combine the oil, garlic, rosemary, and salt in a small dish. Spread the mixture on the top of the mushroom caps as well as on the stem sides. Grill the mushrooms stem side up over direct heat for 2 minutes. Move to indirect heat. Grill for 12 minutes, or until juices start to accumulate.

3. Meanwhile, place the roasted pepper in a food processor and process to a smooth puree. Add the tahini and ground red pepper (if using) and pulse to combine. With the machine running, drizzle in enough of the warm water to make the mixture smooth and fluffy.

4. Carefully transfer the grilled mushrooms to 4 plates. Dollop the roasted pepper–sesame sauce over each mushroom. Garnish with the parsley, if desired.

🕐

MAKE IT AHEAD The roasted pepper–sesame sauce can be prepared and refrigerated up to 3 days in advance. Allow it to come to room temperature before serving.

MAKE IT A FLAT BELLY DIET MEAL: Serve with ½ cup cooked quinoa (111) tossed with 2 tablespoons raisins (62) and 2 tablespoons shredded carrot (6). **Total meal: 409 calories**

Grilled Tofu Cutlets

4 SERVINGS / 234 CALORIES / MUFA: WALNUT OIL

Too often tofu gets a bad rap for bland flavor, but so would chicken breast if it weren't seasoned. This dish should set the record straight on tofu's ability to taste great.

25 MINUTES

¼ large yellow or red bell pepper, finely chopped

4 scallions, white and green parts, finely chopped

2 small celery ribs, finely chopped

2 garlic cloves, minced

4 tablespoons walnut oil

1 container (14 ounces) extra-firm tofu, drained and sliced into 4 pieces

1 teaspoon salt-free seasoning blend of your choice

2 teaspoons red wine vinegar

¼ teaspoon salt

¼ teaspoon ground black pepper

1 package (5 ounces) shredded red cabbage (about 2 cups)

Nutrition per serving

○ 234 calories
○ 10 g protein
○ 9 g carbohydrates
○ 19 g fat
○ 2.5 g saturated fat
○ 0 mg cholesterol
○ 180 mg sodium
○ 3 g fiber

1. Preheat the grill to medium.

2. Combine the bell pepper, scallions, celery, garlic, and 1 tablespoon of the oil in a 13″ x 9″ shallow disposable aluminum baking pan. Stir to mix. Scrape the vegetables to the edges of the pan and set the tofu slices in the center. Sprinkle with ½ teaspoon of the seasoning blend and 1½ teaspoons of the oil. Flip and sprinkle with the remaining ½ teaspoon seasoning blend and 1½ teaspoons of the oil.

3. Place the pan over direct heat and grill, turning the tofu once and stirring the vegetables occasionally, for 15 minutes, or until hot and sizzling.

4. Meanwhile, whisk together the remaining 2 tablespoons oil, the vinegar, salt, and black pepper in a medium bowl. Add the cabbage and toss. Serve the cabbage topped with the tofu and vegetables.

🕐 **MAKE IT AHEAD** The recipe can be completed through step 2 up to 3 days ahead of grilling. Cover the pan with foil and refrigerate. Bring to room temperature and remove the foil before grilling.

MAKE IT A FLAT BELLY DIET MEAL: Serve with ½ cup steamed edamame (122) and ¼ cup cooked wild rice (41). Total meal: 397 calories

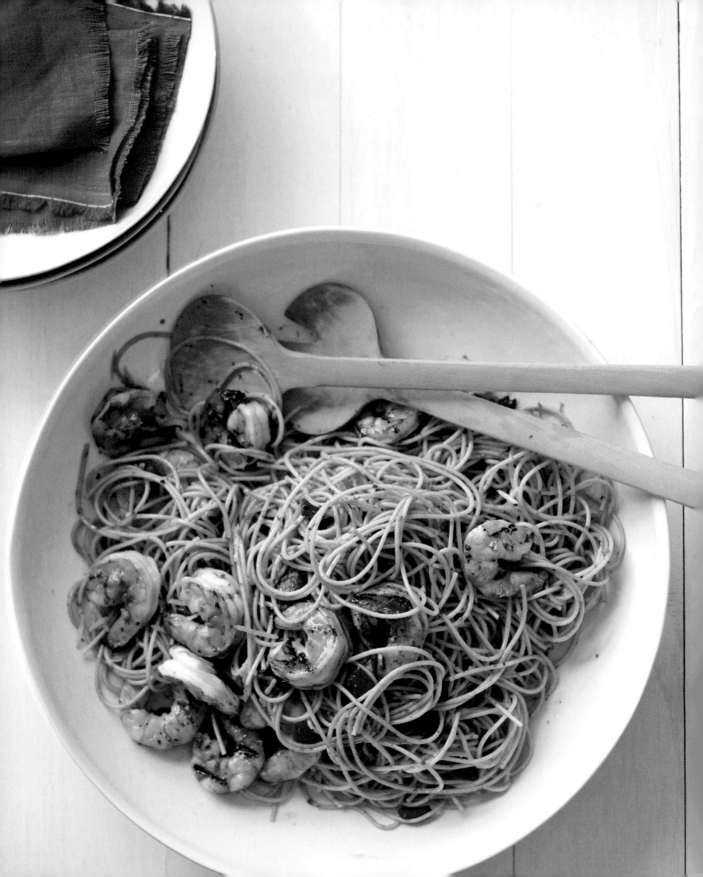

Lemon Shrimp with Roasted Peppers

4 SERVINGS / 391 CALORIES / MUFA: PESTO SAUCE

This recipe is perfect for outdoor grilling and so fast you can probably get the shrimp cooked before your pasta cooking water comes to a boil.

30 MINUTES

- 1 pound peeled and deveined large shrimp
- 2 tablespoons fresh lemon juice
- 1 tablespoon extra-virgin olive oil
- ½ teaspoon salt
- ¼ teaspoon ground black pepper
- 6 ounces multigrain spaghetti
- 1 roasted pepper, rinsed, patted dry, and chopped (about ½ cup)
- ¼ cup pesto sauce
- ½ teaspoon grated lemon zest

Nutrition per serving
- ○ 391 calories
- ○ 34 g protein
- ○ 33 g carbohydrates
- ○ 13 g fat
- ○ 3 g saturated fat
- ○ 175 mg cholesterol
- ○ 670 mg sodium*
- ○ 4 g fiber

1. Combine the shrimp, lemon juice, and oil in a bowl. Refrigerate until ready to grill, but no more than 30 minutes.

2. Preheat the grill to medium-high. Remove the shrimp from the marinade (discard the marinade) and sprinkle with ¼ teaspoon of the salt and ⅛ teaspoon of the pepper. Thread the shrimp onto metal skewers or coat a grill basket with cooking spray. Grill the shrimp 2½ to 3 minutes per side, or until opaque. Transfer to a plate and keep warm.

3. Meanwhile, bring a large pot of water to a boil. Cook the spaghetti according to package directions. Drain and transfer to a large bowl. Toss with the grilled shrimp, roasted pepper, pesto, lemon zest, and remaining ¼ teaspoon salt and ⅛ teaspoon pepper.

* Limit saturated fat to no more than 10 percent of total calories—about 17 grams per day for most women or 21 grams for most men—and sodium intake to no more than 2,500 milligrams.

MAKE IT A FLAT BELLY DIET MEAL: A single serving of this recipe counts as a Flat Belly Diet Meal without any add-ons!

Grilled Shrimp and Zucchini Tostadas

4 SERVINGS / 372 CALORIES / MUFA: AVOCADO

These tostadas are really loaded with flavor. If you find it difficult to get everything onto 1 tortilla, add another to your plate (but don't use extra oil). They're only about 60 calories each, so you'll still be in the ballpark for a Flat Belly Diet meal.

45 MINUTES

- 4 **corn tortillas (6")**
- 3 **tablespoons olive oil**
- ¾ **pound peeled and deveined large shrimp**
- 2 **teaspoons fresh lime juice**
- ¾ **teaspoon salt**
- 1 **zucchini (½ pound), cut crosswise on the diagonal into 12 slices**
- ½ **fresh pineapple, cored and cut into 8 half-round slices**
- ½ **red onion, cut into 3 (¼") slices**
- 1 **cup shredded romaine**
- 1 **Hass avocado, cut into 16 slices**
- 4 **tablespoons fat-free sour cream**

Nutrition per serving
- ○ 372 calories
- ○ 21 g protein
- ○ 35 g carbohydrates
- ○ 18 g fat
- ○ 2.5 g saturated fat
- ○ 130 mg cholesterol
- ○ 600 mg sodium*
- ○ 5 g fiber

1. Preheat the oven to 425°F. Preheat the grill to medium-high. Coat a large baking sheet with cooking spray.

2. Brush the tortillas with 2 teaspoons of the oil and set on the baking sheet. Bake for 11 to 12 minutes, or until crisp. Remove from the oven and cool.

3. Meanwhile, toss the shrimp with 1 tablespoon of the oil, the lime juice, and ¼ teaspoon of the salt. Thread the shrimp onto metal skewers or coat a grill basket with cooking spray. Grill the shrimp for 2½ to 3 minutes per side, or until opaque. Transfer to a plate and keep warm.

4. Brush the zucchini, pineapple, and onion slices with the remaining 4 teaspoons oil and sprinkle with the remaining ½ teaspoon salt. Set on a grill rack (or grill basket if your grates are widely spaced) coated with cooking spray and grill until well marked and tender, 4 minutes per side for the zucchini and pineapple slices, 5 to 6 minutes per side for the onion. Separate the onion slices into rings after grilling.

5. To assemble: Top each tortilla with ¼ cup of the lettuce, 2 pineapple slices, one-fourth of the onion rings, 3 zucchini slices, one-fourth of the shrimp, 4 avocado slices, and 1 tablespoon sour cream.

Limit saturated fat to no more than 10 percent of total calories—about 17 grams per day for most women or 21 grams for most men—and sodium intake to no more than 2,300 milligrams.

MAKE IT A FLAT BELLY DIET MEAL: A single serving of this recipe counts as a Flat Belly Diet Meal without any add-ons!

Grilled Shrimp Rolls

4 SERVINGS / 341 CALORIES / MUFA: CANOLA OIL MAYONNAISE

Taking a cue from the must-have summer sandwich in New England, the classic lobster roll, these grilled creations are easy to put together and just as delicious.

15 MINUTES

- ¾ pound peeled and deveined medium shrimp
- 1 tablespoon extra-virgin olive oil
- 1 garlic clove, minced
- ¼ teaspoon salt
- ¼ teaspoon ground black pepper
- ¼ cup canola oil mayonnaise
- 1 celery rib, finely chopped
- 2 tablespoons finely chopped red onion
- 4 whole wheat hot dog buns

Nutrition per serving
- ○ 341 calories
- ○ 21 g protein
- ○ 24 g carbohydrates
- ○ 18 g fat
- ○ 1.5 g saturated fat
- ○ 135 mg cholesterol
- ○ 580 mg sodium
- ○ 4 g fiber

1. Preheat the grill to medium-high.

2. Combine the shrimp, oil, and garlic in a bowl. Let stand for 10 minutes. Sprinkle the shrimp with the salt and pepper. Thread the shrimp onto metal skewers or coat a grill basket with cooking spray. Grill 2½ to 3 minutes per side, or until opaque. Transfer to a cutting board and let cool for 10 minutes.

3. Coarsely chop the shrimp and transfer to a bowl. Stir in the mayonnaise, celery, and onion. Toast the hot dog buns and divide the shrimp mixture evenly among them.

MAKE IT A FLAT BELLY DIET MEAL: Serve with ½ cup each watermelon balls (23) and cantaloupe balls (30). Total meal: 394 calories

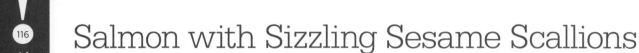

Salmon with Sizzling Sesame Scallions

4 SERVINGS / 318 CALORIES / MUFA: SESAME SEEDS

This simple yet elegant seafood dish is special enough for guests and easy enough for everyday when salmon is on sale.

25 MINUTES

2 tablespoons fresh lemon juice
1 tablespoon honey
¼ teaspoon salt
4 skinless salmon fillets (4 ounces each)
8 scallions, white and green parts, halved lengthwise, then cut on the diagonal into 1″ pieces
½ cup sesame seeds

Nutrition per serving
○ 318 calories
○ 25 g protein
○ 9 g carbohydrates
○ 20 g fat
○ 3.5 g saturated fat
○ 65 mg cholesterol
○ 220 mg sodium
○ 3 g fiber

1. Preheat the grill to medium. Coat an 11″ x 7″ shallow disposable aluminum baking pan with cooking spray.

2. Whisk together the lemon juice, honey, and salt in the baking pan. Dip the salmon in the mixture to coat and set on 1 side of the pan. Stir the scallions and sesame seeds into the remaining honey mixture, then push to the opposite side. Arrange the salmon in the middle of the pan with most of the sesame mixture surrounding it.

3. Place the pan over direct heat and grill for 5 to 6 minutes per side, stirring the sesame mixture occasionally, until the salmon flakes easily with a fork and the sesame seeds have toasted. If necessary, transfer the salmon to a platter and continue grilling the sesame mixture for 1 to 2 minutes longer to brown the seeds. Serve the salmon topped with the sesame mixture.

🕐
MAKE IT AHEAD Grill and chill to serve as a main-dish salad. Flake the salmon and scatter over a bed of mixed greens. Top with the sesame mixture.

MAKE IT A FLAT BELLY DIET MEAL: Serve with ½ cup cooked broccoli florets (22) and ½ cup whole wheat couscous (70). **Total meal: 410 calories.** To serve as part of another FBD meal, omit the sesame seeds (227).

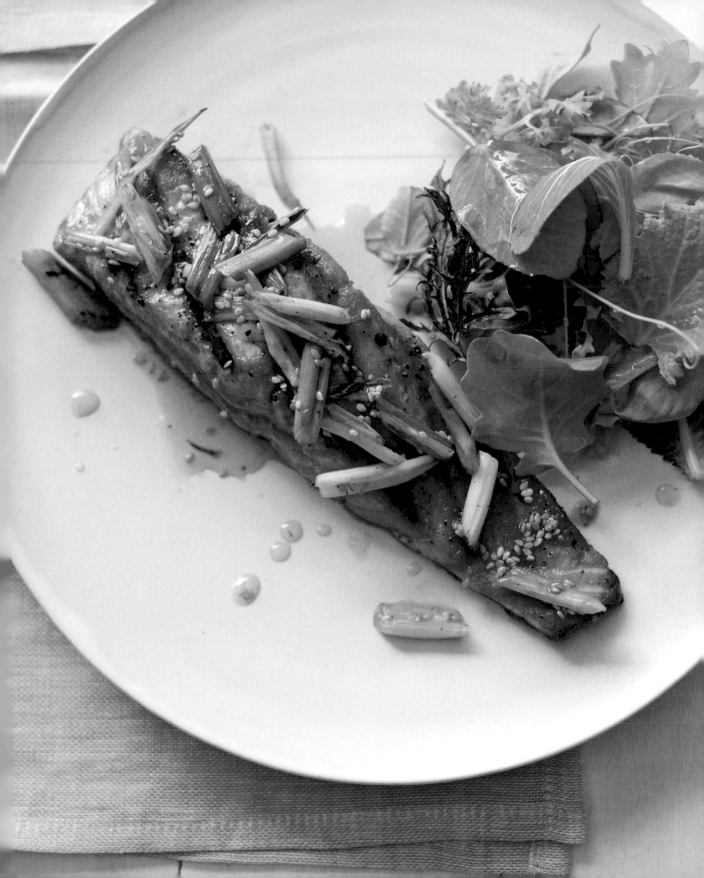

Grilled Tilapia with Balsamic Vinaigrette

4 SERVINGS / 303 CALORIES / MUFA: OLIVE OIL

Tilapia, a firm whitefish that is quite versatile in the kitchen, is usually farm-raised, making it a very sustainable seafood choice.

15 MINUTES

- 1 tablespoon balsamic vinegar
- 1 tablespoon orange juice
- 1 tablespoon thinly sliced fresh basil
- 1 teaspoon Dijon mustard
- ½ teaspoon salt
- ¼ teaspoon ground black pepper
- 4 tablespoons extra-virgin olive oil
- 4 tilapia fillets (6 ounces each)
- 4 cups mixed baby greens

1. Preheat the grill to medium-high.

2. Combine the vinegar, orange juice, basil, mustard, ¼ teaspoon of the salt, and ⅛ teaspoon of the pepper in a small bowl. Slowly whisk in 3 tablespoons of the oil and set aside.

3. Brush the tilapia fillets with the remaining 1 tablespoon oil and sprinkle with the remaining ¼ teaspoon salt and ⅛ teaspoon pepper. Set the fillets on a grill rack that has been coated with cooking spray. Grill for 3½ to 4 minutes per side, or until the fish flakes easily with a fork. Serve the fish on a bed of greens topped with the vinaigrette.

Nutrition per serving
- 303 calories
- 35 g protein
- 3 g carbohydrates
- 17 g fat
- 3 g saturated fat
- 85 mg cholesterol
- 410 mg sodium
- 1 g fiber

MAKE IT A FLAT BELLY DIET MEAL: Serve with a 6″ whole wheat pita (120). Total meal: 423 calories

Grilled Chicken Breasts with Pan-Roasted Tomatoes and Olives

4 SERVINGS / 363 CALORIES / MUFA: OLIVES

Here's a quick and easy way to use your grill to make a perfect pasta sauce to go with your chicken. If you happen to have some precooked chicken on hand, you can whip up this dish indoors in no time flat.

20 MINUTES

6 ounces multigrain penne pasta

2 teaspoons olive oil

1 pound boneless, skinless chicken breasts

½ teaspoon salt

Ground black pepper

1 pint grape tomatoes, halved

40 pitted black olives

2 garlic cloves, smashed

1 sprig fresh rosemary or thyme

Chopped parsley, for garnish

Nutrition per serving

○ 363 calories
○ 35 g protein
○ 35 g carbohydrates
○ 9 g fat
○ 1.5 g saturated fat
○ 65 mg cholesterol
○ 770 mg sodium*
○ 5 g fiber

1. Bring a large pot of water to a boil. Add the pasta and cook according to package directions. Drain and cover to keep warm while you're grilling.

2. Preheat the grill to medium-high.

3. Drizzle 1 teaspoon of the oil over the chicken. Sprinkle with the salt and pepper to taste.

4. Combine the remaining 1 teaspoon oil, the tomatoes, olives, garlic, and rosemary in an ovenproof skillet (cast iron is ideal).

5. Arrange the skillet and chicken on the grill. Cook the chicken for 3 to 4 minutes per side, or until a thermometer inserted in the thickest part registers 165°F. Meanwhile, cook the tomatoes until fragrant and juicy. Remove the chicken from the grill and let rest for 5 minutes. Cook the tomatoes a few minutes longer, if desired. Discard the rosemary sprig.

6. Slice the chicken into thin strips and toss with the pasta and tomato sauce. Garnish with chopped parsley.

Limit saturated fat to no more than 10 percent of total calories—about 17 grams per day for most women or 21 grams for most men—and sodium intake to no more than 2,300 milligrams.

MAKE IT A FLAT BELLY DIET MEAL: Serve with 2 cups chopped romaine (16) mixed with ½ cup chopped carrots (26) and tossed with 1 tablespoon balsamic vinegar (14). Total meal: 419 calories

Mediterranean Chicken Kebabs with Lemon-Tahini Sauce

4 SERVINGS / 273 CALORIES / MUFA: TAHINI

Once opened, your jar of tahini should be refrigerated in a tightly sealed container to prevent rancidity. Use within 3 months.

30 MINUTES

- 2 **teaspoons olive oil**
- 2 **teaspoons minced garlic**
  Juice of 1 lemon
- 1 **pound boneless, skinless chicken breasts, cut into 24 pieces**
- 1 **red bell pepper, cut into 8 pieces**
- 2 **small zucchini (about ¾ pound), cut crosswise into 12 pieces**
- ½ **red onion, quartered**
- ¼ **cup tahini**

Nutrition per serving
- ○ 273 calories
- ○ 30 g protein
- ○ 11 g carbohydrates
- ○ 12 g fat
- ○ 2 g saturated fat
- ○ 65 mg cholesterol
- ○ 90 mg sodium
- ○ 3 g fiber

1. Preheat the grill to high. If using bamboo skewers, soak them in water while you prepare other ingredients.

2. Combine the oil, 1 teaspoon of the garlic, and half of the lemon juice in a small bowl. Drizzle half of the lemon mixture over the chicken and the other half over the pepper, zucchini, and onion. Toss to coat and then thread equal amounts of chicken and vegetables onto skewers.

3. Stir together the tahini, ¼ cup water, remaining 1 teaspoon oil, and remaining lemon juice in a small bowl.

4. Grill the kebabs over indirect heat for 8 to 10 minutes, turning to ensure even browning, until the chicken is cooked through and the vegetables are tender.

5. To serve, drizzle each kebab with one-fourth of the lemon-tahini sauce.

MAKE IT A TEAM EFFORT Once you've assembled the cut-up ingredients, enlist an older child to thread the skewers while you prepare the lemon-tahini sauce. Do the first one together until you're sure your child can handle the sharp skewers.

MAKE IT A FLAT BELLY DIET MEAL: Serve with 1 cup whole wheat couscous (140).
Total meal: 413 calories

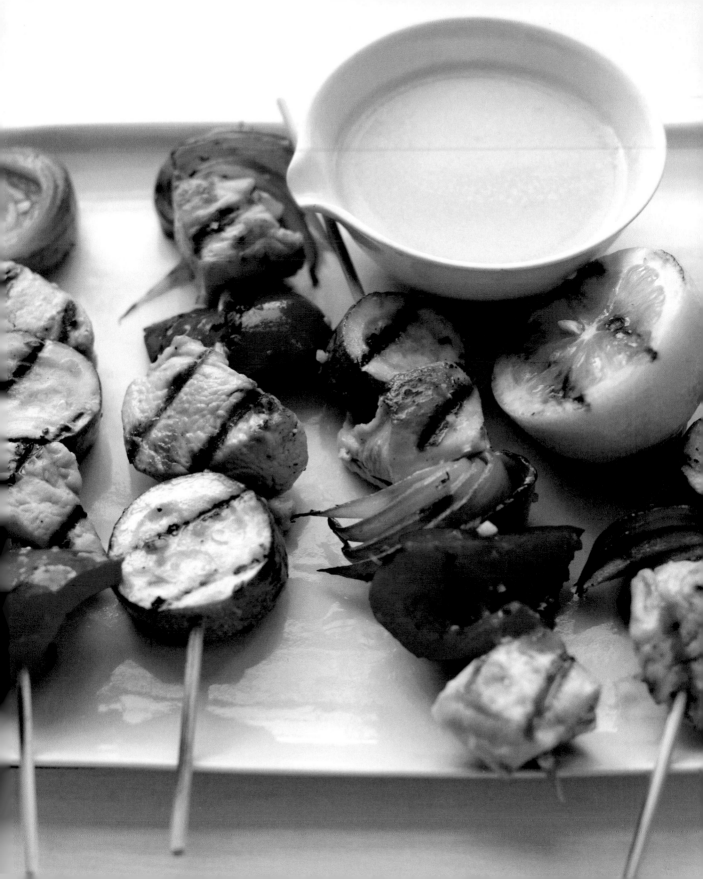

Tandoori Chicken Thighs

4 SERVINGS / 328 CALORIES / MUFA: WALNUTS

This popular Indian chicken dish tastes just as good cooked on a hot grill versus a tandoor, a traditional clay oven that can reach temperatures of 900°F.

45
MINUTES +
MARINATING
TIME

- 4 **bone-in skinless chicken thighs (6 ounces each)**
- 2 **containers (5.3 ounces each) fat-free plain Greek yogurt**
- 2 **tablespoons lemon juice**
- 2 **garlic cloves, minced**
- 1 **tablespoon minced fresh ginger**
- 1 **teaspoon paprika**
- ½ **teaspoon ground coriander**
- ½ **teaspoon ground cumin**
- ¼ **teaspoon ground cinnamon**
- ¼ **teaspoon ground red pepper**
- ½ **cup walnuts**
- 2 **teaspoons honey**
- 2 **teaspoons grated orange zest**
- ¾ **teaspoon salt**

Nutrition per serving

- 328 calories
- 39 g protein
- 9 g carbohydrates
- 15 g fat
- 2.5 g saturated fat
- 140 mg cholesterol
- 600 mg sodium*
- 1 g fiber

1. Combine the chicken, 1 container of the yogurt, the lemon juice, garlic, ginger, paprika, coriander, cumin, cinnamon, and red pepper in a large zip-top bag. Shake well to mix and coat. Refrigerate overnight.

2. Preheat the grill to medium-high.

3. Meanwhile, cook the walnuts in a medium skillet over medium-high heat, shaking the pan often, for 3 to 5 minutes, or until lightly toasted. Transfer to a cutting board. When cool enough to handle, coarsely chop and combine with the remaining container of yogurt, the honey, orange zest, and ¼ teaspoon of the salt. Set aside.

4. Remove the chicken from the marinade and sprinkle with the remaining ½ teaspoon salt. Set on a grill rack that has been coated with cooking spray. Grill 12 to 13 minutes per side, or until a thermometer inserted in the thickest part of the thigh registers 165°F.

5. Serve the chicken with the walnut sauce.

* Limit saturated fat to no more than 10 percent of total calories—about 17 grams per day for most women or 21 grams for most men—and sodium intake to no more than 2,300 milligrams.

MAKE IT A FLAT BELLY DIET MEAL: Serve with 1 cup cooked green beans (44) and half of a 6" whole grain pita (60). **Total meal: 432 calories.** To serve as part of another FBD meal, omit the walnuts (246).

Barbecue Turkey Burgers with Avocado Mash

4 SERVINGS / 358 CALORIES / MUFA: AVOCADO

Unlike many grilled turkey burgers, which have a tendency to be dry, these tasty burgers draw great barbecue flavor from the sauce inside. If you're new to Peppadew peppers, look for them in the olive bar at your grocery; their sweet-peppery flavor offers a perfect way to perk up an otherwise mild avocado.

25 MINUTES

1 Hass avocado, mashed

2 tablespoons finely chopped Peppadew peppers

1 pound 93% lean ground turkey

½ red onion, finely chopped

¼ cup barbecue sauce

4 whole wheat buns

Nutrition per serving

○ 358 calories
○ 27 g protein
○ 34 g carbohydrates
○ 14 g fat
○ 3 g saturated fat
○ 65 mg cholesterol
○ 500 mg sodium
○ 6 g fiber

1. Preheat the grill to high.

2. Combine the avocado and peppers in a small bowl. Set aside.

3. Combine the turkey, onion, and barbecue sauce in a large bowl. Mix with clean hands until thoroughly combined. Form the mixture into 4 patties about ½" thick. Grill the patties for 3 to 4 minutes, or until the bottom is well browned (do not turn sooner or the burgers might fall apart). Turn and grill for 3 to 4 minutes on the second side, or until a thermometer inserted sideways registers 165°F.

4. Serve the burgers on whole wheat buns topped with equal amounts of the avocado mixture.

MAKE IT A FLAT BELLY DIET MEAL: Serve with 1 wedge (one-eighth of a melon) honeydew (58).
Total meal: 416 calories

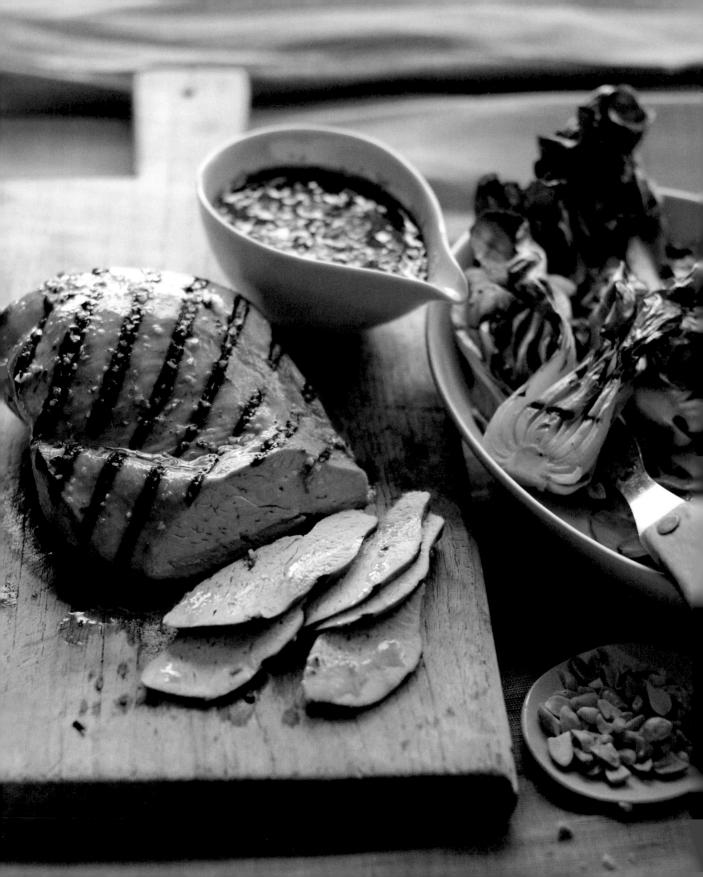

Grilled Turkey and Bok Choy with Chile-Garlic Sauce

4 SERVINGS / 370 CALORIES / MUFA: CANOLA OIL

Chile oil is an important ingredient in many Asian recipes, but you can make your own garlicky version for a fraction of the cost with this easy recipe.

40 MINUTES

¼ cup canola oil

½ teaspoon crushed red-pepper flakes

2 heaping teaspoons minced garlic

1 pound boneless, skinless turkey breast

2 tablespoons oyster sauce

1 tablespoon reduced-sodium soy sauce

2 scallions, thinly sliced

2½ pounds bok choy, halved lengthwise and rinsed under cold water

¼ cup dry-roasted unsalted peanuts, chopped

Nutrition per serving
- 370 calories
- 35 g protein
- 13 g carbohydrates
- 20 g fat
- 2 g saturated fat
- 70 mg cholesterol
- 840 mg sodium*
- 4 g fiber

1. Preheat the grill to medium-high.

2. Meanwhile, heat the canola oil in a small pan over medium heat. Add the red-pepper flakes and cook until the oil begins to sizzle. Remove from the heat and stir in the garlic. Let cool for a few minutes.

3. Rub 2 teaspoons of the chile-garlic oil over the turkey. Add the oyster sauce, soy sauce, and scallions to the chile-garlic oil remaining in the pan. Stir until well combined and set aside.

4. Grill the turkey and bok choy for 20 to 25 minutes, or until a thermometer inserted in the thickest part of the breast registers 155°F and the bok choy is tender. Remove from the heat, cover, and let rest for 10 minutes.

5. Coarsely chop the bok choy and slice the turkey into thin pieces. Pour the reserved chile-garlic sauce over the mixture and toss to coat. Serve topped with peanuts.

Limit saturated fat to no more than 10 percent of total calories—about 17 grams per day for most women or 21 grams for most men—and sodium intake to no more than 2,300 milligrams.

MAKE IT A FLAT BELLY DIET MEAL: Serve with ½ navel orange (35). Total meal: 405 calories

Spice-Rubbed Pork Tenderloin with Avocado, Cucumber, and Onion Salad

4 SERVINGS (¼ PORK, 1 TORTILLA, AND 1½ CUPS SALAD EACH) / 313 CALORIES / MUFA: AVOCADO

Tenderloin is one of the leanest cuts of pork you can buy. But because it doesn't have much fat, it needs a little extra seasoning to make it work—just make sure to use a mild chili powder in your dish if you prefer less spicy dishes.

40 MINUTES

2 teaspoons light brown sugar
1 teaspoon chili powder
1 teaspoon ground cumin
¼ teaspoon garlic powder
¾ teaspoon salt
¼ teaspoon ground black pepper
1 pound well-trimmed pork tenderloin
1 cucumber
2 tomatoes
1 Hass avocado
1 small white onion, thinly sliced
1½ tablespoons olive oil
1 tablespoon fresh lime juice
4 corn tortillas (6")

Nutrition per serving

○ 313 calories
○ 27 g protein
○ 21 g carbohydrates
○ 14 g fat
○ 2.5 g saturated fat
○ 75 mg cholesterol
○ 510 mg sodium
○ 5 g fiber

1. Preheat the grill to medium-high.

2. Combine the brown sugar, chili powder, cumin, garlic powder, ½ teaspoon of the salt, and the pepper in a small bowl. Rub the mixture over the pork. Set the pork on a grill rack that has been coated with cooking spray. Grill, turning occasionally, for 22 to 24 minutes, or until a thermometer inserted in the center of the pork registers 155°F. Transfer to a cutting board and let rest for 10 minutes.

3. Meanwhile, peel the cucumber and cut in half lengthwise. Chop the cucumber into ½"-thick slices. Chop the tomatoes and avocado into 1" chunks. Combine the cucumber, tomatoes, avocado, onion, oil, lime juice, and remaining ¼ teaspoon salt in a bowl.

4. Warm the tortillas on the grill for 30 seconds per side. Slice the pork and serve with the avocado salad and tortillas.

MAKE IT A FLAT BELLY DIET MEAL: Serve with 1 cup sliced mango (108). Total meal: 421 calories

Barbecued Pork Tenderloin

4 SERVINGS / 328 CALORIES / MUFA: PEANUT BUTTER

This main course is so rich and indulgent that all you'll need on the side is steamed spinach—and perhaps some ice-cold watermelon to end the meal.

45 MINUTES

½ cup natural unsalted creamy peanut butter
Juice and zest of ½ lime
2 garlic cloves, minced
1½ teaspoons Cajun seasoning
¼ teaspoon garlic powder
1 pound well-trimmed pork tenderloin
2 tablespoons minced fresh cilantro

Nutrition per serving
○ 328 calories
○ 31 g protein
○ 8 g carbohydrates
○ 18 g fat
○ 3 g saturated fat
○ 75 mg cholesterol
○ 380 mg sodium
○ 2 g fiber

1. Preheat the grill to medium.

2. Combine the peanut butter, lime juice and zest, garlic, Cajun seasoning, and garlic powder in a 13" x 9" shallow disposable aluminum baking pan. Stir until smooth. Pat the tenderloin dry and spread evenly with the peanut butter mixture. Grill in the pan over indirect heat for 30 minutes, or until a thermometer inserted in the center registers 155°F. Transfer to a cutting board and let rest for 10 minutes.

3. Carve the pork into very thin slices. Fan out onto 4 plates. Sprinkle with the cilantro.

MAKE IT A FLAT BELLY DIET MEAL: Serve with 1 cup steamed spinach (41) and 1 cup watermelon balls (46). Total meal: 415 calories

Caramelized Onion and Swiss Burgers

4 SERVINGS / 434 CALORIES / MUFA: TAPENADE

Who needs to pay for a pricey night out for fancy burgers when you can make your own so easily? This recipe is sure to make your weekly request list.

35 MINUTES

- 1 tablespoon olive oil
- 2 yellow onions, thinly sliced
- $\frac{1}{2}$ teaspoon salt
- $\frac{1}{4}$ teaspoon ground black pepper
- 1 pound 93% lean ground beef
- $\frac{1}{4}$ cup black olive tapenade
- 4 slices ($\frac{3}{4}$ ounce each) reduced-fat Swiss cheese
- 4 multigrain English muffins, toasted
- $\frac{1}{2}$ tomato, cut into 4 slices

Nutrition per serving

- 434 calories
- 37 g protein
- 31 g carbohydrates
- 22 g fat
- 6 g saturated fat*
- 80 mg cholesterol
- 500 mg sodium
- 9 g fiber

1. Preheat the grill to medium-high.

2. Heat the oil in a medium nonstick skillet over medium-high heat. Cook the onions, stirring occasionally, for 8 to 9 minutes, or until golden brown. Remove from the heat and season with $\frac{1}{4}$ teaspoon of the salt and $\frac{1}{8}$ teaspoon of the pepper.

3. Meanwhile, gently combine the beef, 2 tablespoons of the tapenade, and the remaining $\frac{1}{4}$ teaspoon salt and $\frac{1}{8}$ teaspoon pepper in a bowl. Form the mixture into 4 patties $\frac{1}{2}$" thick. Set on a grill rack coated with cooking spray. Grill for 5 minutes without turning. Turn and grill for 4 minutes, or until a thermometer inserted sideways registers 160°F. Transfer the burgers to a plate. Top each burger with 1 slice of cheese and let rest 1 to 2 minutes to melt the cheese.

4. Spread the bottom half of each English muffin with $1\frac{1}{2}$ teaspoons of the remaining tapenade. Top each with 1 tomato slice, one-fourth of the onions, and a burger. Top each burger with 1 of the the remaining English muffin halves.

Limit saturated fat to no more than 10 percent of total calories—about 17 grams per day for most women or 21 grams for most men—and sodium intake to no more than 2,300 milligrams.

MAKE IT A FLAT BELLY DIET MEAL: A single serving of this recipe counts as a Flat Belly Diet Meal without any add-ons!

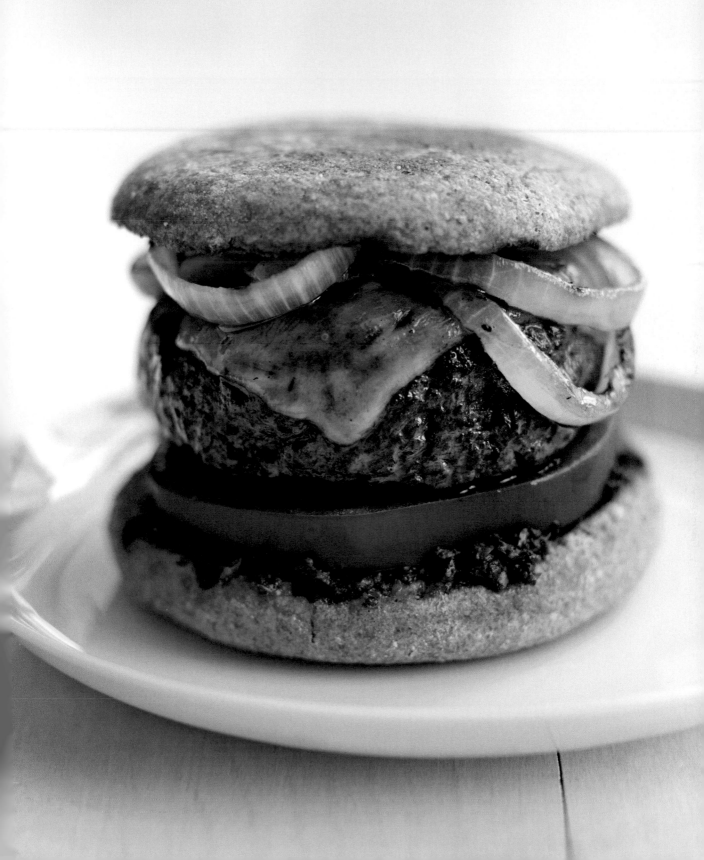

Grilled Flank Steak with Chimichurri Sauce

4 SERVINGS / 294 CALORIES / MUFA: OLIVE OIL

Similar to a pesto with its bright green color, the vibrant flavors of this chimichurri sauce take an ordinary flank steak to new heights.

35 MINUTES + MARINATING TIME

- 1 pound well-trimmed flank steak
- 2½ teaspoons minced garlic
- 5 teaspoons fresh lime juice
- ¼ cup extra-virgin olive oil
- 1 tablespoon red wine vinegar
- ¼ cup chopped parsley
- ¼ cup chopped fresh basil
- 3 tablespoons chopped fresh cilantro
- ½ teaspoon ground cumin
- ¾ teaspoon salt
- ¼ teaspoon ground black pepper

Nutrition per serving

- ○ 294 calories
- ○ 25 g protein
- ○ 2 g carbohydrates
- ○ 20 g fat
- ○ 4.5 g saturated fat*
- ○ 35 mg cholesterol
- ○ 500 mg sodium
- ○ 0 g fiber

1. Combine the flank steak, 2 teaspoons of the garlic, 3 teaspoons of the lime juice, and 1 teaspoon of the oil in a bowl. Toss well to coat and refrigerate for 1 hour.

2. Meanwhile, combine the remaining ½ teaspoon garlic, 2 teaspoons lime juice, 3 tablespoons + 2 teaspoons oil, the vinegar, parsley, basil, cilantro, cumin, ¼ teaspoon of the salt, and ⅛ teaspoon of the pepper. Set the chimichurri sauce aside.

3. Preheat the grill to medium-high.

4. Sprinkle the flank steak with the remaining ½ teaspoon salt and ⅛ teaspoon pepper. Set on a grill rack coated with cooking spray. Grill for 8 to 9 minutes for medium-rare or longer for desired doneness. Turn halfway through cooking time. Transfer to a cutting board and let rest for 5 minutes.

5. Thinly slice the steak across the grain. Serve topped with the chimichurri sauce.

* Limit saturated fat to no more than 10 percent of total calories—about 17 grams per day for most women or 21 grams for most men—and sodium intake to no more than 2,300 milligrams.

MAKE IT A FLAT BELLY DIET MEAL: Serve with 1 medium baked sweet potato (103).
Total meal: 397 calories

Marinated Beef Tip Roast

6 SERVINGS / 270 CALORIES / MUFA: OLIVE OIL

Don't fear the amount of garlic in the recipe. The cloves mellow out while simmering in the marinade to make the sauce. It's common to find eye of round roasts in 3-pound packages, so buy that size, if necessary, and use the other half for the Oven-Baked Pot Roast recipe on page 197.

40 MINUTES + MARINATING TIME

6 tablespoons olive oil
Juice and zest of 1 lemon
1 teaspoon dried thyme
8 garlic cloves, halved
½ teaspoon salt
¼ teaspoon ground black pepper
1½ pounds well-trimmed boneless beef eye of round roast

Nutrition per serving
○ 270 calories
○ 26 g protein
○ 2 g carbohydrates
○ 17 g fat
○ 3 g saturated fat
○ 45 mg cholesterol
○ 260 mg sodium
○ 0 g fiber

1. Combine the oil, lemon juice and zest, thyme, garlic, salt, and pepper in a large zip-top bag. Place the roast in the bag. Massage the marinade into the roast. Seal and refrigerate, turning and massaging occasionally, for 12 to 24 hours.

2. Preheat the grill to medium.

3. Working over a small saucepan, snip a bottom corner of the marinade bag to make a small hole. Squeeze all of the marinade and the garlic cloves into the pan. Remove the roast from the bag, oil a grill rack, and place the roast over direct heat. Grill for 10 minutes, turning to sear all sides of the roast. Move the roast to indirect heat and grill for 30 minutes, or until a thermometer inserted in the center registers 145°F for medium-rare/160°F for medium/165°F for well done. Transfer to a plate and let rest for 10 minutes.

4. Meanwhile, cover the saucepan and bring the marinade to a simmer over medium-low heat. Reduce the heat and simmer for 15 minutes. Turn off the heat and allow to sit while the roast cooks.

5. Reheat the marinade briefly. Transfer to a mini food processor or blender. Process for 2 to 3 minutes, or until the sauce is thickened and lighter in color. Add any juices that have accumulated on the beef roast plate. Transfer the beef to a cutting board and carve into thin slices. Serve with the sauce.

🕐 MAKE IT **AHEAD** If you are serving only 4 for dinner, save the 2 leftover portions for recipes that call for cooked roast beef.

MAKE IT A FLAT BELLY DIET MEAL: Serve with Haricots Verts (page 220), but omit the olive oil (131).
Total meal: 401 calories

QUICK-FIX PANTRY RESCUES

Salmon Salad with Avocado-Lime Dressing

Place ¼ cup mashed **Hass avocado** (96) and 1 tablespoon fresh lime juice (4) in a blender; process, adding spoonfuls of water until as thin as a salad dressing. Flake 4 ounces grilled salmon fillet (207) over 2 cups baby spinach (20) and top with the dressing. Serve with 8 thin whole wheat crackers (70) on the side. **Total Calories = 397**

Grilled Shrimp and Tapenade Pita

Combine 3 ounces grilled shrimp (84), ½ cup grape tomatoes (15), ¼ cup chopped cucumber (4), and 2 tablespoons **black olive tapenade** (88) in a 6″ whole wheat pita (120). Serve with 1 orange (69). **Total Calories = 380**

Grilled Chicken with Italian Mashed Beans

Rinse and drain ½ cup canned cannellini beans (100), then mash with 1 tablespoon **olive oil** (120), ½ teaspoon minced garlic (8), and a dash of dried oregano (0). Warm in the microwave until heated through. Serve with 3 ounces grilled chicken breast (122) and ½ cup steamed broccoli (22). **Total Calories = 372**

Cheesy Chicken Quesadilla

Heat 1 tablespoon **olive oil** (120) in a nonstick skillet over medium-high heat. Place 2 ounces chopped grilled chicken (81) and ¼ cup shredded reduced-fat Cheddar cheese (80) on 1 side of an 8″ whole wheat tortilla (106); fold over and cook for 2 to 3 minutes per side, or until crispy. **Total Calories = 387**

Grilled Eggplant Pasta with Garlic Oil

Coat ½ pound Japanese eggplant (53) with ½ teaspoon olive oil (20) and ¼ teaspoon salt (0). Grill over indirect heat for 4 to 5 minutes, or until tender. Meanwhile, cook 2 ounces multigrain pasta (202). Drain and toss with 1 tablespoon **olive oil** (120), 1 teaspoon minced garlic (15), ¼ teaspoon crushed red-pepper flakes (0), and 1 tablespoon Parmesan cheese (22). Chop the eggplant into bite-size pieces and toss with the pasta. **Total Calories = 432**

Menu for a Perfect Summer Cookout

Mixed grill of Barbecued Pork Tenderloin (page 127)
and grilled boneless, skinless chicken breasts
5-Bean Salad (page 205)
Sliced beefsteak tomatoes
Cucumber Coleslaw (below)
Blueberry Pie (page 276)

SERVES 8

⊙ **The night before:** Make Blueberry Pie and a double-batch of 5-Bean Salad. Cover and refrigerate the salad.

⊙ **About 2 hours before serving:** Prepare Cucumber Coleslaw by combining ¼ cup canola oil, 2 tablespoons cider vinegar, 1 tablespoon Dijon mustard, and 2 teaspoons honey in a large bowl. Thinly slice 1 head of cabbage and peel and seed 3 cucumbers. Grate the cucumbers and squeeze to remove as much water as possible. Add the cucumbers and cabbage to the oil mixture and toss to coat. Season to taste with salt and pepper. Refrigerate until ready to serve.

⊙ **About 1 hour before serving:** Grill the pork tenderloin along with some chicken breasts for those who prefer less seasoned dishes.

⊙ **About 15 minutes before serving:** Slice the tomatoes and sprinkle with salt and pepper.

MAKE IT A FLAT BELLY DIET MEAL: Enjoy *either* the pork tenderloin (328) with coleslaw on the side (105) or a 3-ounce piece of grilled chicken (122) with the bean salad (254) and a few tomato slices (12). **Total meal = 433 calories (pork and coleslaw) or 388 calories (chicken and bean salad).** Later in the day, enjoy a slice of pie as your FBD snack (435). **Total meal = 435 calories**

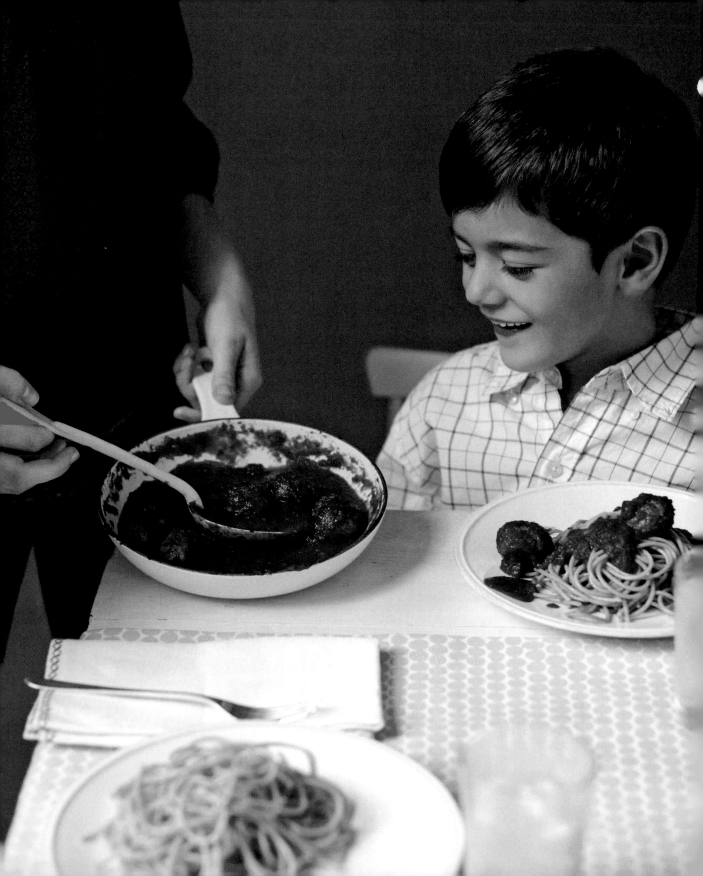

7

STOVETOP
Standards

- Butternut Squash Ravioli
- Mushroom, Onion, and Avocado Quesadillas
- Cashew, Tofu, and Broccoli Stir-Fry
- Penne with Cherry Tomatoes
- Chickpea Ragu with Polenta
- Pan-Seared Shrimp Tacos
- Shrimp and Broccoli with Peanut BBQ Sauce
- Spaghetti with White Clam Sauce
- Halibut with Chopped Olive Salad
- Sesame-Crusted Tuna Steaks
- Pan-Seared Chicken Breasts with Walnuts and Apples
- Chicken Cutlets Topped with Turkey Bacon and Avocado

- Thai Basil-Coconut Chicken
- Indian Chicken in Cashew-Cilantro Sauce
- Chicken and Bok Choy with Almonds
- Chinese BBQ Chicken Patties
- Chicken Tenders with Two Dips
- Chicken Cacciatore
- Chicken Picadillo
- Chicken Thighs with Green Beans
- Pork and Sweet Potato Skillet
- Lebanese Beef Patties
- Spaghetti and Meatballs
- Stovetop Meat Loaf with Mushroom Gravy
- Beefsteak Stuffed with Olives

Butternut Squash Ravioli

4 SERVINGS / 398 CALORIES / MUFA: WALNUTS

An ordinary serving of packaged cheese ravioli can have over 330 calories—hardly enough room for a sauce and MUFA serving! But with this easy-to-prepare recipe, you're in control of the ingredients.

45 MINUTES

1 package (12 ounces) frozen butternut squash puree
½ cup walnuts
1 egg yolk
½ cup grated Parmesan cheese
½ teaspoon salt
¼ teaspoon ground black pepper
⅛ teaspoon ground nutmeg
24 wonton wrappers
1 tablespoon unsalted butter
2 tablespoons extra-virgin olive oil
1 tablespoon chopped fresh sage
1 tablespoon fresh lemon juice

Nutrition per serving

○ 398 calories
○ 13 g protein
○ 41 g carbohydrates
○ 22 g fat
○ 6 g saturated fat*
○ 70 mg cholesterol
○ 690 mg sodium*
○ 4 g fiber

1. Place squash in a microwaveable bowl and cook on high power for 5 minutes. Stir until smooth and allow to cool 5 minutes.

2. Meanwhile, place the walnuts in a medium skillet and cook over medium-high heat, shaking the pan often, for 3 to 5 minutes, or until lightly toasted. Transfer to a cutting board to cool, then finely chop. Transfer the nuts to the bowl with the squash and stir in the egg yolk, ¼ cup of the cheese, ¼ teaspoon of the salt, ⅛ teaspoon of the pepper, and the nutmeg. Mix well.

3. Arrange 12 wonton wrappers on a work surface. Drop 2 slightly rounded teaspoons of filling onto the center of each. Wet the edge of the wrapper with a finger dipped in water. Fold 1 corner of the wrapper diagonally over the filling to form a triangle. Gently press out any air and squeeze the edges to seal. Repeat with the remaining filling and wrappers.

4. Melt the butter in a small skillet over medium-high heat. Cook, shaking the pan occasionally, until the butter begins to brown and smell nutty. Add the olive oil and sage and cook for 1 minute. Turn the heat to low and add the lemon juice and remaining ¼ teaspoon salt and ⅛ teaspoon pepper. Keep warm.

5. Bring a large pot of water to a gentle boil. Add the ravioli a few at a time and cook for 2 minutes. Drain, transfer to a large bowl, and immediately pour in the butter mixture. Toss well to coat. Sprinkle with the remaining ¼ cup cheese and serve.

* Limit saturated fat to no more than 10 percent of total calories—about 17 grams per day for most women or 21 grams for most men—and sodium intake to no more than 2,300 milligrams.

MAKE IT A FLAT BELLY DIET MEAL: Serve with 2 cups romaine (16) and 1 tablespoon balsamic vinegar (14). Total meal: 428 calories

Mushroom, Onion, and Avocado Quesadillas

4 SERVINGS / 381 CALORIES / MUFA: AVOCADO

If your family is addicted to taco night, switch things up and try a quesadilla night instead. These meaty-tasting mushrooms are so satisfying you're likely to have a new tradition on your hands.

40
MINUTES

1 tablespoon olive oil
1 large onion, chopped
1 package (8 ounces) sliced mushrooms
¼ teaspoon salt
4 garlic cloves, minced
1 Hass avocado, mashed with a fork
2 tablespoons chopped fresh cilantro
4 flour tortillas (8")
1 cup (4 ounces) shredded reduced-fat sharp Cheddar cheese

1. Heat the oil in a large nonstick skillet over medium-high heat. Add the onion, mushrooms, and salt. Cook, stirring occasionally, for 9 to 10 minutes, or until browned. Stir in the garlic and cook for 2 minutes longer. Remove from the heat.

2. Combine the avocado and cilantro in a bowl. Arrange the tortillas in a single layer on a work surface. Spread the bottom half of each tortilla with one-fourth of the avocado mixture. Top each with 2 tablespoons of the cheese and one-fourth of the onion mixture. Sprinkle each with 2 tablespoons of the remaining cheese. Fold the top half of each tortilla over the filling.

3. Wipe out the skillet and place over medium heat. Add 2 quesadillas and cook for 3 to 4 minutes per side, or until the filling is hot and the outside is lightly browned. Repeat with the remaining quesadillas. Transfer to a cutting board and cut each in half before serving.

Nutrition per serving

- 381 calories
- 14 g protein
- 36 g carbohydrates
- 22 g fat
- 6 g saturated fat*
- 20 mg cholesterol
- 680 mg sodium*
- 7 g fiber

Limit saturated fat to no more than 10 percent of total calories—about 17 grams per day for most women or 21 grams for most men—and sodium intake to no more than 2,300 milligrams.

MAKE IT A FLAT BELLY DIET MEAL: A single serving of this recipe counts as a Flat Belly Diet Meal without any add-ons!

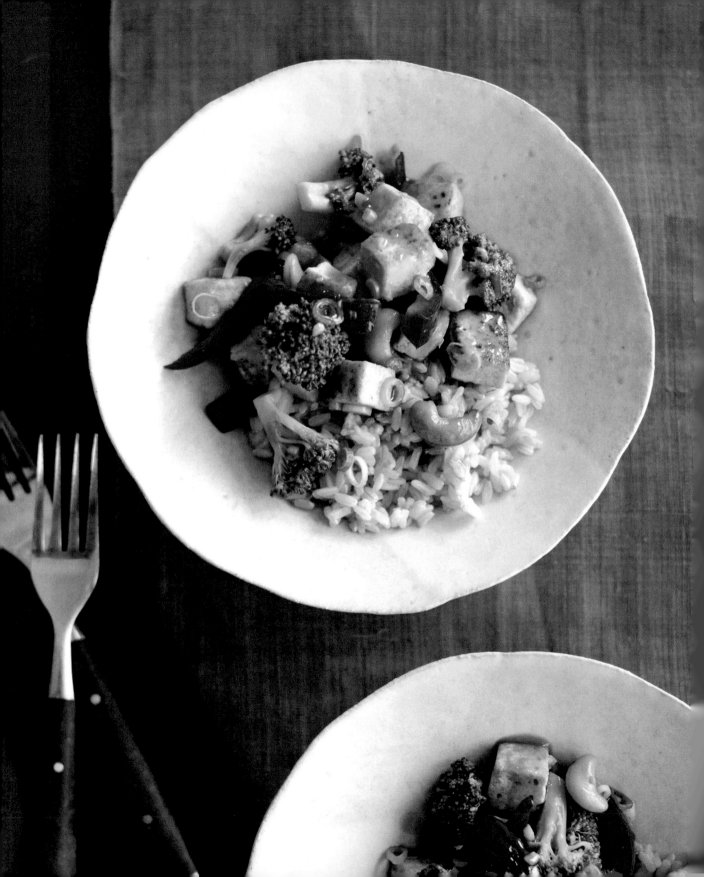

Cashew, Tofu, and Broccoli Stir-Fry

4 SERVINGS (1¼ CUPS EACH) / 382 CALORIES / MUFA: CASHEWS

When you calculate the time spent driving to and from the restaurant, this dish is probably faster than regular takeout. And with your own fresh ingredients and only 1 tablespoon of oil in the mix, it's surely a lot healthier.

20 MINUTES

1 container (14 ounces) firm light tofu
2 tablespoons reduced-sodium soy sauce
2 tablespoons honey
1 tablespoon rice vinegar
1 teaspoon cornstarch
3 cups broccoli florets
3 teaspoons toasted sesame oil
1 red bell pepper, chopped
1 tablespoon minced fresh ginger
3 garlic cloves, minced
½ cup unsalted cashews
3 scallions, chopped
2 cups cooked brown rice

Nutrition per serving
○ 382 calories
○ 16 g protein
○ 48 g carbohydrates
○ 15 g fat
○ 2.5 g saturated fat
○ 0 mg cholesterol
○ 510 mg sodium
○ 6 g fiber

1. Place the tofu on a paper towel set on a dinner plate. Top with a second paper towel and another dinner plate. Place a can or other similar weight on the upper plate and leave for 20 minutes to press excess water from the tofu.

2. Meanwhile, bring a medium pot of water to a boil. Combine the soy sauce, honey, vinegar, and cornstarch in a small bowl.

3. Add the broccoli to the boiling water, return to a boil, and cook for 1 minute, or until bright green. Drain and set aside.

4. Transfer the tofu to a cutting board and cut into ½" to ¾" cubes. Heat 2 teaspoons of the sesame oil in a large nonstick skillet over medium-high heat. Add the tofu and cook, stirring occasionally, for 4 to 5 minutes, or until lightly golden. Transfer the tofu to a plate and set aside.

5. Heat the remaining 1 teaspoon oil in the skillet. Add the pepper and cook, stirring occasionally, for 1 minute. Add the ginger and garlic and cook for 30 seconds, or until fragrant. Stir in the broccoli and tofu, and cook for 1½ minutes, or until hot. Stir the soy sauce mixture to recombine and add to the skillet along with the cashews. Cook, stirring, for 1 minute. Remove from the heat and stir in the scallions. Serve over the rice.

MAKE IT A FLAT BELLY DIET MEAL: A single serving of this recipe counts as a Flat Belly Diet Meal without any add-ons!

Penne with Cherry Tomatoes

4 SERVINGS (1¼ CUPS EACH) / 371 CALORIES / MUFA: OLIVE OIL

Your kitchen will smell like the best Italian restaurant in town when you have this easy sauce simmering on the stove. For busy weeknights, make the pasta ahead of time, toss with ½ teaspoon olive oil, and refrigerate in a zip-top plastic bag. Do that and you can have this dish on the table in 10 minutes or less.

25
MINUTES

- 8 **ounces multigrain penne pasta**
- ¼ **cup extra-virgin olive oil**
- 6 **garlic cloves, sliced**
- ⅛ **teaspoon crushed red-pepper flakes**
- 2 **cups cherry or grape tomatoes, halved**
- ¼ **cup chopped fresh basil**
- ¼ **cup grated Parmesan cheese**
- ½ **teaspoon salt**

Nutrition per serving
○ 371 calories
○ 10 g protein
○ 47 g carbohydrates
○ 17 g fat
○ 3 g saturated fat
○ 5 mg cholesterol
○ 370 mg sodium
○ 3 g fiber

1. Bring a large pot of water to a boil. Add the pasta and cook according to package directions. Drain and set aside.

2. Heat the oil in a large skillet over medium-high heat. Add the garlic and red-pepper flakes and cook, stirring often, for 1 minute, or until the garlic begins to brown. Stir in the tomatoes and cook, stirring often, for 1 to 1½ minutes, or until starting to wilt. Add the pasta and toss while cooking for 1 minute longer. Remove from the heat and stir in the basil, cheese, and salt. Serve hot or at room temperature.

MAKE IT A FLAT BELLY DIET MEAL: Serve with 2 cups mixed greens (18) and 1 tablespoon balsamic vinegar (10). Total meal: 399 calories

Chickpea Ragu with Polenta

4 SERVINGS (¾ CUP RAGU AND ½ CUP POLENTA EACH) / 428 CALORIES / MUFA: TAPENADE

Cheesy, soft polenta makes the perfect base for this hearty chickpea stew. If you're in the mood for cooking ahead, make some extra polenta while you're at it, and enjoy Pan-Fried Cheddar Polenta (page 66) the next morning.

20 MINUTES

- 2 **tablespoons olive oil**
- 1 **onion, finely chopped**
- 1 **teaspoon dried oregano**
- 3 **garlic cloves, minced**
- 1 **can (15 ounces) no-salt-added chickpeas, rinsed and drained**
- 1 **can (14.5 ounces) no-salt-added diced tomatoes**
- ½ **cup tapenade**
- 2 **cups 1% milk**
- ½ **teaspoon salt**
- ½ **cup instant polenta**
- ¼ **cup grated Parmesan cheese**

Nutrition per serving
- ○ 428 calories
- ○ 13 g protein
- ○ 45 g carbohydrates
- ○ 20 g fat
- ○ 3.5 g saturated fat
- ○ 10 mg cholesterol
- ○ 870 mg sodium*
- ○ 6 g fiber

1. Heat the oil in a large nonstick skillet over medium-high heat. Add the onion and oregano, and cook, stirring occasionally, for 2 to 3 minutes, or until the onion begins to soften. Stir in the garlic and cook for 30 seconds. Add the chickpeas and cook for 3 minutes. Stir in the tomatoes and cook for 3 to 4 minutes, or until starting to thicken. Reduce the heat to low, stir in the tapenade, and keep warm.

2. Combine the milk, 1 cup water, and salt in a medium saucepan. Bring the mixture to a boil over medium-high heat and whisk in the polenta in a steady stream. Cook, stirring occasionally, for 3 to 5 minutes, or until the polenta thickens. Remove from the heat and whisk in the cheese. Serve the chickpea ragu on top of the polenta.

* Limit saturated fat to no more than 10 percent of total calories—about 17 grams per day for most women or 21 grams for most men—and sodium intake to no more than 2,300 milligrams.

MAKE IT A FLAT BELLY DIET MEAL: A single serving of this recipe counts as a Flat Belly Diet Meal without any add-ons!

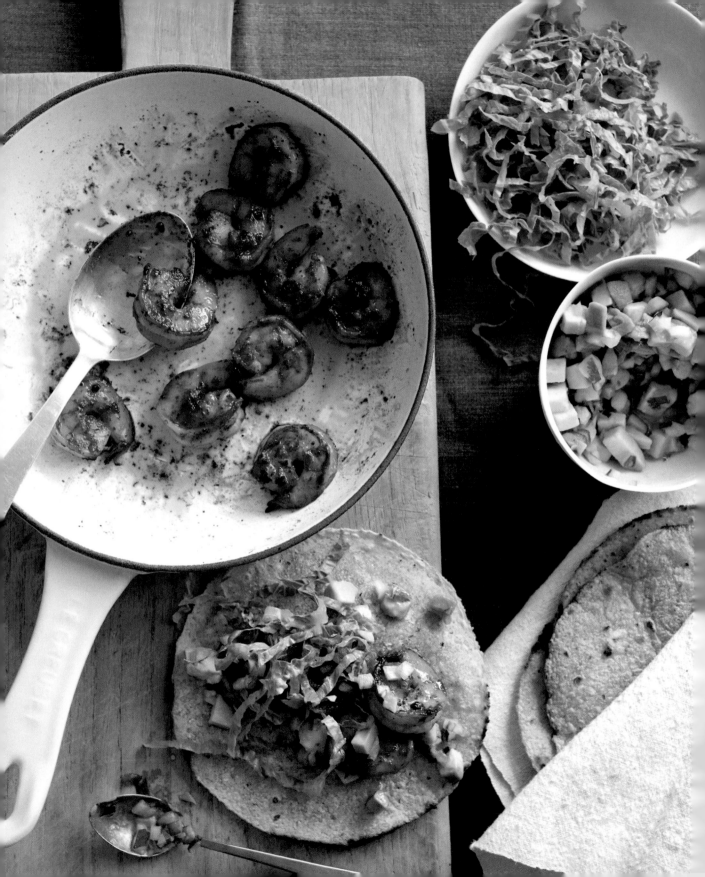

Pan-Seared Shrimp Tacos

4 SERVINGS (2 TACOS EACH) / 320 CALORIES / MUFA: AVOCADO

Not batter-dipped or deep-fried, as many fish tacos are, these leaner tacos are loaded with heart-healthy MUFAs from the avocado topping.

15 MINUTES

1 Hass avocado, cubed

3 tablespoons finely chopped red onion

2 tablespoons chopped fresh cilantro

$\frac{1}{2}$ jalapeño pepper, finely chopped

1 tablespoon fresh lime juice

$\frac{1}{2}$ teaspoon salt

1 pound peeled and deveined medium shrimp

$1\frac{1}{2}$ teaspoons chile powder

1 tablespoon olive oil

8 corn tortillas (6")

1 cup shredded romaine

1. Combine the avocado, onion, cilantro, pepper, lime juice, and $\frac{1}{4}$ teaspoon of the salt in a bowl and set aside. Combine the shrimp, chile powder, and remaining $\frac{1}{4}$ teaspoon salt in a separate bowl.

2. Heat the oil in a large nonstick skillet over medium-high heat. Add the shrimp and cook for $2\frac{1}{2}$ to 3 minutes per side, or until opaque. Transfer to a plate and keep warm.

3. Heat the tortillas in a dry skillet over medium-high heat for about 30 seconds per side, or according to package directions, until hot and lightly toasted. Dividing evenly, top each tortilla with the romaine, avocado mixture, and shrimp. Serve hot.

Nutrition per serving

○ 320 calories
○ 27 g protein
○ 27 g carbohydrates
○ 12 g fat
○ 2 g saturated fat
○ 170 mg cholesterol
○ 480 mg sodium
○ 6 g fiber

MAKE IT A FLAT BELLY DIET MEAL: Serve with $\frac{1}{2}$ cup canned juice-packed pineapple chunks (54).
Total meal: 374 calories

Shrimp and Broccoli with Peanut BBQ Sauce

4 SERVINGS (1½ CUPS SHRIMP AND BROCCOLI WITH ¼ CUP SAUCE EACH) / 420 CALORIES / MUFA: PEANUT BUTTER

You'll have no problem getting young ones to finish their broccoli with this sweet and spicy sauce served alongside.

15 MINUTES

- 1 pound peeled and deveined large shrimp
- 1 garlic clove, minced
- 1 tablespoon fresh lime juice
- 1 teaspoon ground cumin
- 1 teaspoon paprika
- ½ cup natural unsalted creamy peanut butter
- ⅓ cup barbecue sauce
- 4 tablespoons water
- ½ small chipotle pepper in adobo sauce, minced
- 1 tablespoon canola oil
- ⅛ teaspoon salt
- 4 cups broccoli florets
- 1 tablespoon fresh lemon juice

1. Combine the shrimp, garlic, lime juice, cumin, and paprika in a bowl and let stand for 10 minutes.

2. Meanwhile, whisk together the peanut butter, barbecue sauce, 3 tablespoons of the water, and the chipotle pepper in a small bowl until smooth. Set the sauce aside.

3. Heat the oil in a large nonstick skillet over medium-high heat. Sprinkle the shrimp with the salt and add to the skillet, in 2 batches if necessary, and cook for 2½ to 3 minutes per side. Transfer to a plate and keep warm.

4. Return the skillet to medium-high heat and add the broccoli along with the remaining 1 tablespoon water. Cover and steam for 2 to 3 minutes, or until bright green and tender. Drizzle the lemon juice over the broccoli and toss to coat. Serve the shrimp and broccoli with Peanut BBQ Sauce.

Nutrition per serving
- 420 calories
- 33 g protein
- 24 g carbohydrates
- 22 g fat
- 2.5 g saturated fat
- 170 mg cholesterol
- 520 mg sodium
- 4 g fiber

MAKE IT A FLAT BELLY DIET MEAL: A single serving of this recipe counts as a Flat Belly Diet Meal without any add-ons!

Spaghetti with White Clam Sauce

4 SERVINGS (³⁄₄ CUP EACH) / 378 CALORIES / MUFA: OLIVE OIL

It's good to have a few dishes that you can put together when you're running low on fresh ingredients, and this is one of them. If necessary, skip the fresh basil—the real flavors come from the clams and garlic.

25 MINUTES

- 6 ounces multigrain spaghetti
- ¼ cup extra-virgin olive oil
- 1 onion, chopped
- 5 garlic cloves, sliced
- ½ teaspoon dried basil
- 1 bottle (8 ounces) clam juice
- 2 cans (6.5 ounces each) chopped clams, drained
- ¼ teaspoon salt
- ¼ teaspoon ground black pepper
- 3 tablespoons thinly sliced fresh basil
- 1 tablespoon trans-free margarine

1. Bring a large pot of water to a boil. Add the spaghetti and cook according to package directions. Drain well.

2. Meanwhile, heat the oil in a large skillet over medium-high heat. Add the onion and cook, stirring occasionally, for 5 to 6 minutes, or until starting to brown. Stir in the garlic and dried basil and cook for 1½ to 2 minutes, or until the garlic begins to brown. Pour in the clam juice and bring the mixture just to a boil. Cook for about 3 minutes, or until the mixture is reduced by one-third. Stir in the clams and cook for 1 minute to heat through.

3. Add the spaghetti, salt, and pepper and cook, tossing, for 1 minute to heat through. Remove from the heat and stir in the fresh basil and margarine, tossing until the margarine melts.

Nutrition per serving
- ○ 378 calories
- ○ 19 g protein
- ○ 35 g carbohydrates
- ○ 18 g fat
- ○ 2.5 g saturated fat
- ○ 30 mg cholesterol
- ○ 360 mg sodium
- ○ 4 g fiber

MAKE IT A FLAT BELLY DIET MEAL: A single serving of this recipe counts as a Flat Belly Diet Meal without any add-ons!

Halibut with Chopped Olive Salad

4 SERVINGS / 325 CALORIES / MUFA: OLIVES

Halibut is an excellent source of magnesium, a mineral that helps regulate blood sugar levels and promotes normal blood pressure.

20 MINUTES

20 **pitted large black olives, chopped**

20 **pitted kalamata olives, chopped**

½ **roasted pepper, finely chopped (about ¼ cup)**

2 **tablespoons finely chopped red onion**

1 **tablespoon chopped fresh basil**

2 **teaspoons balsamic vinegar**

5 **teaspoons olive oil**

4 **halibut fillets (6 ounces each)**

¼ **teaspoon salt**

⅛ **teaspoon ground black pepper**

1. Combine the olives, roasted pepper, onion, basil, vinegar, and 3 teaspoons of the oil in a bowl and set aside.

2. Heat the remaining 2 teaspoons oil in a large nonstick skillet over medium-high heat. Sprinkle the fish with the salt and pepper and cook for 4 to 5 minutes per side, or until the fish flakes easily with a fork. Serve each piece of fish topped with one-fourth of the olive mixture.

* Limit saturated fat to no more than 10 percent of total calories—about 17 grams per day for most women or 21 grams for most men—and sodium intake to no more than 2,300 milligrams.

Nutrition per serving
○ 325 calories
○ 36 g protein
○ 5 g carbohydrates
○ 17 g fat
○ 2.5 g saturated fat
○ 55 mg cholesterol
○ 770 mg sodium*
○ 1 g fiber

MAKE IT A FLAT BELLY DIET MEAL: Serve with ½ cup cooked wild rice (83). Total meal: 408 calories

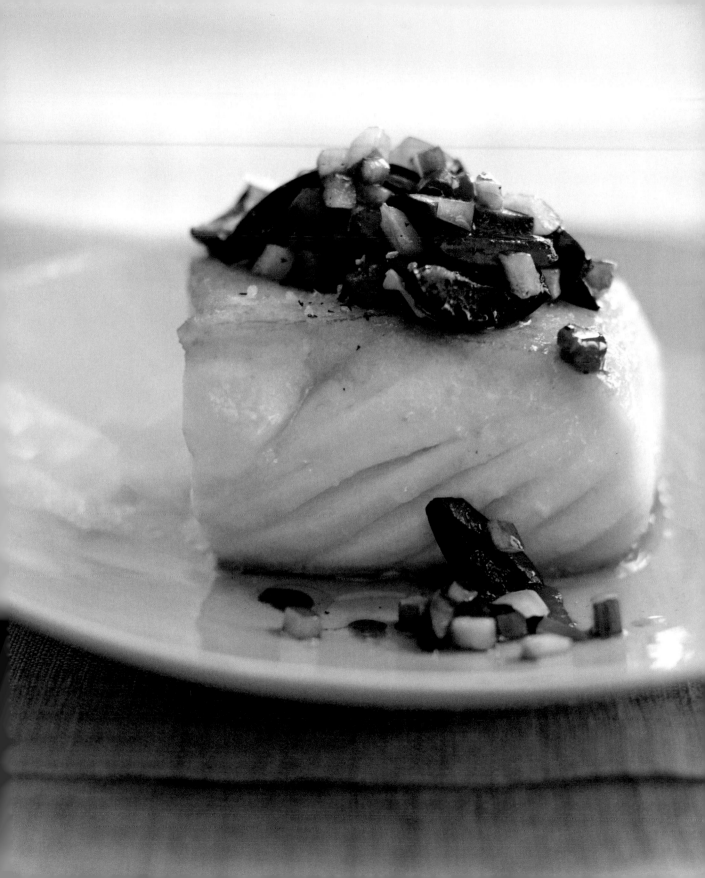

Flat Belly Diet! Family Cookbook

Sesame-Crusted Tuna Steaks

4 SERVINGS / 373 CALORIES / MUFA: SESAME SEEDS

You'll be amazed how easily this restaurant-worthy dish comes together. The sesame seeds impart a nutty flavor and help keep the fish nice and moist.

25 MINUTES

⅓ cup orange juice

4 tablespoons hoisin sauce

4 tuna steaks (5 ounces each)

½ cup sesame seeds

4 teaspoons toasted sesame oil

6 cups shredded Napa cabbage

2 carrots, grated

Nutrition per serving

○ 373 calories
○ 38 g protein
○ 23 g carbohydrates
○ 15 g fat
○ 2.5 g saturated fat
○ 65 mg cholesterol
○ 430 mg sodium
○ 4 g fiber

1. Combine the orange juice and 2 tablespoons of the hoisin sauce in a bowl. Set aside.

2. Pat the tuna dry with paper towels. Spread ¼ cup of the sesame seeds on a small plate and firmly press both sides of each tuna steak onto the seeds to coat. Transfer to a plate.

3. Heat 2 teaspoons of the oil in a large nonstick skillet over medium-high heat. Add the cabbage and carrots and cook, stirring occasionally, for 4 minutes, or until wilted. Stir in the remaining 2 tablespoons hoisin sauce and ¼ cup sesame seeds and cook for 2 minutes longer. Transfer to a bowl and keep warm.

4. Return the skillet to medium-high heat and add the remaining 2 teaspoons oil. Add the tuna steaks and cook for about 3 minutes per side for rare, or longer to desired doneness. Serve the tuna steaks over the cabbage mixture and drizzle the orange sauce on top.

MAKE IT A FLAT BELLY DIET MEAL: Serve with 1 wedge (⅛ melon) cantaloupe (23).
Total meal: 396 calories

Pan-Seared Chicken Breasts with Walnuts and Apples

4 SERVINGS / 317 CALORIES / MUFA: WALNUTS

Steamed asparagus makes an easy, vibrant side vegetable to go with this fruity main dish.

20 MINUTES

½ cup walnuts, chopped

2 teaspoons canola oil

4 boneless, skinless chicken breast halves (5 ounces each)

1 tablespoon all-purpose flour

1 Granny Smith apple, unpeeled, quartered and sliced

1 small red onion, quartered and sliced

¼ teaspoon salt

¼ teaspoon ground black pepper

½ cup apple cider

Nutrition per serving
○ 317 calories
○ 35 g protein
○ 13 g carbohydrates
○ 14 g fat
○ 1.5 g saturated fat
○ 80 mg cholesterol
○ 240 mg sodium
○ 2 g fiber

1. Place the walnuts in a large nonstick skillet and cook over medium-high heat, shaking the pan often, for 3 to 5 minutes, or until lightly toasted. Transfer to a plate.

2. Return the skillet to medium-high heat and add the oil. Lightly dust the chicken with the flour on both sides. Place the chicken smooth side down in the skillet. Cook for 4 to 5 minutes, or until browned on the bottom. Flip and continue cooking for 4 to 5 minutes, or until cooked through. Transfer to a plate.

3. Add the apple, onion, salt, and pepper to the skillet. Toss for about 2 minutes, or until the browned bits in the bottom of the skillet are clinging to the apples. Add the cider. Bring to a boil, then reduce to a brisk simmer. Cook for 4 minutes, or until the cider is reduced by about half. Add the reserved chicken and any accumulated juices on the plate and toss to coat. Serve the chicken with the apple-onion mixture spooned over the top. Sprinkle 2 tablesoons of the toasted walnuts over each serving.

MAKE IT **FASTER** Thinner chicken breasts cook more quickly and evenly. Use a smooth meat pounder or a heavy skillet to flatten breasts before cooking. Place the breasts on a work surface and cover with plastic wrap or parchment paper. If using a skillet, press down firmly while gliding over the surface.

MAKE IT A FLAT BELLY DIET MEAL: Serve with ½ cup cooked pearled barley (97) and 4 ounces steamed asparagus spears (23). Total meal: 437 calories

Chicken Cutlets Topped with Turkey Bacon and Avocado

4 SERVINGS / 210 CALORIES / MUFA: AVOCADO

With a high-quality hard-anodized nonstick skillet, you can brown chicken with a minimum of hot oil. Here's how: Preheat the pan and add the oil, then spread with a silicone brush. Let it heat for 1 minute before adding the chicken.

20 MINUTES

1 Hass avocado

1 small tomato, chopped

1 tablespoon shredded fresh basil

2 teaspoons fresh lemon juice

¼ teaspoon salt

¼ teaspoon ground black pepper

2 boneless, skinless chicken breast halves (8 ounces each)

1 teaspoon canola oil

2 slices natural turkey bacon, chopped

2 tablespoons fat-free reduced-sodium chicken broth or water

Nutrition per serving
○ 210 calories
○ 28 g protein
○ 4 g carbohydrates
○ 9 g fat
○ 1.5 g saturated fat
○ 70 mg cholesterol
○ 300 mg sodium
○ 3 g fiber

1. Mash the avocado in a bowl with a fork. Add the tomato, basil, lemon juice, ⅛ teaspoon of the salt, and ⅛ teaspoon of the pepper. Stir to combine and set aside.

2. Cut each chicken breast in half horizontally by slicing parallel to the work surface. Pound lightly to an even thickness and season with the remaining ⅛ teaspoon salt and ⅛ teaspoon pepper.

3. Heat the oil in a large nonstick skillet over medium-high heat. Cook the chicken for 3 to 4 minutes per side, or until browned and cooked through. Transfer to a plate and set aside.

4. Reduce the heat to medium. Add the bacon and cook, stirring occasionally, for 4 to 5 minutes, or until the bacon is crisp. Transfer to a plate and set aside.

5. Return the skillet to medium heat. Add the broth and cook, scraping the bottom to incorporate any browned bits, until the mixture boils and reduces slightly. Serve the cutlets topped with the reserved avocado mixture and bacon bits. Drizzle with the pan juices.

MAKE IT A FLAT BELLY DIET MEAL: Serve with Garlic Mashed Potatoes (page 226), prepared with 6 ounces fat-free plain Greek yogurt (160) instead of the olive oil, and 1 peach (59). **Total meal: 429 calories**

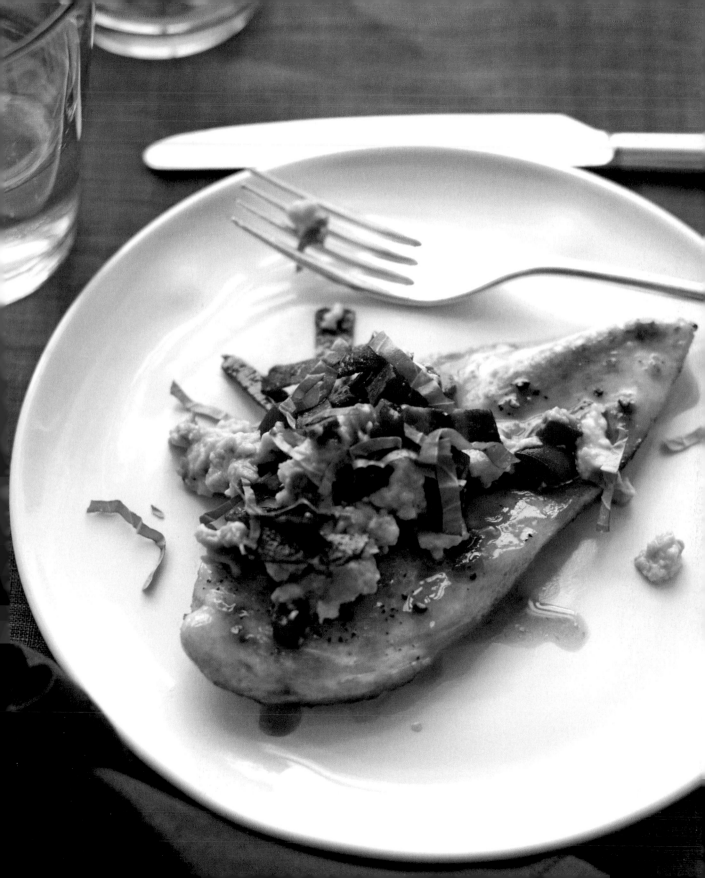

Thai Basil-Coconut Chicken

4 SERVINGS / 313 CALORIES / MUFA: CANOLA OIL

Save money by freezing leftover canned coconut milk in a plastic freezer container; just thaw in the refrigerator before using. Look for fish sauce in the Asian section of the grocery store.

15 MINUTES

½ cup light coconut milk

½ cup fat-free reduced-sodium chicken broth

1 tablespoon reduced-sodium fish sauce

2 teaspoons cornstarch

4 tablespoons canola oil

4 boneless, skinless chicken breast halves (4 ounces each)

½ cup fresh or frozen shelled edamame

½ red bell pepper, thinly sliced

2 garlic cloves, minced

2 tablespoons minced fresh Thai or regular basil

1. Combine the coconut milk, broth, and fish sauce in a small bowl. Whisk in the cornstarch and stir until combined. Set aside.

2. Heat 2 tablespoons of the oil in a large nonstick skillet over medium-high heat. Add the chicken smooth side down and cook for 2 minutes on each side, or until browned. Transfer to a plate and keep warm.

3. Return the skillet to medium heat. Add the remaining 2 tablespoons oil, the edamame, pepper, garlic, and salt. Cook for 30 seconds, or until the garlic is fragrant. Add the reserved coconut-milk mixture. Cook, stirring, for 1 to 2 minutes, or until thickened. Add the reserved chicken and any accumulated juices on the plate. Spoon the sauce over the chicken. Reduce the heat to a simmer, partially cover, and cook for 5 minutes, or until the chicken is cooked through. Stir in the basil.

Nutrition per serving

○ 313 calories
○ 29 g protein
○ 6 g carbohydrates
○ 18 g fat
○ 3 g saturated fat
○ 65 mg cholesterol
○ 370 mg sodium
○ 1 g fiber

MAKE IT A FLAT BELLY DIET MEAL: Serve with 1 cup cooked soba noodles (113).
Total meal: 426 calories

Indian Chicken in Cashew-Cilantro Sauce

4 SERVINGS / 230 CALORIES / MUFA: CASHEWS

You'll be impressed by how a dish with so few ingredients can taste so complex.

35 MINUTES

1 cup packed fresh cilantro
½ cup unsalted roasted cashews
1 cup fat-free reduced-sodium chicken broth
¼ teaspoon salt
1 pound boneless, skinless chicken breast tenders
Juice of 1 lime
Crushed red-pepper flakes (optional)

Nutrition per serving
○ 230 calories
○ 26 g protein
○ 7 g carbohydrates
○ 9 g fat
○ 2 g saturated fat
○ 65 mg cholesterol
○ 340 mg sodium
○ 1 g fiber

1. Place the cilantro and cashews in a food processor or blender and process to a paste. With the machine running, add the broth. The mixture will be runny and grainy.

2. Transfer the mixture to a medium nonstick skillet and add the salt. Bring to a simmer over medium heat. Add the chicken and spoon the sauce over it. Simmer, stirring occasionally, for 12 to 15 minutes, or until the chicken is no longer pink. (Cooking time will depend on the thickness of the tenders.)

3. Remove from the heat. Stir in the lime juice. Serve with red-pepper flakes, if desired, at the table.

MAKE IT A FLAT BELLY DIET MEAL: Serve with ½ cup cooked basmati rice (100) and ½ cup cooked green peas (67). Total meal: 397 calories

Chicken and Bok Choy with Almonds

4 SERVINGS / 250 CALORIES / MUFA: ALMONDS

No MSG and a beneficial serving of MUFA—this is a stir-fry you can look forward to enjoying again and again.

15 MINUTES

- 1 cup fat-free reduced-sodium chicken broth
- 1 tablespoon reduced-sodium soy sauce
- ¾ teaspoon grated fresh ginger
- 1 tablespoon cornstarch
- 2 teaspoons canola oil
- 1 pound boneless, skinless chicken breast tenders, cut into ½″ chunks
- ½ cup slivered almonds
- ½ pound baby bok choy, bulb and leaves, chopped
- ½ small red onion, thinly sliced
- 2 garlic cloves, minced

Nutrition per serving
- ○ 250 calories
- ○ 31 g protein
- ○ 8 g carbohydrates
- ○ 11 g fat
- ○ 1 g saturated fat
- ○ 65 mg cholesterol
- ○ 490 mg sodium
- ○ 2 g fiber

1. Combine the broth, soy sauce, and ginger in a small bowl. Whisk in the cornstarch and stir until combined. Set aside.

2. Heat the oil in a large nonstick skillet over medium-high heat. Add the chicken and almonds. Cook for 1 minute without stirring. Toss the mixture and continue cooking, tossing occasionally, for 3 minutes, or until the chicken begins to brown. Transfer the chicken and almonds to a plate.

3. Return the skillet to medium-high heat and add the bok choy, onion, and garlic. Cook, tossing occasionally, for 3 minutes, or until the bok choy is crisp-tender.

4. Return the chicken, almonds, and any accumulated juices from the plate to the skillet. Stir the reserved broth mixture to recombine, add to the pan, and cook, stirring constantly, for about 1 minute, or until the broth thickens. Reduce the heat to a simmer and cook for 1 to 2 minutes, or until the chicken is cooked through and the flavors have combined.

⧖
MAKE IT **FASTER** The most time-consuming part of a stir-fry is chopping the ingredients. If you do all the cutting up the night before and refrigerate the ingredients, you can practically fly through your next stir-fry.

MAKE IT A FLAT BELLY DIET MEAL: Serve with ½ cup cooked brown rice (109) and ½ cup canned mandarin oranges (36). Total meal: 395 calories

Chinese BBQ Chicken Patties

4 SERVINGS / 404 CALORIES / MUFA: PINE NUTS

Hoisin sauce is spicy, sweet, and thick. Think of it as Chinese barbecue sauce. Store in the refrigerator after opening.

30 MINUTES

2 **scallions**

½ **cup pine nuts**

1 **slice (¼" thick) fresh ginger**

1 **garlic clove**

1 **pound boneless, skinless chicken breasts, cut into large chunks**

¼ **teaspoon ground black pepper**

1 **teaspoon canola oil**

4 **tablespoons hoisin sauce**

4 **ounces dry fine Chinese wheat noodles or angel hair pasta**

¾ **cup fat-free reduced-sodium chicken broth**

Nutrition per serving

○ 404 calories
○ 32 g protein
○ 35 g carbohydrates
○ 15 g fat
○ 1.5 g saturated fat
○ 65 mg cholesterol
○ 520 mg sodium
○ 1 g fiber

1. Bring a covered medium pot of water to a boil over high heat.

2. Meanwhile, cut the white and light green of the scallions into 1" lengths. Cut the tender part of the dark green portions crosswise into thin slices. Set aside.

3. Finely chop the pine nuts in a food processor. Set aside. In the same work bowl, with the processor running, drop the white and light green scallion pieces, ginger, and garlic through the feed tube to mince. Turn the machine off and add the chicken and pepper. Pulse about 12 times, or until the chicken is coarsely chopped. Add the ground pine nuts. Pulse to incorporate. Shape the chicken mixture into 8 patties (½" thick).

4. Heat the oil in a large nonstick skillet over medium-high heat. Place the patties in the skillet. Cook for 3 minutes, or until browned on the bottom. Flip and cook for 3 minutes, or until browned on the second side and cooked through. Spread 1 tablespoon of the hoisin sauce evenly over the patties. Transfer to a plate and keep warm.

5. When the water boils, add the noodles and cook according to package directions. Drain the noodles and add to the skillet. Add the broth and remaining 3 tablespoons hoisin sauce. Toss over low heat to coat. Divide the noodles among 4 plates. Top with the patties and any accumulated juices from the plate. Sprinkle with the reserved scallion greens.

🕐

MAKE IT AHEAD Refrigerate cooked and cooled patties in a plastic storage container for up to 2 days. Reheat in the microwave while preparing noodles.

MAKE IT A FLAT BELLY DIET MEAL: A single serving of this recipe counts as a Flat Belly Diet Meal without any add-ons!

Chicken Tenders with Two Dips

4 SERVINGS / 332 CALORIES / MUFA: OLIVE OIL

Isn't it good to know that the dips you're serving contain no emulsifiers or sweeteners? Only fresh, wholesome ingredients served here!

20 MINUTES

- 1 cup fat-free plain Greek yogurt
- 4 tablespoons olive oil
- 2 tablespoons finely chopped fresh dill
- 2 tablespoons finely chopped scallions (white and green parts)
- 2 teaspoons fresh lemon juice
- ¼ teaspoon salt
- ¼ teaspoon ground black pepper
- 1¼ pounds boneless, skinless chicken breast tenders
- 2 large tomatoes, chopped
- 1 garlic clove, minced
- ½ teaspoon dried oregano

Nutrition per serving
- ○ 332 calories
- ○ 39 g protein
- ○ 7 g carbohydrates
- ○ 16 g fat
- ○ 2.5 g saturated fat
- ○ 80 mg cholesterol
- ○ 260 mg sodium
- ○ 1 g fiber

1. Whisk together the yogurt, 1 tablespoon of the oil, the dill, scallions, lemon juice, ⅛ teaspoon of the salt, and ⅛ teaspoon of the pepper. Set aside.

2. Heat 2 tablespoons of the oil in a large nonstick skillet over medium-high heat. Add the chicken and cook for 10 minutes, turning occasionally, until browned on all sides and cooked through. Transfer to a plate and keep warm.

3. Add the remaining 1 tablespoon oil to the skillet. Reduce the heat to medium. Add the tomatoes, garlic, oregano, remaining ⅛ teaspoon salt, and remaining ⅛ teaspoon pepper. Cook, tossing frequently, for 4 minutes, or until the tomatoes start to release their juices.

4. Serve the tenders with ¼ cup dill sauce and ¼ cup chunky tomato sauce per serving.

MAKE IT A FLAT BELLY DIET MEAL: Serve with ½ cup cooked whole wheat couscous (70). Total meal: 402 calories

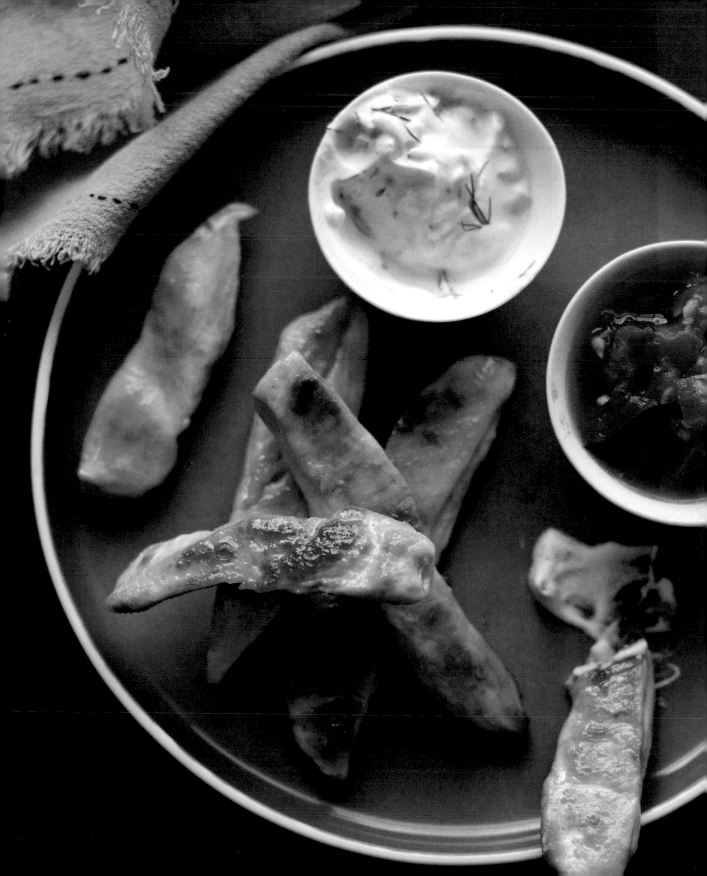

Chicken Cacciatore

4 SERVINGS / 315 CALORIES / MUFA: OLIVES

This dish is a crowd-pleaser, so double the recipe if you're serving company for supper. Brown mushrooms, also known as cremini, are baby portobellos.

20
MINUTES

¾ **pound boneless, skinless chicken breast tenders**

2 **teaspoons olive oil**

1 **package (8 ounces) brown mushrooms (cremini), quartered**

1 **small onion, chopped**

2 **garlic cloves, minced**

¼ **teaspoon salt**

¼ **teaspoon ground black pepper**

1 **can (14.5 ounces) no-salt-added basil-garlic-oregano diced tomatoes**

4 **ounces multigrain rotini pasta**

40 **pitted black olives**

1 **tablespoon minced parsley**

Nutrition per serving

○ 315 calories
○ 28 g protein
○ 32 g carbohydrates
○ 9 g fat
○ 1 g saturated fat
○ 50 mg cholesterol
○ 570 mg sodium
○ 6 g fiber

1. Bring a medium pot of water to a boil over high heat.

2. Meanwhile, cut the chicken into ½" pieces. Heat the oil in a large nonstick skillet over medium-high heat. Add the chicken and cook, turning occasionally, for 4 minutes, or until browned on all sides. Transfer to a plate.

3. Add the mushrooms, onion, garlic, salt, and pepper to the skillet and toss to combine. Reduce the heat to medium, cover, and cook, tossing occasionally, for 3 minutes, or until the mushrooms exude liquid. Uncover and cook to evaporate most of the liquid. Add the tomatoes and the reserved chicken with any accumulated juices from the plate. Reduce the heat to a simmer.

4. When the water boils, add the pasta and cook according to package directions. Drain the pasta and transfer to the skillet. Add the olives and toss gently to combine. Serve sprinkled with the parsley.

MAKE IT A FLAT BELLY DIET MEAL: Serve with a 1-ounce slice of whole grain French bread (90). **Total meal: 405 calories**

Chicken Picadillo

4 SERVINGS / 248 CALORIES / MUFA: BRAZIL NUTS

This Latin-inspired dish comes together in a snap. Because it can land on the table so quickly, it's better to serve with quick-cooking brown rice.

15 MINUTES

- ½ pound boneless, skinless chicken thighs, trimmed of all visible fat
- 2 teaspoons olive oil
- ½ large red bell pepper, finely chopped
- 1 onion, finely chopped
- 2 garlic cloves, minced
- ¼ teaspoon salt
- 1 cup canned no-salt-added diced tomatoes
- 2 tablespoons raisins
- ½ cup chopped blanched Brazil nuts
- 2 tablespoons chopped fresh cilantro

1. Cut the chicken into chunks. Place in a food processor and pulse 8 times to chop coarsely. (The chicken can also be chopped by hand with a large heavy knife.)

2. Heat the oil in a large nonstick skillet over medium-high heat. Add the pepper, onion, garlic, and salt. Cook, stirring, for 2 minutes, or until the vegetables are sizzling and the garlic is fragrant. Add the chicken. Cook, stirring, for 3 minutes, or until the chicken is just beginning to brown. Add the tomatoes and raisins. Reduce the heat and simmer for 5 minutes, or until the chicken is cooked through. Stir in the nuts and cilantro.

Nutrition per serving
- ○ 248 calories
- ○ 15 g protein
- ○ 13 g carbohydrates
- ○ 16 g fat
- ○ 3.5 g saturated fat
- ○ 45 mg cholesterol
- ○ 220 mg sodium
- ○ 3 g fiber

MAKE IT A FLAT BELLY DIET MEAL: Serve with ¾ cup cooked brown rice (163). Total meal: 411 calories

Chicken Thighs with Green Beans

4 SERVINGS / 269 CALORIES / MUFA: PEANUTS

Sweet onion and peanuts give this skillet dish a definite Southern vibe. Add a dash of hot sauce if you like.

20 MINUTES

½ **pound green beans, broken into 1" pieces**

1 **teaspoon canola oil**

½ **red bell pepper, chopped**

½ **sweet onion, chopped**

¼ **teaspoon salt**

¼ **teaspoon ground black pepper**

¾ **pound boneless, skinless chicken thighs, trimmed of all visible fat, cut into chunks**

1 **tablespoon all-purpose flour**

¾ **cup fat-free reduced-sodium chicken broth**

½ **cup unsalted dry-roasted peanuts**

Cider or red wine vinegar

Nutrition per serving

○ 269 calories
○ 22 g protein
○ 11 g carbohydrates
○ 16 g fat
○ 2.5 g saturated fat
○ 70 mg cholesterol
○ 280 mg sodium
○ 4 g fiber

1. Bring 1 cup water to a boil in a medium saucepan over high heat. Add the beans, cover, and boil for 5 minutes, or until crisp-tender. Drain and rinse under cold water. Drain and set aside.

2. Meanwhile, heat the oil in a large nonstick skillet over medium-high heat. Add the bell pepper, onion, salt, and black pepper. Cook, stirring, for 6 minutes, or until the onion is golden. Scrape the vegetables to the sides of the skillet and add the chicken in the center. Cook, stirring, for 4 minutes, or until browned.

3. Place the flour in a small bowl. Whisk in the broth until well blended. Add the mixture to the skillet. Cook, stirring constantly, for about 2 minutes, or until thickened. Add the reserved beans and simmer for 2 to 3 minutes, or until the beans are hot and the chicken is cooked through. Sprinkle with the peanuts. Splash with vinegar, if desired.

MAKE IT A FLAT BELLY DIET MEAL: Serve with ¼ pound boiled red potatoes (73) tossed with 2 teaspoons trans-free margarine (53). **Total meal: 395 calories**

Pork and Sweet Potato Skillet

4 SERVINGS (1¾ CUPS PORK AND 3 TABLESPOONS SAUCE EACH) / 302 CALORIES / MUFA: AVOCADO

Younger taste buds may find the heat in this dish to be a little intense. If so, substitute 1 tablespoon of your favorite mild chili powder in place of the chipotle.

25 MINUTES

3 teaspoons olive oil
1 pound well-trimmed pork tenderloin, cut into 1" pieces
2 large sweet potatoes
1 red onion
1 red bell pepper
¾ cup water
1 tablespoon honey
1 chipotle pepper in adobo sauce, minced
Juice of 1 lime
1 Hass avocado
¼ cup chopped fresh cilantro
1 tablespoon chopped yellow or white onion
¼ teaspoon salt

Nutrition per serving
○ 302 calories
○ 26 g protein
○ 24 g carbohydrates
○ 11 g fat
○ 2 g saturated fat
○ 75 mg cholesterol
○ 260 mg sodium
○ 6 g fiber

1. Heat 1 teaspoon of the oil in a large nonstick skillet over medium-high heat. Add the pork and cook for 5 to 7 minutes, or until browned. Transfer to a plate and keep warm.

2. Add the sweet potatoes, onion, bell pepper, and ½ cup of the water to the skillet. Cover and cook for 5 minutes, or until the sweet potatoes are tender.

3. Remove from the heat and stir in the honey, chipotle pepper, and half of the lime juice. Return the pork to the skillet and toss to combine.

4. Place the avocado, 2 tablespoons of the cilantro, the onion, salt, remaining lime juice, remaining ¼ cup water, and remaining 2 teaspoons oil in a blender. Process for 1 minute to make a sauce.

5. Serve the pork and vegetables sprinkled with the remaining 2 tablespoons cilantro and the avocado sauce on the side.

MAKE IT A FLAT BELLY DIET MEAL: Serve with a 1-ounce whole wheat dinner roll (77). Total meal: 379 calories

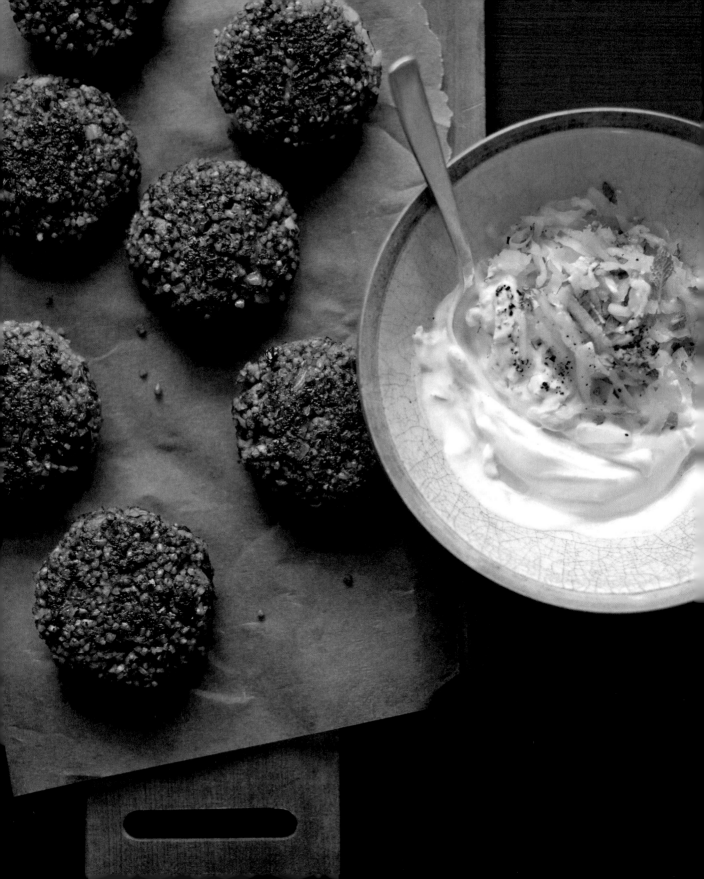

Lebanese Beef Patties

4 SERVINGS (3 PATTIES AND ½ CUP SAUCE EACH) / 420 CALORIES / MUFA: OLIVE OIL

If you can't find bulgur wheat in the bulk section of your grocery, look for a box of tabbouleh mix, which usually contains just the right amount for this recipe (save the seasoning packet for another use).

35 MINUTES

- ¾ cup medium-coarse bulgur wheat
- 1 cup fresh mint leaves, chopped
- 1 small yellow onion, finely chopped
- 1 teaspoon ground cumin
- 1 teaspoon ground allspice
- 1 teaspoon salt
- ¾ teaspoon ground black pepper
- 1 pound 95% lean ground beef
- 4 tablespoons olive oil
- 1 cucumber
- 1 cup fat-free plain Greek yogurt

Nutrition per serving

- ○ 420 calories
- ○ 33 g protein
- ○ 27 g carbohydrates
- ○ 20 g fat
- ○ 4.5 g saturated fat*
- ○ 70 mg cholesterol
- ○ 400 mg sodium
- ○ 6 g fiber

1. Place 1 cup of water in a small microwaveable bowl and bring to a boil in the microwave. Add the bulgur and let sit while you prepare the other ingredients.

2. Combine ¾ cup of the mint, the onion, cumin, allspice, salt, and ½ teaspoon of the pepper in a large bowl. Add the beef and bulgur and mix with clean hands until thoroughly combined. Shape into 12 patties about ¾" thick.

3. Heat 1 tablespoon of the oil in a large nonstick skillet over medium-high heat. Add half of the patties and cook for 5 minutes per side, or until browned and crispy. When the patties are cooked through, transfer to a plate and keep warm. Repeat with the remaining patties and 1 tablespoon of the oil.

4. Meanwhile, peel, seed, and grate the cucumber. Stir in the yogurt, remaining ¼ cup mint, remaining 2 tablespoons oil, and remaining ¼ teaspoon pepper. Serve the patties with the yogurt sauce on the side.

* Limit saturated fat to no more than 10 percent of total calories—about 17 grams per day for most women or 21 grams for most men—and sodium intake to no more than 2,300 milligrams.

⧖ MAKE IT **FASTER** If you're pressed for time, use 2 skillets to cook both batches of patties at once.

MAKE IT A FLAT BELLY DIET MEAL: A single serving of this recipe counts as a Flat Belly Diet Meal without any add-ons!

Spaghetti and Meatballs

8 SERVINGS / 410 CALORIES / MUFA: OLIVE OIL

This recipe makes a generous amount of tasty sauce, so if your family is not following the FBD serving sizes exactly, feel free to make some extra pasta for them. Simply measure out ½ cup of cooked pasta and ½ cup of sauce for yourself beforehand. And don't forget the meatballs!

25 MINUTES

- 12 **ounces multigrain spaghetti**
- 4 **tablespoons olive oil**
- 1 **slice whole wheat bread, torn into bite-sized pieces**
- ¼ **cup whole milk**
- 1 **large egg**
- 1 **tablespoon salt-free Italian seasoning**
- 1 **pound 95% lean ground beef**
- 1 **tablespoon minced garlic**
- 1 **can (28 ounces) crushed tomatoes**
- ¼ **cup chopped parsley (optional)**

Nutrition per serving
- ○ 410 calories
- ○ 23 g protein
- ○ 40 g carbohydrates
- ○ 18 g fat
- ○ 3.5 g saturated fat
- ○ 60 mg cholesterol
- ○ 480 mg sodium
- ○ 5 g fiber

1. Bring a large pot of water to a boil. Add the spaghetti and cook according to package directions. Drain and toss with 1 tablespoon of the oil. Cover to keep warm until the meatballs and sauce are ready.

2. Meanwhile, place the bread in a large bowl and cover with the milk. Wait until the bread absorbs most of the milk (about 1 minute), then add the egg and Italian seasoning. Mix with a fork until smooth (a few pieces of crust may remain). Add the beef and mix until thoroughly combined. With clean hands, shape into 24 meatballs.

3. Heat 1 tablespoon of the oil in a large nonstick skillet over medium-high heat. Add half of the meatballs and cook, turning to ensure even browning, for 5 to 7 minutes, or until cooked through. Transfer to a plate and repeat with the remaining meatballs and 1 tablespoon of the oil.

4. Add the garlic and remaining 1 tablespoon oil to the skillet. Cook for 30 seconds, or until fragrant. Add the tomatoes, reduce the heat, and cook for 5 minutes to blend the flavors. Serve the spaghetti topped with the sauce and meatballs. Sprinkle with the parsley, if desired.

🕐
MAKE IT **AHEAD** Prepare the meatballs and sauce ahead of time and dinner's ready in the time that it takes to cook the pasta.

MAKE IT A FLAT BELLY DIET MEAL: A single serving of this recipe counts as a Flat Belly Diet Meal without any add-ons!

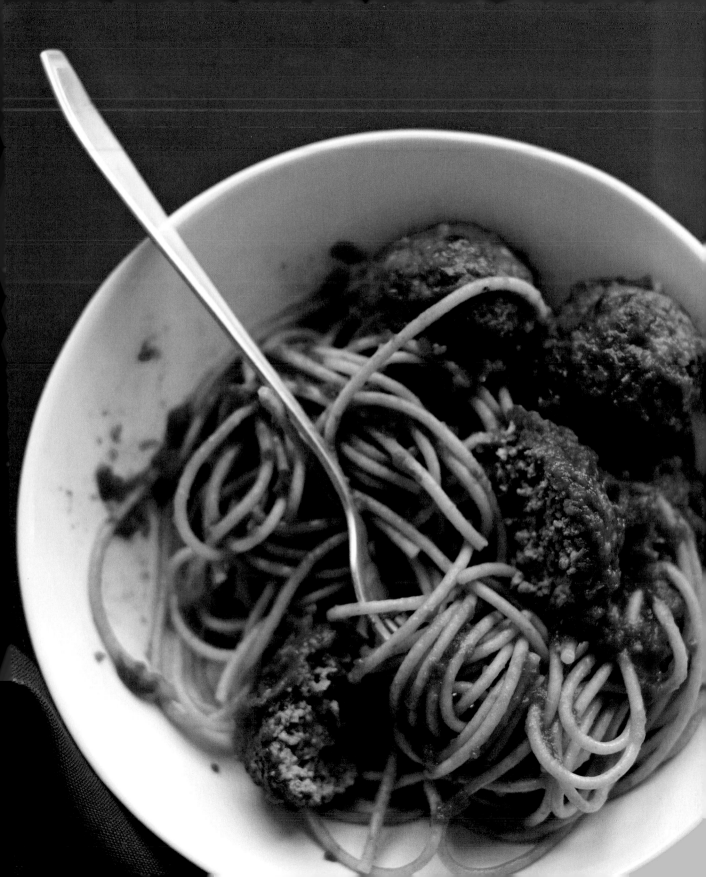

Stovetop Meat Loaf with Mushroom Gravy

4 SERVINGS / 342 CALORIES / MUFA: WALNUTS

These individual meat loaves come together in considerably less time because they cook faster on the stovetop than in the oven.

35 MINUTES

½ cup walnuts
½ onion, coarsely chopped
1 package (8 ounces) sliced brown mushrooms (cremini)
1 large egg
2 tablespoons ketchup
½ teaspoon ground thyme
½ teaspoon salt
1 pound 95% lean ground beef
¾ cup panko bread crumbs
1 teaspoon olive oil
¼ cup fat-free plain Greek yogurt

Nutrition per serving
○ 342 calories
○ 32 g protein
○ 15 g carbohydrates
○ 17 g fat
○ 4 g saturated fat*
○ 125 mg cholesterol
○ 510 mg sodium
○ 2 g fiber

1. Place the walnuts in a medium skillet and cook over medium-high heat, shaking the pan often, for 3 to 5 minutes, or until lightly toasted. Transfer the nuts to a food processor and let cool slightly.

2. Add the onion and half of the mushrooms to the processor and pulse 4 or 5 times, or until finely chopped.

3. Combine the egg, ketchup, thyme, and salt in a large bowl. Beat lightly with a fork until smooth. Add the mushroom-onion mixture and the beef and mix well. Add the bread crumbs and mix with clean hands until thoroughly combined. Shape into 4 loaves 5" long and 1½" wide.

4. Heat the oil in a large nonstick skillet over medium-high heat. Add the loaves and cook for 3 minutes on each side, or until browned. Top with the remaining mushrooms and pour ¼ cup water into the center of the skillet. Cover, reduce the heat to low, and cook for 15 minutes, or until a thermometer inserted in the center of a loaf registers 165°F.

5. Transfer the loaves to a plate and stir the yogurt into the mushroom mixture in the skillet. Serve the loaves with the sauce spooned on top.

Limit saturated fat to no more than 10 percent of total calories—about 17 grams per day for most women or 21 grams for most men—and sodium intake to no more than 2,300 milligrams.

MAKE IT A FLAT BELLY DIET MEAL: Serve with ½ cup cooked corn (66). Total meal: 408 calories

Beefsteak Stuffed with Olives

4 SERVINGS / 333 CALORIES / MUFA: OLIVES

Because it's so lean, top round can be a relatively bland cut of beef, but in this dish, it's practically bursting with flavor from the intense olive and tomato combination inside. Be careful not to overcook, as it will toughen considerably.

35 MINUTES

2 **thin top round steaks,**
    ³/₄ **pound each**
40 **pitted kalamata olives**
½ **cup sun-dried tomatoes**
    (not oil-packed)
1 **teaspoon minced garlic**
1 **teaspoon dried oregano**
¼ **teaspoon ground black**
    pepper
1 **tablespoon olive oil**
2 **tablespoons balsamic**
    vinegar

Nutrition per serving
○ 333 calories
○ 38 g protein
○ 19 g carbohydrates
○ 19 g fat
○ 4 g saturated fat*
○ 75 mg cholesterol
○ 840 mg sodium*
○ 1 g fiber

1. Pound the meat to an even thickness (about ¼") between 2 sheets of parchment paper using a meat mallet or the bottom of a heavy skillet. Score the steaks on 1 side with a sharp knife in a crosshatch pattern.

2. Combine the olives, tomatoes, garlic, oregano, and pepper in a food processor and pulse until evenly combined.

3. Divide the olive mixture between the 2 steaks and spread evenly, leaving a ½" border along the sides. Starting on a long side, roll the steaks up tightly. Tie with kitchen twine or secure with toothpicks.

4. Heat the oil in a large nonstick skillet over medium-high heat. Cook the beef for 5 minutes, turning to brown on all sides. Transfer to a plate. Add the vinegar to the skillet and let reduce by half. Pour the vinegar reduction over the steak. Cover loosely with foil and let rest for 10 minutes before slicing into 1" pieces.

Limit saturated fat to no more than 10 percent of total calories—about 17 grams per day for most women or 21 grams for most men—and sodium intake to no more than 2,300 milligrams.

MAKE IT A FLAT BELLY DIET MEAL: Serve with ½ cup whole wheat couscous (70).
Total meal: 403 calories

QUICK-FIX PANTRY RESCUES

Middle Eastern Couscous

Cook ⅓ cup whole wheat couscous (140) according to package directions to make 1 cup. Meanwhile, combine 1 tablespoon **olive oil** (119), 1 tablespoon fresh lemon juice (4), 1 teaspoon chopped garlic (15), and ½ teaspoon chopped fresh oregano (0). When the couscous is done, toss with ½ cup rinsed and drained (130) canned chickpeas ¼ cup chopped roasted pepper (15), and the lemon juice mixture. **Total Calories = 423**

Cupboard Pasta

Cook 2 ounces multigrain pasta (203) according to package directions. Drain and toss with ½ cup water-packed chopped artichoke hearts (45), 1 tablespoon **olive oil** (119), and 1 teaspoon chopped garlic (15). Top with 1 tablespoon grated Parmesan cheese (22). **Total Calories = 404**

Spicy Spaghetti

Cook 2 ounces multigrain spaghetti (203) according to package directions. Drain and toss with 3 ounces water-packed light tuna (105), 10 pitted **black olives** (50), 1 teaspoon chopped garlic (15), 1 teaspoon olive oil (40), and a pinch of red-pepper flakes (0). **Total Calories = 413**

Pesto Polenta

Spread 1 tablespoon **pesto sauce** (80) over 4 ounces of precooked sliced polenta (50) and top with 3 ounces precooked chicken breast (122), 1 chopped plum tomato (11), and ¼ cup shredded part-skim mozzarella cheese (71). Cover and microwave on high power for 2 to 3 minutes, or until heated through. Serve with 1 orange (69). **Total Calories = 403**

Mexican Eggs

Cook 1 tablespoon chopped red onion (4) in 1 teaspoon canola oil (40) in a nonstick skillet over medium heat until soft. Add ½ cup canned hominy (59), ⅛ teaspoon salt (0), and ¼ teaspoon chili powder (2) and toss to combine. Beat 2 large eggs (156) and pour over the hominy mixture. Reduce the heat to low and cook for 3 to 5 minutes, or until the bottom has begun to set. Flip and cook for 2 to 3 minutes longer, or until completely set. Garnish with ¼ cup mashed **Hass avocado** (96) and 1 tablespoon salsa (5). Serve with ½ cup sliced mango (54). **Total Calories = 417**

Menu for a Weekend Brunch

Indian Chicken in Cashew-Cilantro Sauce (page 153)

Golden Rice Pilaf (page 227)

Whole wheat pita

Carrot Salad (below)

Mango Tart with Macadamia Crust (page 277)

NOTE: Double all recipes except for Carrot Salad and Mango Tart.

SERVES 8

⊙ **Early in the day:** Make Mango Tart. Let sit at room temperature until ready to serve.

⊙ **About 90 minutes before serving:** Make Indian Chicken. Cover and keep warm while the rest of the meal comes together.

⊙ **About 1 hour before serving:** Prepare Carrot Salad by using a vegetable peeler to slice 2 pounds of carrots into thin ribbons. Chop ¼ cup fresh mint and set aside. Stir together 1 tablespoon honey, 1 tablespoon fresh lemon juice, and 1 tablespoon olive oil and toss with the carrots. Season to taste with salt and pepper. Set aside.

⊙ **About 35 minutes before serving:** Start Golden Rice Pilaf.

⊙ **About 15 minutes before serving:** Brush the pita (6") lightly with olive oil, rub with a halved garlic clove, and wrap in foil. Warm in a 350°F oven.

MAKE IT A FLAT BELLY DIET MEAL: Enjoy the Indian chicken (230) with *either* the salad (68) and a pita (120) or the rice pilaf (omit the pistachios) (187). **Total meal: 418 calories (with salad and pita) or 417 calories (with rice).** Later in the evening, enjoy mango tart (336) as your FBD snack with a large cappuccino made with ¾ cup fat-free milk (62). **Total meal: 398 calories (tart)**

8

Comforting
CASSEROLES,
STEWS,
AND MORE

- Corn and Potato Chowder
- Italian Lentil-Broccoli Stew
- Vegetarian Lasagna with Tofu
- Florentine Baked Beans
- Fish Nuggets with Tartar Sauce
- Crunchy Crust Mac and Cheese
- Tuna Noodle Casserole
- Southern-Style Baked Shrimp
- Shrimp and Ham Jambalaya
- Chicken and Yellow Rice Casserole

- Mexican Corn Soup
- Chicken and Almond Dumplings
- Broccoli Chicken Casserole
- Chicken Tortilla Casserole
- Turkey Potpies
- Rosemary Pork and Rice Bake
- Mexican Pork Stew
- Chipotle Beef and Bean Chili
- Beef Goulash Noodle Casserole
- Oven-Baked Pot Roast

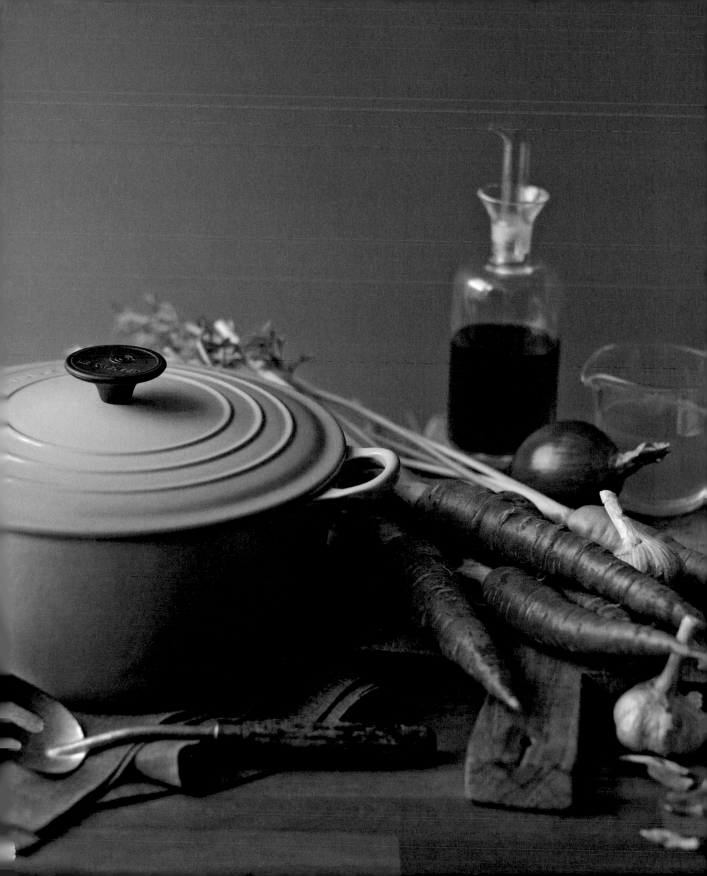

Corn and Potato Chowder

4 SERVINGS (1½ CUPS EACH) / 276 CALORIES / MUFA: WALNUTS

Pureed cooked cauliflower adds a lush texture to this soup—without unwanted calories. Crispy toasted walnuts take the place of croutons.

20 MINUTES

½ cup walnuts

3 cups cauliflower florets

2 cups reduced-sodium vegetable broth or water

1 onion

1 small green bell pepper

1 teaspoon canola oil

½ pound small red potatoes, cut into ½" cubes

1½ cups fat-free milk

¾ teaspoon dried thyme

¼ teaspoon salt

¼ teaspoon ground black pepper

1 cup fresh or frozen corn kernels

1 tablespoon chopped parsley

Nutrition per serving

○ 276 calories

○ 11 g protein

○ 37 g carbohydrates

○ 12 g fat

○ 1 g saturated fat

○ 0 mg cholesterol

○ 450 mg sodium

○ 7 g fiber

1. Place the walnuts in a large nonstick skillet and cook over medium-high heat, shaking the pan often, for 3 to 5 minutes, or until lightly toasted. Transfer to a plate and let cool. Coarsely chop and set aside.

2. Combine the cauliflower and broth in the same skillet. Cover and set over high heat until the liquid comes to a boil. Reduce to a brisk simmer and cook for 15 minutes, or until the cauliflower is very tender.

3. Meanwhile, finely chop the onion and bell pepper. Warm the oil in a large saucepan over medium-low heat and add the onion and bell pepper. Cover and cook, stirring occasionally, for 3 minutes, or until the vegetables start to soften. Add the potatoes, milk, thyme, salt, and black pepper. Bring almost to a boil. Reduce to a simmer and cook for 12 minutes, or until the potatoes are tender.

4. When the cauliflower is tender, transfer it and any cooking liquid to a blender or food processor. Puree for 2 to 3 minutes, or until very smooth. Add to the potato mixture along with the corn and parsley. Simmer for a few minutes, just until the corn is hot. Serve sprinkled with the walnuts.

🕐 **MAKE IT AHEAD** Soups are so easy on cooks. They can be refrigerated for several days and portions reheated as needed.

MAKE IT A FLAT BELLY DIET MEAL: Serve with ½ cup canned juice-packed pineapple chunks (54) and Asian Snack Mix (page 235), but omit the peanuts (70). **Total meal: 400 calories**

Italian Lentil-Broccoli Stew

4 SERVINGS (1½ CUPS EACH) / 219 CALORIES / MUFA: OLIVES

Lentils and other legumes can be as satisfying as meat when they are prepared in well-seasoned recipes.

35 MINUTES

1 stalk broccoli (8 ounces)
1 small carrot, finely chopped
1 small onion, finely chopped
2 garlic cloves, minced
2 teaspoons olive oil
¾ cup dried green or brown lentils
2 cups reduced-sodium vegetable broth or water
1 teaspoon dried oregano
¼ teaspoon ground black pepper
  Pinch of salt
40 pitted large green olives, slivered
½ ounce shaved or coarsely shredded Parmesan cheese

Nutrition per serving
○ 219 calories
○ 10 g protein
○ 28 g carbohydrates
○ 9 g fat
○ 0 g saturated fat
○ 0 mg cholesterol
○ 580 mg sodium
○ 8 g fiber

1. Cut the florets from the broccoli stalk. Peel and cut the stalk into small chunks, and cut the florets into like-size pieces. Set aside.

2. Stir together the carrot, onion, garlic, and oil in a medium saucepan. Cover and cook over medium heat for 5 minutes, or until the vegetables start to soften.

3. Stir in the lentils, broth, oregano, pepper, and salt. Cover and bring to a brisk simmer. Reduce to a low simmer and cook for 20 minutes.

4. Stir in the reserved broccoli. Re-cover and simmer for 5 minutes, or until the lentils are tender and the broccoli is crisp-tender. Stir in the olives. Add more water, if necessary, to thin the stew to the desired consistency. Serve garnished with the cheese.

🕐
MAKE IT **AHEAD** Stews taste delicious when made ahead, and this one is no exception.

MAKE IT A FLAT BELLY DIET MEAL: Serve half a 6″ whole wheat pita (60) and Fall Fruit Salad (page 208), but reduce the walnut oil to 2 tablespoons (122). **Total meal: 401 calories**

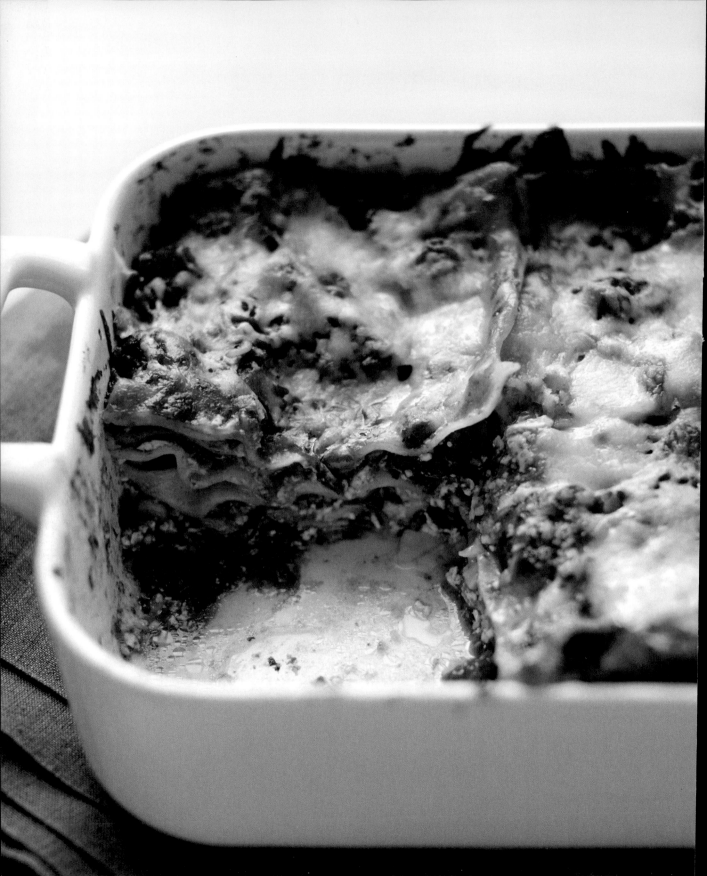

Vegetarian Lasagna with Tofu

4 SERVINGS / 363 CALORIES / MUFA: PESTO SAUCE

Yes, you can eat your lasagna and have a flat belly, too! This lightened-up version relies on tofu instead of ricotta cheese.

1 HOUR 15 MIN

- 2 cans (14.5 ounces each) no-salt-added basil-oregano-garlic diced tomatoes
- 1 package (12 ounces) soft silken tofu
- 6 no-boil lasagna noodles (4 ounces)
- ¼ cup pesto sauce
- 4 cups baby spinach
- 1 cup (4 ounces) shredded reduced-fat Italian cheese blend
- ¼ teaspoon salt
- ¼ teaspoon ground black pepper

Nutrition per serving
- ○ 363 calories
- ○ 14 g protein
- ○ 38 g carbohydrates
- ○ 14 g fat
- ○ 5 g saturated fat*
- ○ 20 mg cholesterol
- ○ 610 mg sodium*
- ○ 6 g fiber

1. Preheat the oven to 375°F. Coat an 8" x 8" baking dish with cooking spray.

2. Cook the tomatoes in a small nonstick skillet over medium heat until slightly thickened, about 10 minutes.

3. Place a strainer over the sink or a bowl and crumble in the tofu, squeezing it dry of excess liquid. Set aside.

4. Spread one-third of the tomatoes over the bottom of the baking dish. Layer ingredients in this order: 2 noodles, 2 table-spoons pesto, half the tofu, 2 cups spinach, ⅓ cup cheese, and ⅛ teaspoon each salt and pepper. Spread one-third of the toma-toes over the top. Repeat a second layer: 2 noodles, the remaining 2 tablespoons pesto, the remaining tofu, the remaining 2 cups spinach, ⅓ cup of the cheese, and the remaining ⅛ teaspoon each salt and pepper. Place the remaining 2 noodles on top. Cover with the remaining tomatoes. Set the remaining ⅓ cup cheese aside. Cover the dish tightly with foil.

5. Bake for 30 minutes, or until hot and bubbling. Carefully remove the foil and, with a spatula, gently press down the corners of the noodles to submerge in sauce. Sprinkle with the reserved cheese. Bake uncovered for 20 minutes, or until the top is slightly browned. Remove and let rest for 10 minutes before cutting.

* Limit saturated fat to no more than 10 percent of total calories—about 17 grams per day for most women or 21 grams for most men—and sodium intake to no more than 2,300 milligrams.

MAKE IT A FLAT BELLY DIET MEAL: Serve with 2 cups mixed salad greens (18) tossed with 1 cup chopped cucumber (16), 1 cup sliced mushrooms (15), and 1 tablespoon balsamic vinegar (14). **Total meal:** 426 calories

Florentine Baked Beans

4 SERVINGS / 240 CALORIES / MUFA: OLIVE OIL

Crusty whole grain bread and steamed kale are all you need to make a meal of these savory Italian beans.

40 MINUTES

1 can (14.5 ounces) no-salt-added cannellini or Great Northern beans, rinsed and drained

1 cup drained canned no-salt-added diced tomatoes

¼ cup olive oil

½ small carrot, chopped

¼ small red onion, chopped

1 teaspoon crumbled dried sage

¼ teaspoon ground black pepper

⅛ teaspoon salt

2 tablespoons grated Romano cheese

1. Preheat the oven to 375°F. Coat an 8″ x 8″ baking dish with cooking spray.

2. Place the beans, tomatoes, oil, carrot, onion, sage, pepper, and salt in the dish. Stir to mix. Sprinkle with the cheese.

3. Bake for 30 minutes, or until bubbling and golden. Allow to rest for 5 minutes before serving.

Nutrition per serving

○ 240 calories
○ 7 g protein
○ 20 g carbohydrates
○ 15 g fat
○ 2.5 g saturated fat
○ 0 mg cholesterol
○ 190 mg sodium
○ 5 g fiber

MAKE IT A FLAT BELLY DIET MEAL: Serve with 1-ounce slice whole grain French bread (90) and 1 cup cooked kale (36) tossed with 1 teaspoon trans-free margarine (26). **Total meal: 392 calories**

Fish Nuggets with Tartar Sauce

4 SERVINGS (1 TABLESPOON SAUCE EACH) / 403 CALORIES / MUFA: CANOLA OIL MAYONNAISE

No minced fish or fillers in this dish! Just the light clean taste of cod that's sure to please adults and kids alike.

25 MINUTES

¼ cup canola oil mayonnaise
1 tablespoon chopped onion
1 teaspoon capers, chopped
1 teaspoon sweet pickle relish
1 teaspoon fresh lemon juice
2 tablespoons all-purpose flour
½ teaspoon salt
¼ teaspoon ground black pepper
2 large eggs, lightly beaten
2 cups panko bread crumbs
1½ pounds cod fillets, fresh or thawed if frozen, cut into 20 equal pieces

Nutrition per serving
○ 403 calories
○ 38 g protein
○ 24 g carbohydrates
○ 16 g fat
○ 1.5 g saturated fat
○ 185 mg cholesterol
○ 630 mg sodium*
○ 1 g fiber

1. Preheat the oven to 400°F. Line a baking sheet with parchment paper and set aside.

2. Combine the mayonnaise, onion, capers, pickle relish, and lemon juice in a small bowl. Set the tartar sauce aside.

3. Arrange 3 shallow bowls or pie plates side by side. Fill the first with the flour, salt, and pepper; put the eggs in the second bowl and the bread crumbs in the third. Dredge each piece of fish first in the flour, then the eggs, and finally the bread crumbs.

4. Arrange the coated fish pieces on the baking sheet so that the pieces don't touch. Coat generously with cooking spray and bake for 5 minutes. Remove the baking sheet, turn the pieces over, and coat again with cooking spray. Bake for 5 minutes, or until the fish flakes easily with a fork. Serve with the tartar sauce.

* Limit saturated fat to no more than 10 percent of total calories—about 17 grams per day for most women or 21 grams for most men—and sodium intake to no more than 2,300 milligrams.

MAKE IT A FLAT BELLY DIET MEAL: Serve with ½ cup cooked carrots (27). Total meal: 430 calories

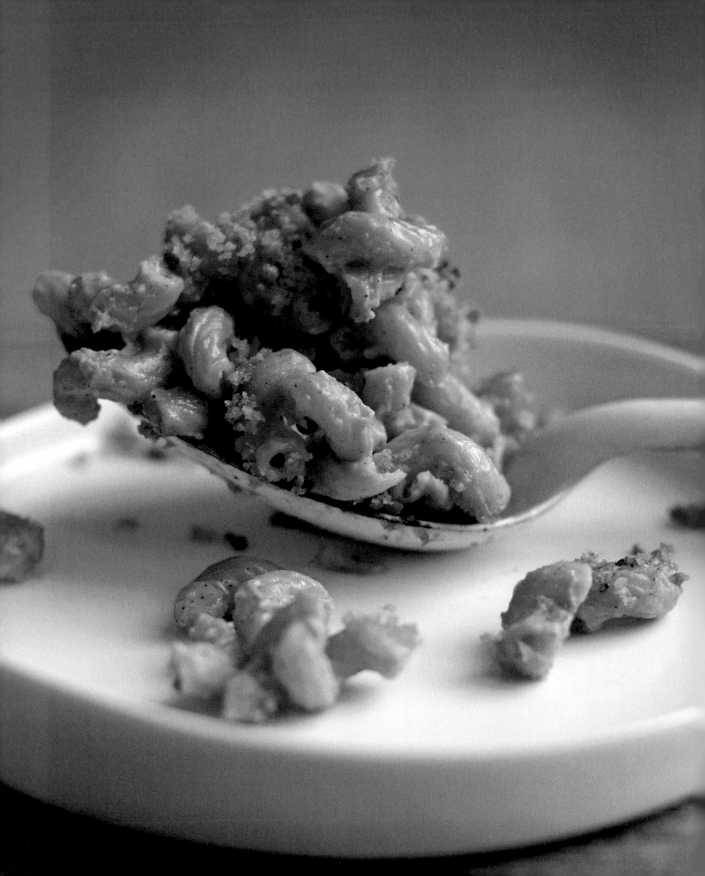

Crunchy Crust Mac and Cheese

4 SERVINGS / 328 CALORIES / MUFA: OLIVE OIL

You probably won't have any trouble enticing your family to eat this creamy macaroni and cheese casserole. You can even keep the MUFA a secret, if you want.

50 MINUTES

- 4 ounces multigrain elbow macaroni
- 3 tablespoons panko bread crumbs
- 4 tablespoons olive oil
- 2 tablespoons all-purpose flour
- ½ teaspoon paprika
- ½ teaspoon salt
- ⅛ teaspoon ground black pepper
- 2 cups fat-free milk
- ½ cup (2 ounces) shredded reduced-fat Cheddar cheese

Nutrition per serving
- 328 calories
- 14 g protein
- 31 g carbohydrates
- 17 g fat
- 3.5 g saturated fat*
- 15 mg cholesterol
- 480 mg sodium
- 2 g fiber

1. Preheat the oven to 350°F. Coat an 8" x 8" baking dish with cooking spray.

2. Bring a medium pot of water to a boil. Add the macaroni and cook according to package directions. Drain, rinse with cold water, and drain again. Set aside.

3. Combine the bread crumbs and 2 teaspoons of the oil and stir with a fork to evenly coat.

4. Add the remaining 3 tablespoons + 1 teaspoon oil to a large saucepan. Set over medium-high heat. Whisk in the flour, paprika, salt, and pepper until smooth. Gradually add the milk, whisking constantly. Cook, whisking, for 5 minutes, or until thickened. Remove from the heat. Stir in the cheese until it melts. Stir in the macaroni. Pour into the baking dish. Top evenly with the crumb mixture.

5. Bake for 15 minutes, or until bubbling and golden. Allow to rest for 10 minutes before serving.

Limit saturated fat to no more than 10 percent of total calories—about 17 grams per day for most women or 21 grams for most men—and sodium intake to no more than 2,300 milligrams.

MAKE IT A FLAT BELLY DIET MEAL: Serve with 1 cup steamed broccoli (44) tossed with 1 teaspoon trans-free margarine (26). Total meal: 398 calories

Tuna Noodle Casserole

4 SERVINGS / 403 CALORIES / MUFA: CANOLA OIL MAYONNAISE

This isn't your old-fashioned casserole. Lightened up with the sunny flavors of lemon and artichoke, this dish also gets a healthy dose of fiber from whole grain egg noodles.

50 MINUTES

6 ounces whole wheat egg noodles

1 pouch (6.4 ounces) light tuna

1 can (14 ounces) water-packed artichoke hearts, drained and chopped

½ cup frozen green peas

¼ cup canola oil mayonnaise

¼ cup grated Parmesan cheese

1 teaspoon capers, chopped

Zest of 1 lemon +
1 tablespoon juice

½ cup panko bread crumbs

Nutrition per serving

○ 403 calories
○ 23 g protein
○ 45 g carbohydrates
○ 14 g fat
○ 1.5 g saturated fat
○ 25 mg cholesterol
○ 700 mg sodium*
○ 5 g fiber

1. Preheat the oven to 350°F. Coat an 8" x 8" baking dish with cooking spray.

2. Bring a large pot of water to a boil. Add the noodles and cook according to package directions. Drain and set aside.

3. Combine the tuna, artichokes, peas, mayonnaise, 2 tablespoons of the cheese, the capers, and lemon zest and juice in a large bowl. Toss gently until thoroughly mixed. Stir in the noodles and spread the mixture evenly in the baking dish.

4. Scatter the bread crumbs and remaining 2 tablespoons cheese evenly over the top and bake for 30 minutes, or until heated through.

* Limit saturated fat to no more than 10 percent of total calories—about 17 grams per day for most women or 21 grams for most men—and sodium intake to no more than 2,300 milligrams.

MAKE IT **FASTER** If you prepare the noodles ahead of time, you can have this dish ready to pop in the oven as soon as the oven is finished preheating.

MAKE IT A FLAT BELLY DIET MEAL: A single serving of this recipe counts as a Flat Belly Diet Meal without any add-ons!

Southern-Style Baked Shrimp

4 SERVINGS / 322 CALORIES / MUFA: OLIVE OIL

Just a hint of honey provides a nice balance to the slight spiciness of these shrimp. Make sure to serve with something that can soak up the delicious MUFA-rich sauce.

40 MINUTES

¼ cup olive oil

2 tablespoons fresh lemon juice

2 teaspoons Cajun seasoning

2 teaspoons minced garlic

2 teaspoons honey

2 teaspoons reduced-sodium soy sauce

1½ pounds peeled and deveined large shrimp

2 tablespoons chopped parsley

1. Preheat the oven to 350°F.

2. Meanwhile, combine the oil, lemon juice, Cajun seasoning, garlic, honey, and soy sauce in an 8" x 8" baking dish. Add the shrimp and toss gently to coat. Let sit for 15 minutes.

3. Bake for 15 to 18 minutes, or until the shrimp are opaque throughout. Serve sprinkled with the parsley.

* Limit saturated fat to no more than 10 percent of total calories—about 17 grams per day for most women or 21 grams for most men—and sodium intake to no more than 2,300 milligrams.

Nutrition per serving
○ 322 calories
○ 35 g protein
○ 6 g carbohydrates
○ 17 g fat
○ 2.5 g saturated fat
○ 260 mg cholesterol
○ 610 mg sodium*
○ 0 g fiber

MAKE IT A FLAT BELLY DIET MEAL: Serve with ½ cup cooked lentils (115). Total meal: 437 calories

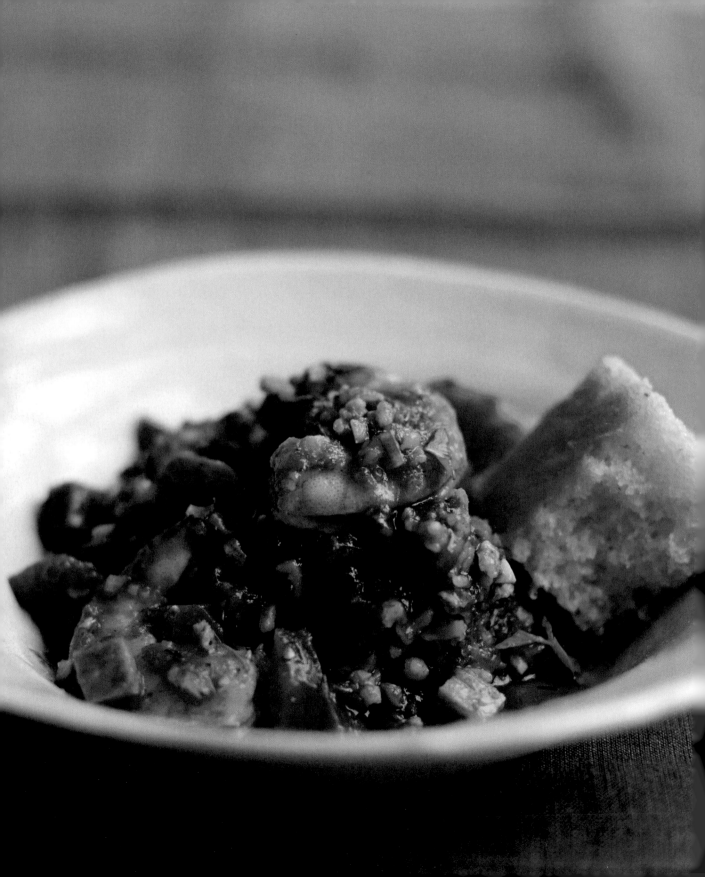

Shrimp and Ham Jambalaya

4 SERVINGS (1 CUP EACH) / 282 CALORIES / MUFA: OLIVE OIL

The appeal of many one-pot meals is that they cook unattended, and this jambalaya straight from the Big Easy is one such dish.

45 MINUTES

¼ cup olive oil
1 small onion, chopped
½ large red bell pepper, chopped
2 garlic cloves, minced
1½ teaspoons Cajun seasoning
¼ teaspoon salt
1 can (14.5 ounces) no-salt-added plum tomatoes, chopped (with juice)
¼ cup instant brown rice
2 ounces reduced-fat smoked ham, diced
¾ pound peeled and deveined medium shrimp
¼ cup chopped parsley
Hot-pepper sauce (optional)

1. Preheat the oven to 375°F.

2. Heat the oil in a large Dutch oven over medium-high heat. Add the onion, bell pepper, garlic, Cajun seasoning, and salt. Cook, stirring, for 4 minutes, or until the onion begins to soften. Stir in the tomatoes (with juice), rice, and ham. Cover and bake for 10 minutes.

3. Carefully uncover the dish. Stir in the shrimp, making sure they are buried in the sauce. Re-cover and bake for 5 minutes. Remove from the oven and allow to rest for 5 minutes. Stir in the parsley and serve with hot-pepper sauce at the table, if desired.

Nutrition per serving
○ 282 calories
○ 22 g protein
○ 14 g carbohydrates
○ 16 g fat
○ 2 g saturated fat
○ 135 mg cholesterol
○ 490 mg sodium
○ 3 g fiber

MAKE IT A FLAT BELLY DIET MEAL: Serve with a small piece of cornbread (75) and ½ cup cooked greens (25). Total meal: 382 calories

Chicken and Yellow Rice Casserole

4 SERVINGS (1½ CUPS EACH) / 364 CALORIES / MUFA: OLIVES

Chicken thighs impart more flavor than breast meat, making them ideal for this cozy dish. Though we like combining two different types of olives, by all means use just one if you have a strong preference for one over the other.

50 MINUTES

3 teaspoons olive oil
¾ pound boneless, skinless chicken thighs
1 onion, chopped
1 red bell pepper, chopped
1 green bell pepper, chopped
4 garlic cloves, minced
1 teaspoon dried oregano
¾ cup long-grain white rice
¼ teaspoon saffron threads, lightly crushed
1¾ cups fat-free reduced-sodium chicken broth
1 can (8 ounces) no-salt-added tomato sauce
20 pitted Manzanilla olives
20 pitted large black olives

Nutrition per serving

○ 364 calories
○ 22 g protein
○ 41 g carbohydrates
○ 12 g fat
○ 2 g saturated fat
○ 70 mg cholesterol
○ 730 mg sodium*
○ 4 g fiber

1. Preheat the oven to 400°F.

2. Trim the chicken thighs of all visible fat and cut into ½" chunks.

3. Heat 2 teaspoons of the oil in a large ovenproof nonstick skillet over medium-high heat. Add the chicken and cook, stirring occasionally, for 4 minutes, or until lightly browned. Transfer the chicken to a plate.

4. Add the remaining 1 teaspoon oil to the skillet. Stir in the onion, bell peppers, garlic, and oregano. Cook, stirring occasionally, for 3 to 4 minutes, or until the vegetables soften. Stir in the rice and saffron and cook, stirring, for 1 minute. Return the chicken and any accumulated juices from the plate to the skillet. Add the broth, tomato sauce, and olives. Bring to a boil, cover, and transfer to the oven.

5. Bake for 23 to 25 minutes, or until the liquid is absorbed and the rice is tender. Remove from the oven and let rest for 5 minutes. Stir well before serving.

* Limit saturated fat to no more than 10 percent of total calories—about 17 grams per day for most women or 21 grams for most men—and sodium intake to no more than 2,300 milligrams.

MAKE IT A FLAT BELLY DIET MEAL: Serve with 6 steamed asparagus spears (19). Total meal: 383 calories

Mexican Corn Soup

4 SERVINGS (1 CUP EACH) / 252 CALORIES / MUFA: AVOCADO

Just half a jalapeño provides a little kick in this soup. Wash your hands thoroughly after handling a jalapeño, and don't touch your eyes or lips until you do.

45 MINUTES

1 tablespoon olive oil
1 onion, chopped
3 garlic cloves, minced
½ jalapeño pepper, finely chopped
1 teaspoon ground cumin
1 teaspoon dried oregano
4 cups fat-free reduced-sodium chicken broth
4 cups fresh corn kernels (5 ears), cobs reserved
¾ teaspoon salt
1 Hass avocado, diced
1 red bell pepper, chopped
2 tablespoons chopped fresh cilantro
1 tablespoon fresh lime juice

1. Heat the oil in a large saucepan over medium-high heat. Add the onion, garlic, jalapeño pepper, cumin, and oregano. Cook, stirring occasionally, for 3 to 4 minutes, or until starting to soften. Add the broth, 1 cup water, and corn cobs. Bring to a boil, reduce to a simmer, cover, and cook for 15 minutes. Discard the cobs and stir in the corn kernels and ½ teaspoon of the salt. Return to a simmer and cook for 10 to 11 minutes, or until tender. Remove from the heat and let cool 15 minutes.

2. Meanwhile, combine the avocado, bell pepper, cilantro, lime juice, and remaining ¼ teaspoon salt in a small bowl.

3. Puree the soup, in batches, in a blender. Divide among 4 bowls and top each with one-fourth of the avocado mixture.

* Limit saturated fat to no more than 10 percent of total calories—about 17 grams per day for most women or 21 grams for most men—and sodium intake to no more than 2,300 milligrams.

Nutrition per serving
○ 252 calories
○ 8 g protein
○ 38 g carbohydrates
○ 11 g fat
○ 1.5 g saturated fat
○ 0 mg cholesterol
○ 630 mg sodium*
○ 8 g fiber

MAKE IT A FLAT BELLY DIET MEAL: Serve with a 1-ounce whole wheat dinner roll (77) spread with 2 teaspoons trans-free margarine (53). **Total meal: 382 calories**

Chicken and Almond Dumplings

4 SERVINGS (1 CUP SOUP AND 3 DUMPLINGS EACH) / 409 CALORIES / MUFA: ALMONDS

For best results, make sure the almonds are finely ground. Nuts provide a nice firmness to the dumplings, but you don't want to detect any little pieces.

1 HOUR 20 MIN

1 tablespoon olive oil

3 carrots, cut into ½" pieces

2 celery ribs, chopped

1 onion, finely chopped

2 garlic cloves, minced

½ teaspoon dried thyme

3 cups fat-free reduced-sodium chicken broth

1 pound boneless, skinless chicken breasts, chopped

½ cup almonds

¾ cup all-purpose flour

½ teaspoon baking powder

¼ teaspoon baking soda

¼ teaspoon salt

1 tablespoon trans-free margarine

6 tablespoons low-fat buttermilk

Nutrition per serving

○ 409 calories

○ 35 g protein

○ 31 g carbohydrates

○ 17 g fat

○ 2 g saturated fat

○ 65 mg cholesterol

○ 870 mg sodium*

○ 5 g fiber

1. Heat the oil in a large saucepan over medium-high heat. Add the carrots, celery, onion, garlic, and thyme. Cook, stirring occasionally, for 2 to 3 minutes, or until just starting to soften. Stir in the broth and 1 cup of water. Add the chicken. Bring to a boil, reduce to a simmer, cover, and cook for 30 minutes.

2. Meanwhile, bring a large pot of water to a simmer. Place the almonds in a medium skillet and cook over medium-high heat, shaking the pan often, for 3 to 5 minutes, or until lightly toasted. Transfer to a plate to cool for 5 minutes. Place the almonds in a food processor or blender and process to a fine meal.

3. Combine the ground almonds, flour, baking powder, baking soda, and salt in a bowl. With a pastry blender or 2 knives used scissor fashion, cut the margarine into the flour mixture until it resembles coarse crumbs. Stir in the buttermilk until a soft dough forms.

4. Place the dough on a lightly floured surface and pat to a ½" thickness. Cut the dough into 12 equal pieces. Drop into the simmering water and cook, turning once, for 17 to 18 minutes, or until the dumplings are cooked through. Remove with a slotted spoon and transfer to the pan with the chicken mixture. Simmer gently for 5 minutes. Divide among 4 bowls.

* Limit saturated fat to no more than 10 percent of total calories—about 17 grams per day for most women or 21 grams for most men—and sodium intake to no more than 2,300 milligrams.

MAKE IT A FLAT BELLY DIET MEAL: A single serving of this recipe counts as a Flat Belly Diet Meal without any add-ons!

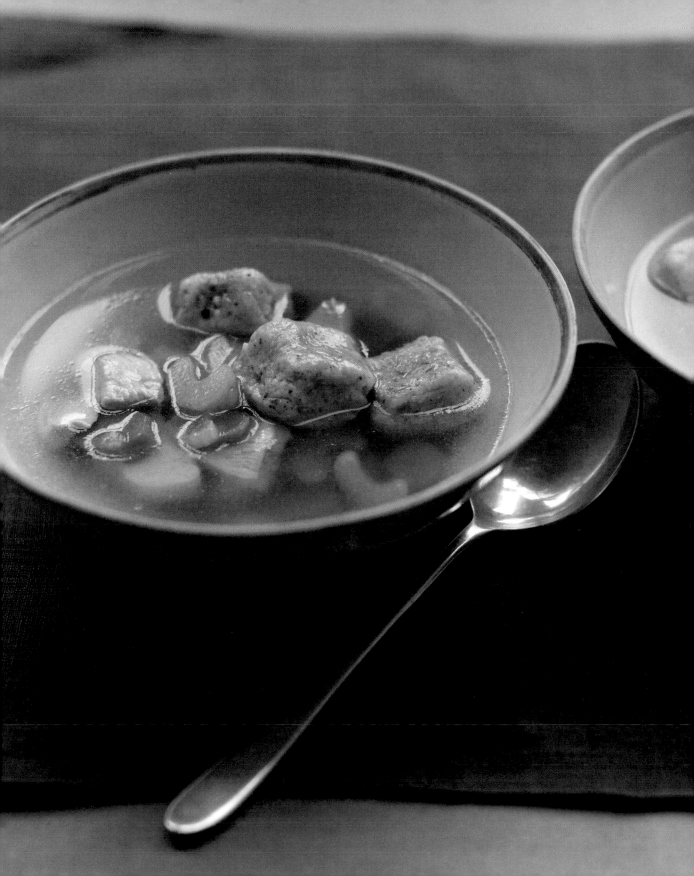

Broccoli Chicken Casserole

4 SERVINGS / 410 CALORIES / MUFA: ALMONDS

Chicken breast tenders are great to have on hand for a dish like this because they don't require as much preparation. However, they can be more expensive than regular boneless, skinless chicken breasts, so feel free to use those if you prefer.

1
HOUR

- 2 **tablespoons olive oil**
- 1 **pound boneless, skinless chicken breast tenders, cut into 1" chunks**
- ½ **onion, chopped**
- ¼ **cup all-purpose flour**
- 1 **tablespoon Dijon mustard**
- 1½ **cups fat-free reduced-sodium chicken broth**
- 2 **cups broccoli florets**
- 1 **cup instant brown rice**
- ½ **cup sliced almonds**
- ½ **cup (2 ounces) shredded reduced-fat Cheddar cheese**

Nutrition per serving

- ○ 410 calories
- ○ 37 g protein
- ○ 29 g carbohydrates
- ○ 17 g fat
- ○ 3.5 g saturated fat
- ○ 75 mg cholesterol
- ○ 400 mg sodium
- ○ 4 g fiber

1. Preheat the oven to 350°F. Coat an 8″ x 8″ baking dish with cooking spray.

2. Heat the oil in a large nonstick skillet over medium-high heat. Add the chicken and onion. Cook for 7 to 10 minutes, stirring occasionally, until the chicken and onion are browned. Sprinkle the flour over the chicken mixture and cook for 1 to 2 minutes, or until browned. Stir in the mustard. Slowly add the broth, stirring constantly to make a smooth sauce. Stir in the broccoli and rice.

3. Transfer the mixture to the baking dish and sprinkle the almonds and cheese evenly over the top.

4. Cover with foil and bake for 20 minutes. Uncover and bake for 10 minutes, or until the top is golden. Let rest for 10 minutes before serving.

MAKE IT A FLAT BELLY DIET MEAL: A single serving of this recipe counts as a Flat Belly Diet Meal without any add-ons!

Chicken Tortilla Casserole

4 SERVINGS / 421 CALORIES / MUFA: AVOCADO

If you like, assemble this dish the night before you plan to serve it, cover, and refrigerate. Just pop it in the oven and you're done!

55 MINUTES

1 tablespoon olive oil

1 onion, chopped

2 garlic cloves, minced

1 orange bell pepper, chopped

1 jalapeño pepper, minced

12 ounces precooked boneless, skinless chicken breast, shredded (see page 86)

1 cup corn and black bean salsa

2 ounces baked tortilla chips

1 cup (4 ounces) shredded reduced-fat Mexican blend cheese

1 Hass avocado, cut into 16 slices

1. Preheat the oven to 350°F. Coat an 8″ x 8″ baking dish with cooking spray.

2. Heat the oil in a large nonstick skillet over medium-high heat. Add the onion, garlic, and peppers. Cook, stirring occasionally, for 4 to 5 minutes, or until softened. Remove from the heat and stir in the chicken and ½ cup of the salsa.

3. Line the bottom of the baking dish with half of the tortilla chips. Top with the chicken mixture, then spoon the remaining ½ cup salsa on top. Sprinkle with ½ cup of the cheese. Coarsely crumble the remaining chips over the top. Sprinkle with the remaining ½ cup cheese. Transfer to the oven and bake for 18 to 20 minutes, or until the cheese melts and the filling is hot. Remove from the oven and let rest for 5 minutes. Cut into 4 servings and top each with 4 avocado slices.

* Limit saturated fat to no more than 10 percent of total calories—about 17 grams per day for most women or 21 grams for most men—and sodium intake to no more than 2,300 milligrams.

Nutrition per serving

○ 421 calories

○ 38 g protein

○ 28 g carbohydrates

○ 18 g fat

○ 6 g saturated fat*

○ 90 mg cholesterol

○ 650 mg sodium*

○ 5 g fiber

MAKE IT A FLAT BELLY DIET MEAL: A single serving of this recipe counts as a Flat Belly Diet Meal without any add-ons!

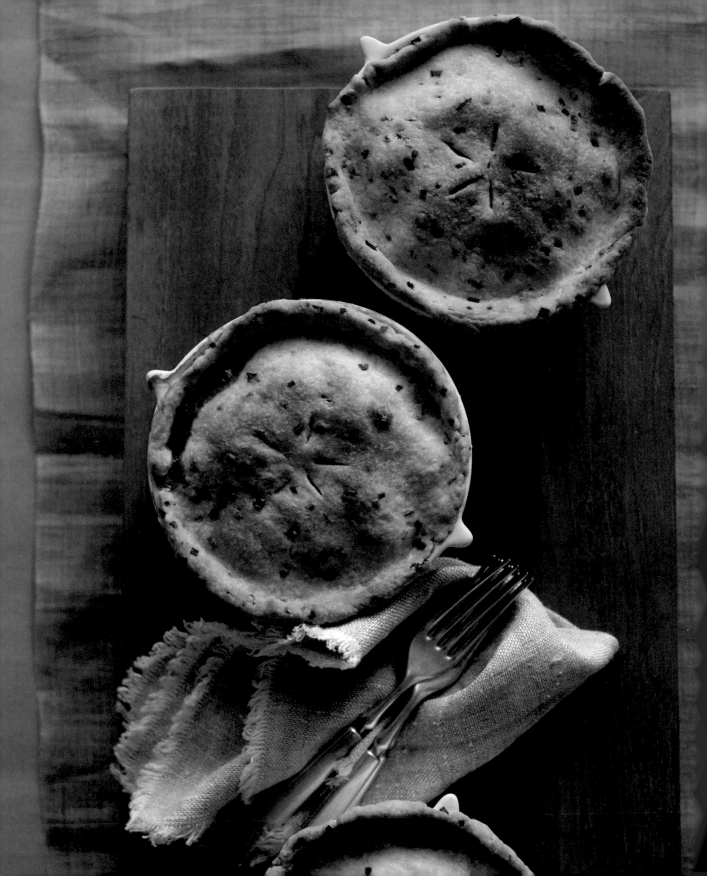

Turkey Potpies

6 SERVINGS / 357 CALORIES / MUFA: SAFFLOWER OIL

These delicious potpies can be baked in a 9″ deep-dish pie plate, too. Just divide your portions carefully to avoid disagreements over who gets the most crust!

1
HOUR
5 MIN

1½ cups all-purpose flour
3 tablespoons chopped fresh chives
¾ teaspoon salt
6 tablespoons safflower oil
1 onion, chopped
1 package (8 ounces) sliced mushrooms
1 teaspoon chopped fresh thyme leaves
2 celery ribs, chopped
1 cup frozen peas and carrots
1½ cups fat-free reduced-sodium chicken broth
1 pound precooked boneless, skinless turkey breast, cut into ½″ pieces

Nutrition per serving
○ 357 calories
○ 28 g protein
○ 28 g carbohydrates
○ 15 g fat
○ 1 g saturated fat
○ 65 mg cholesterol
○ 680 mg sodium*
○ 2 g fiber

1. Combine 1¼ cups of the flour, the chives, and ¼ teaspoon of the salt in a bowl. Add 5 tablespoons of the oil and 3 tablespoons water. Stir with a fork until a rough dough begins to form. Knead the dough in the bowl 4 or 5 times until smooth, then press into a 4″-diameter disk. Let rest for 20 minutes.

2. Meanwhile, preheat the oven to 400°F. Coat six 1-cup or larger ramekins with cooking spray.

3. Heat the remaining 1 tablespoon oil in a large nonstick skillet over medium-high heat. Add the onion, mushrooms, and thyme. Cook, stirring occasionally, for 5 to 6 minutes, or until the mushrooms start to brown. Stir in the celery and peas and carrots. Cook for 2 minutes. Whisk together the remaining ¼ cup flour and ½ teaspoon salt in a small bowl. Whisk in the broth until smooth. Pour the broth mixture into the skillet and cook, stirring occasionally, for 2 minutes, or until thickened. Season with pepper. Remove from the heat and stir in the turkey. Divide the mixture among the ramekins.

4. Divide the dough into 6 equal pieces and place on a lightly floured surface. Roll each piece into a 5″ circle, large enough to cover a ramekin. Set the dough over the filling and decoratively crimp the dough edges, if desired. Pierce the dough 4 or 5 times with the tip of a sharp knife. Arrange the ramekins on a baking sheet and bake for 25 to 30 minutes, or until the tops are lightly browned and the filling is bubbling. Remove from the oven and let rest 5 to 10 minutes before serving.

Limit saturated fat to no more than 10 percent of total calories—about 17 grams per day for most women or 21 grams for most men—and sodium intake to no more than 2,300 milligrams.

MAKE IT A FLAT BELLY DIET MEAL: Serve with 2 cups baby spinach (20) tossed with ½ cup sliced strawberries (27) and 1 tablespoon balsamic vinegar (14). **Total meal: 418 calories**

Rosemary Pork and Rice Bake

4 SERVINGS / 346 CALORIES / MUFA: PINE NUTS

Rosemary is a classic companion for pork, but if you don't have it on hand, replace it with dried sage or poultry seasoning.

45 MINUTES

1½ cups baby carrots

1½ cups small white onions

½ pound well-trimmed pork tenderloin, cut into 1" pieces

6 tablespoons instant brown rice

2 garlic cloves, minced

¾ teaspoon finely chopped fresh rosemary

¼ teaspoon salt

¼ teaspoon ground black pepper

½ cup no-salt-added tomato sauce

½ cup fat-free reduced-sodium chicken broth

½ cup pine nuts, finely ground

1 tablespoon minced parsley

1. Preheat the oven to 350°F. Coat a 13" x 9" baking dish with cooking spray.

2. Slice the carrots in half lengthwise. Cut the onions into quarters.

3. Place the carrots, onions, pork, rice, garlic, rosemary, salt, and pepper in the baking dish. Stir together the tomato sauce and broth in a measuring cup. Pour over the pork mixture. Top evenly with the pine nuts. Cover tightly with foil.

4. Bake for 30 minutes, or until the mixture is bubbling and the carrots are tender. Remove the foil carefully to avoid hot steam. If desired, broil 6" from the heat for 2 to 3 minutes, or until the nuts are golden. Allow to rest for 5 minutes. Serve sprinkled with the parsley.

* Limit saturated fat to no more than 10 percent of total calories—about 17 grams per day for most women or 21 grams for most men—and sodium intake to no more than 2,300 milligrams.

Nutrition per serving

○ 346 calories

○ 19 g protein

○ 21 g carbohydrates

○ 20 g fat

○ 4.5 g saturated fat*

○ 35 mg cholesterol

○ 460 mg sodium

○ 5 g fiber

MAKE IT A FLAT BELLY DIET MEAL: Serve with 1 cup cooked brussels sprouts (56).
Total meal: 402 calories To serve as part of another FBD meal, omit the pine nuts (146).

Mexican Pork Stew

4 SERVINGS (1¼ CUPS STEW AND 3 TABLESPOONS AVOCADO CREAM EACH) / 348 CALORIES / MUFA: AVOCADO

Hominy is hulled corn kernels that have been stripped of the bran, so if you want even more fiber in this dish, substitute 1 can chickpeas instead.

50 MINUTES

- 4 teaspoons olive oil
- 1 pound well-trimmed pork tenderloin, cut into ¾" pieces
- 1 onion
- 1 carrot
- 1 celery rib
- 3 garlic cloves, minced
- 1 teaspoon ground cumin
- ½ teaspoon dried basil
- 2 cups fat-free reduced-sodium chicken broth
- 1 can (15 ounces) white hominy, rinsed and drained
- 1 tomato
- 3 tablespoons fresh cilantro
- ½ teaspoon salt
- 1 cup mashed Hass avocado
- ¼ cup fat-free sour cream

Nutrition per serving
- ○ 348 calories
- ○ 28 g protein
- ○ 22 g carbohydrates
- ○ 17 g fat
- ○ 2.5 g saturated fat
- ○ 75 mg cholesterol
- ○ 760 mg sodium*
- ○ 7 g fiber

1. Heat 2 teaspoons of the oil in a Dutch oven over medium-high heat. Add the pork and cook, stirring occasionally, for 6 minutes, or until lightly browned. Transfer to a plate and set aside.

2. Chop the onion, carrot, and celery. Seed and chop the tomato and set aside. Tear or chop the cilantro into small pieces and set aside.

3. Reduce the heat to medium and add the remaining 2 teaspoons oil. Stir in the onion, carrot, celery, garlic, cumin, and basil. Cook, stirring occasionally, for 6 to 7 minutes, or until softened. Add the broth, hominy, and reserved pork. Increase the heat to medium-high and bring to boil. Reduce to a simmer, cover, and cook for 18 to 20 minutes, or until the pork is tender. Stir in the tomato, cilantro, and salt.

4. Divide the stew among 4 bowls. Whisk together the avocado and sour cream in a medium bowl. Spoon the mixture into the center of each bowl and serve.

* Limit saturated fat to no more than 10 percent of total calories—about 17 grams per day for most women or 21 grams for most men   and sodium intake to no more than 2,300 milligrams.

MAKE IT A FLAT BELLY DIET MEAL: Serve with 2 cups arugula (14) tossed with 1 tablespoon Parmesan cheese (22) and lemon juice, salt, and pepper to taste. **Total meal: 384 calories**

Chipotle Beef and Bean Chili

4 SERVINGS (1 CUP EACH) / 371 CALORIES / MUFA: PUMPKIN SEEDS

If you enjoy the crunch of a few tortilla chips crumbled over your chili, you'll be pleased by how well MUFA-laden pumpkin seeds provide a similar experience.

35 MINUTES

1 onion
1 green bell pepper
3 garlic cloves
1 tablespoon canola oil
½ pound 95% lean ground beef
1 chipotle pepper in adobo sauce, minced
4 teaspoons chili powder
2 teaspoons ground cumin
1 teaspoon dried oregano
1 can (14.5 ounces) fire-roasted diced tomatoes
1 can (15 ounces) no-salt-added black beans, rinsed and drained
½ teaspoon salt
½ cup shelled unsalted dry-roasted pumpkin seeds

1. Finely chop the onion, bell pepper, and garlic. Set aside.

2. Heat the oil in a Dutch oven over medium-high heat. Add the beef and cook for 3 to 4 minutes, breaking into smaller pieces with a wooden spoon, until no longer pink. Stir in the onion, bell pepper, and garlic. Cook, stirring occasionally, for 4 to 5 minutes, or until starting to soften. Add the chipotle pepper, chili powder, cumin, and oregano and cook for 1 minute. Stir in the tomatoes and cook for 1 minute. Add the beans and ¼ cup water, if necessary, and bring to a boil. Reduce to a simmer, cover, and cook for 15 minutes.

3. Remove from the heat and stir in the salt. Divide among 4 bowls and top each with 2 tablespoons pumpkin seeds.

* Limit saturated fat to no more than 10 percent of total calories—about 17 grams per day for most women or 21 grams for most men—and sodium intake to no more than 2,300 milligrams.

Nutrition per serving
○ 371 calories
○ 28 g protein
○ 25 g carbohydrates
○ 19 g fat
○ 4 g saturated fat*
○ 35 mg cholesterol
○ 590 mg sodium
○ 7 g fiber

MAKE IT A FLAT BELLY DIET MEAL: Serve topped with 2 tablespoons shredded reduced-fat Cheddar cheese (40). Total meal: 411 calories

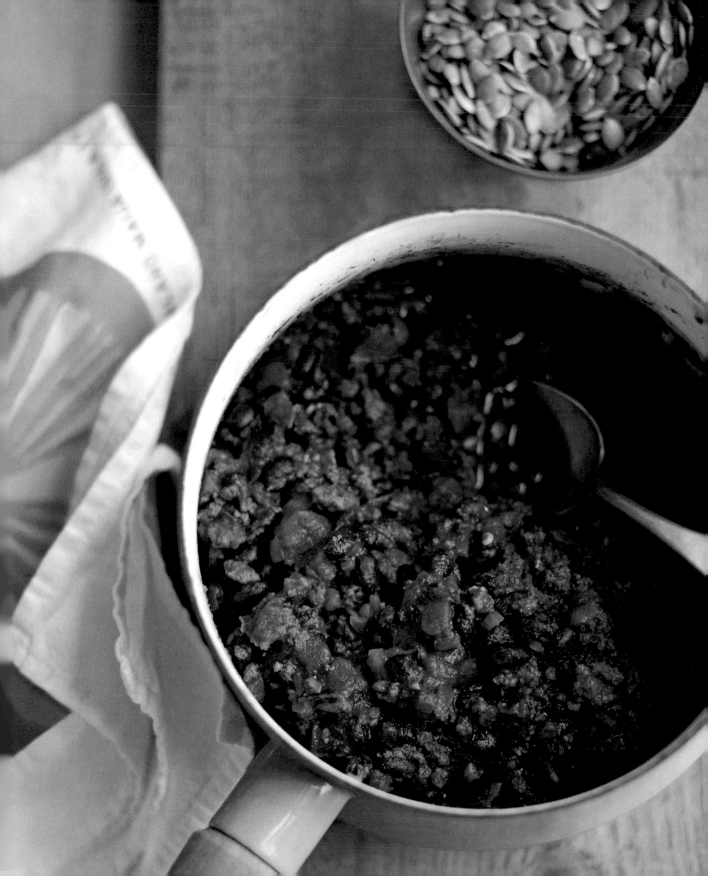

Beef Goulash Noodle Casserole

4 SERVINGS (1 CUP EACH) / 363 CALORIES / MUFA: CANOLA OIL

We liked baking this dish because it makes it easy to leave a meal cooking unattended. However, you could keep it on the stove if you prefer; just keep the lid on tight and turn the heat down to low.

45 MINUTES

¼ cup canola oil
1 onion, chopped
½ red bell pepper, chopped
1¼ teaspoons paprika
1 teaspoon dried thyme
¾ pound 95% lean ground beef
1 can (14.5 ounces) no-salt-added petite diced tomatoes
3 ounces dried whole wheat noodles
½ cup fat-free reduced-sodium chicken broth
½ teaspoon ground black pepper
¼ teaspoon salt
¼ cup fat-free sour cream
1½ tablespoons all-purpose flour

Nutrition per serving
○ 363 calories
○ 24 g protein
○ 24 g carbohydrates
○ 19 g fat
○ 3 g saturated fat
○ 55 mg cholesterol
○ 240 mg sodium
○ 3 g fiber

1. Preheat the oven to 350°F.

2. Heat the oil in a Dutch oven over medium-high heat. Add the onion, bell pepper, paprika, and thyme. Cook, stirring, for 3 minutes. Crumble the beef into the pan. Cook, stirring, for 4 minutes, or until the beef is no longer pink. Stir in the tomatoes, noodles, broth, black pepper, and salt.

3. Cover tightly and bake for 15 minutes. Carefully remove the cover and stir. Bake, uncovered, for 10 minutes. Remove from the oven, cover, and let sit for 10 minutes, or until the noodles are tender.

4. Meanwhile, whisk the sour cream and flour in a small bowl. Whisk into the casserole. Stir over low heat for 1 to 2 minutes, or until thickened.

🕐 **MAKE IT AHEAD** This baked dish can be cooled and refrigerated in an airtight container. Reheat individual portions on a microwaveable plate covered with waxed paper.

MAKE IT A FLAT BELLY DIET MEAL: Serve with 1 cup cooked carrots (54). Total meal: 417 calories

Oven-Baked Pot Roast

6 SERVINGS / 360 CALORIES / MUFA: OLIVE OIL

Eye of round roasts rarely come in 1½-pound packages, so go ahead and buy a 3-pound roast for this dish; freeze half of it for another meal later in the month.

3 HOURS 30 MIN

¼ cup all-purpose flour
1 teaspoon ground coriander
1 teaspoon dried oregano
¾ teaspoon salt
½ teaspoon dried thyme
½ teaspoon ground black pepper
1½ pounds boneless beef eye of round roast, trimmed of visible fat
6 tablespoons olive oil
3 onions, thinly sliced
½ cup red wine (optional)
1 can (14.5 ounces) fat-free reduced-sodium beef broth
2 tablespoons Dijon mustard

Nutrition per serving
○ 360 calories
○ 27 g protein
○ 10 g carbohydrates
○ 18 g fat
○ 3 g saturated fat
○ 50 mg cholesterol
○ 530 mg sodium
○ 1 g fiber

1. Preheat the oven to 425°F.

2. Combine the flour, coriander, oregano, salt, thyme, and pepper in a large bowl. Add the roast and turn to coat. Heat 2 tablespoons of the oil in a Dutch oven over medium-high heat. Add the roast (set aside the flour mixture) and cook, turning occasionally, for 8 minutes, or until browned. Transfer to a plate.

3. Add the remaining 4 tablespoons oil to the Dutch oven. Stir in the onions and cook, stirring occasionally, for 17 to 19 minutes, or until golden. Pour in the wine and, if using, cook for 2 to 3 minutes, or until reduced by about half. Whisk in the broth, 1 cup of water, the mustard, and reserved flour mixture and cook for 30 seconds.

4. Add the beef, cover, and transfer to the oven. Bake for 2 hours. Turn the roast and stir in another ½ cup water if the sauce looks too thick. Cover and bake for 40 to 45 minutes, or until the beef is tender. Let the roast rest for 10 minutes, then transfer to a cutting board and cut into 12 slices. Serve 2 slices per person, with sauce.

MAKE IT A FLAT BELLY DIET MEAL: Serve with ½ cup roasted baby potatoes (70). **Total calories:** 430 calories

QUICK-FIX PANTRY RESCUES

Easy Creamy Bean Soup

Rinse and drain 1 cup canned cannellini beans (200) and puree with $\frac{1}{2}$ cup fat-free reduced-sodium chicken broth (3), 1 teaspoon fresh lemon juice (1), 1 teaspoon chopped garlic (15), $\frac{1}{8}$ teaspoon ground black pepper (0), and a pinch of dried rosemary (0). Add water if a thinner soup is desired. Cook until warmed through. Drizzle with 1 tablespoon **olive oil** (120) and serve with a 1-ounce slice of Italian bread (77). **Total Calories = 416**

Quick Peanut Stew

Peel and chop 1 baked medium sweet potato (103) and combine with 1 tablespoon grated fresh ginger (5) and 1 cup fat-free reduced-sodium chicken broth (5). Cook until warmed through. Stir in 2 tablespoons creamy **peanut butter** (188). Serve with 1 piece reduced-fat mozzarella string cheese (80). **Total Calories = 381**

Walnut Chicken

Combine 1 cup cooked brown rice (218), 2 ounces chopped precooked chicken breast (81), 1 tablespoon dried cranberries (23), 1 chopped scallion (5), and 2 tablespoons chopped **walnuts** (82) in a small baking dish. Cover and bake in a 350°F oven for 20 minutes, or until heated through. **Total Calories = 409**

Cheesy Baked Pasta

Arrange 1 cup cooked multigrain pasta (174) in the bottom of a small baking dish. Top with $\frac{1}{4}$ cup fat-free ricotta cheese (45), $\frac{1}{3}$ cup marinara sauce (48), and 2 tablespoons shredded reduced-fat mozzarella cheese (35). Drizzle 1 tablespoon **olive oil** (120) over the top. Cover and bake in a 350°F oven for 15 minutes. Uncover and bake for another 5 minutes, or until the cheese is bubbling. **Total Calories = 422**

Fast Tamale Casserole

Combine $\frac{1}{2}$ cup frozen meatless crumbles (60), $\frac{1}{2}$ cup frozen corn (72), and 2 tablespoons salsa (10). Place in a small baking dish. Cover with 4 ounces sliced precooked polenta (50) and $\frac{1}{4}$ cup shredded reduced-fat Cheddar cheese (80). Cover and bake in a 350°F oven for 15 minutes. Uncover and bake another 5 minutes, or until the cheese is bubbling. Top with $\frac{1}{4}$ cup mashed **Hass avocado** (96) and 1 tablespoon reduced-fat sour cream (20). **Total Calories = 388**

Menu for Watching the "Big Game"

Fruit, vegetable, and cheese platter
Southern-Style Baked Shrimp (page 181)
Shrimp and Ham Jambalaya (page 183)
Cornbread (below)

NOTE: Double all recipes except for the cornbread.

SERVES 8

🕐 **The night before:** Assemble the vegetable, fruit, and cheese platter, prepping all ingredients that won't discolor before serving. Peel and devein the shrimp, if necessary.

🕐 **About 3 hours before serving:** Start Jambalaya. Keep warm.

🕐 **About 2 hours before serving:** Prepare Cornbread by brushing a 9" pie plate or 10" cast-iron skillet with 1 tablespoon canola oil and preheating the oven to 425°F. Combine 1 cup buttermilk with ⅓ cup water, 1 egg white, 2 tablespoons canola oil, and 3 tablespoons packed brown sugar in a small bowl. Mix 1¼ cups yellow cornmeal, 1 cup all-purpose flour, 2 teaspoons baking powder, and ½ teaspoon salt in a large bowl. Stir the buttermilk mixture into the cornmeal mixture until combined. Pour into the skillet and bake for 15 minutes. When cool, cut into 8 wedges.

🕐 **About 30 minutes before serving:** Start Baked Shrimp. Finish preparing and set out the vegetable, fruit, and cheese platter for an appetizer.

MAKE IT A FLAT BELLY DIET MEAL: Enjoy ½ wedge of cornbread (104) with either the baked shrimp (322) or the jambalaya (282) with 1 cup raw vegetables from the appetizer platter (30). **Total meal = 416 calories (jambalaya) or 426 calories (shrimp)**

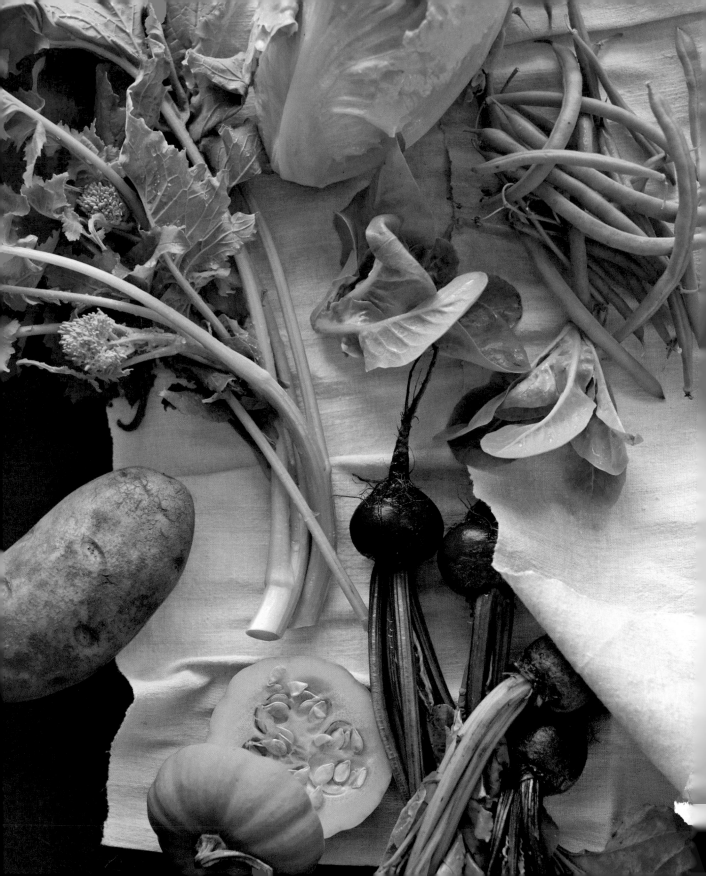

Amazing
Sides and
SALADS

9

- Chilean Avocado, Bean, and Corn Salad
- Tomato-Olive Salad
- 5-Bean Salad
- Roasted Beet Salad
- Fall Fruit Salad
- Green Bean and Pumpkin Seed Salad
- Roasted Pepper–Corn Pasta Salad
- Pasta Salad with Caramelized Onions and Zucchini
- Broccoli Pasta Salad
- Sicilian Tuna Salad
- Thai Peanut Slaw
- Spinach-Avocado Caesar Salad
- Creamy Sesame Greens
- Broccoli Rabe with Toasted Garlic
- Haricots Verts
- Roasted Carrots and Hazelnuts
- Mexican Grilled Corn on the Cob
- Salt and Pepper Oven Fries
- Garlic Mashed Potatoes
- Golden Rice Pilaf

Chilean Avocado, Bean, and Corn Salad

4 SERVINGS (¾ CUP EACH) / 196 CALORIES / MUFA: AVOCADO

When you choose minimally processed canned and frozen ingredients, healthy meals become quicker and easier to bring to the table.

5 MINUTES

Whisk the oil, vinegar, garlic, paprika, and salt in a bowl. Add the beans, avocado, and corn. Toss. Serve sprinkled with paprika.

MAKE IT **A TEAM EFFORT**

Let young helpers pitch in by rinsing the beans and draining the corn.

  2 teaspoons extra-virgin olive oil
  2 teaspoons red wine vinegar
  1 small garlic clove, minced
 ¼ teaspoon paprika + some for garnish
 ⅛ teaspoon salt
1½ cups canned no-salt-added navy beans, rinsed and drained
  1 Hass avocado, cut into chunks
 ½ cup fresh or frozen corn kernels

Nutrition per serving
○ 196 calories
○ 7 g protein
○ 26 g carbohydrates
○ 8 g fat
○ 1 g saturated fat
○ 0 mg cholesterol
○ 250 mg sodium
○ 10 g fiber

MAKE IT A FLAT BELLY DIET MEAL: Serve with Salmon with Sizzling Sesame Scallions (page 116), but omit the sesame seeds (227). **Total meal: 423 calories**

Tomato-Olive Salad

4 SERVINGS (1½ CUPS EACH) / 184 CALORIES / MUFA: OLIVES

Fennel is the secret ingredient in this summery salad. Look for it near the leafy greens in your grocery's produce section. For extra flavor, chop some of the delicate, dill-like fronds and toss them into the salad, too.

10 MINUTES

Combine the romaine, tomatoes, cucumber, olives, fennel, and onion in a large bowl. Add the oil, vinegar, salt, and pepper and toss well.

Limit saturated fat to no more than 10 percent of total calories—about 17 grams per day for most women or 21 grams for most men—and sodium intake to no more than 2,300 milligrams.

- 4 cups shredded romaine
- 2 cups grape tomatoes, halved
- 1 cucumber, halved lengthwise and thinly sliced crosswise
- 20 pitted large black olives, sliced
- 20 pitted kalamata olives, sliced
- ½ fennel bulb, thinly sliced
- ½ small red onion, thinly sliced
- 2 tablespoons extra-virgin olive oil
- 4 teaspoons balsamic vinegar
- ¼ teaspoon salt
- ¼ teaspoon ground black pepper

Nutrition per serving
- 184 calories
- 2 g protein
- 12 g carbohydrates
- 15 g fat
- 2 g saturated fat
- 0 mg cholesterol
- 670 mg sodium*
- 4 g fiber

MAKE IT A FLAT BELLY DIET MEAL: Serve with a 3-ounce turkey burger (169) on a 1-ounce whole grain hamburger bun (75). Total meal: 428 calories

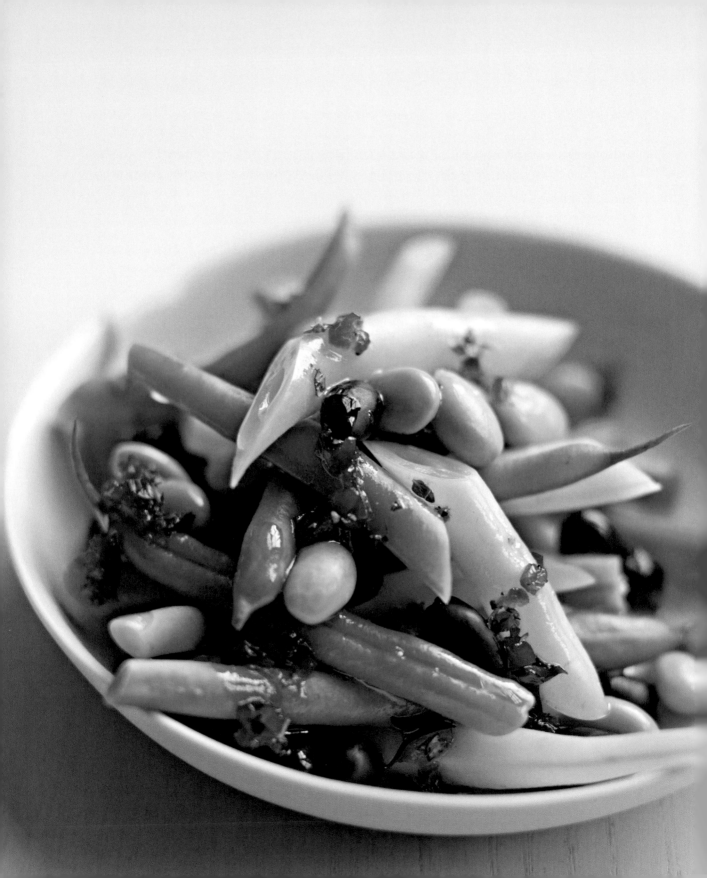

5-Bean Salad

4 SERVINGS (1 CUP EACH) / 254 CALORIES / MUFA: CANOLA OIL

Here's a potluck favorite that's quick to put together. Look for Peppadews in the olive bar at your grocery. They're about the size of a cherry pepper, only much sweeter.

10 MINUTES

¼ cup canola oil

2 tablespoons seasoned rice vinegar

2 tablespoons chopped Peppadew peppers

¼ teaspoon dried thyme
Ground black pepper

1 cup frozen green beans

½ cup frozen shelled edamame

1 can (14.5 ounces) cut wax beans, rinsed and drained

½ cup canned dark red kidney beans, rinsed and drained

½ cup canned black beans, rinsed and drained

1. Combine the oil, vinegar, papper, and thyme in a large bowl. Season with black pepper to taste.

2. Rinse the green beans and edamame under hot water until thawed. Add to the dressing along with the wax beans, kidney beans, and black beans. Toss to coat.

Nutrition per serving
- 254 calories
- 8 g protein
- 21 g carbohydrates
- 16 g fat
- 1 g saturated fat
- 0 mg cholesterol
- 320 mg sodium
- 7 g fiber

MAKE IT A FLAT BELLY DIET MEAL: Serve with 1 ounce baked multigrain tortilla chips (118).
Total meal: 372 calories

Roasted Beet Salad

4 SERVINGS (1¼ CUPS EACH) / 301 CALORIES / MUFA: WALNUTS

The addition of lightly cooked pears to this classic salad combination will likely make this already sweet vegetable more palatable to even the pickiest of eaters.

1 HOUR 35 MIN

4 **medium beets (about 1½ pounds), ends trimmed**
½ **cup balsamic vinegar**
2 **tablespoons sugar**
½ **cup walnuts, coarsely chopped**
2 **teaspoons olive oil**
2 **pears, peeled, cored, and cut into 8 wedges each**
½ **teaspoon salt**
¼ **teaspoon ground black pepper**
2 **cups arugula (optional)**
4 **tablespoons (1 ounce) crumbled blue cheese**

Nutrition per serving
○ 301 calories
○ 7 g protein
○ 42 g carbohydrates
○ 13 g fat
○ 2.5 g saturated fat
○ 5 mg cholesterol
○ 550 mg sodium
○ 8 g fiber

1. Preheat the oven to 425°F.

2. Wrap the beets in foil and set on a baking sheet. Bake for 1 hour, or until a knife easily pierces the beets. Remove from the oven and let cool for 30 minutes. Peel the beets, cut each into 8 wedges (wear disposable rubber gloves if you're concerned about the beets staining on your hands), and transfer to a bowl.

3. Meanwhile, combine the vinegar and sugar in a small saucepan. Bring the mixture to a boil over medium-high heat and cook for 5 to 6 minutes, or until reduced by about half and thick enough to coat the back of a spoon. Set aside.

4. Place the walnuts in a large nonstick skillet and cook over medium-high heat, shaking the pan often, for 2 to 3 minutes, or until lightly toasted. Transfer to the bowl with the beets.

5. Add the oil to the skillet and return to medium-high heat. Add the pears and cook for 2 minutes per side, or until lightly browned. Remove from the heat.

6. Add the reserved vinegar mixture, the salt, and pepper to the beets, tossing to coat well. Place ½ cup arugula (if using) on each of 4 plates and top with the beet mixture and pears. Sprinkle each serving with 1 tablespoon blue cheese.

MAKE IT A FLAT BELLY DIET MEAL: Serve with 2 ounces broiled flank steak (105).
Total meal: 406 calories

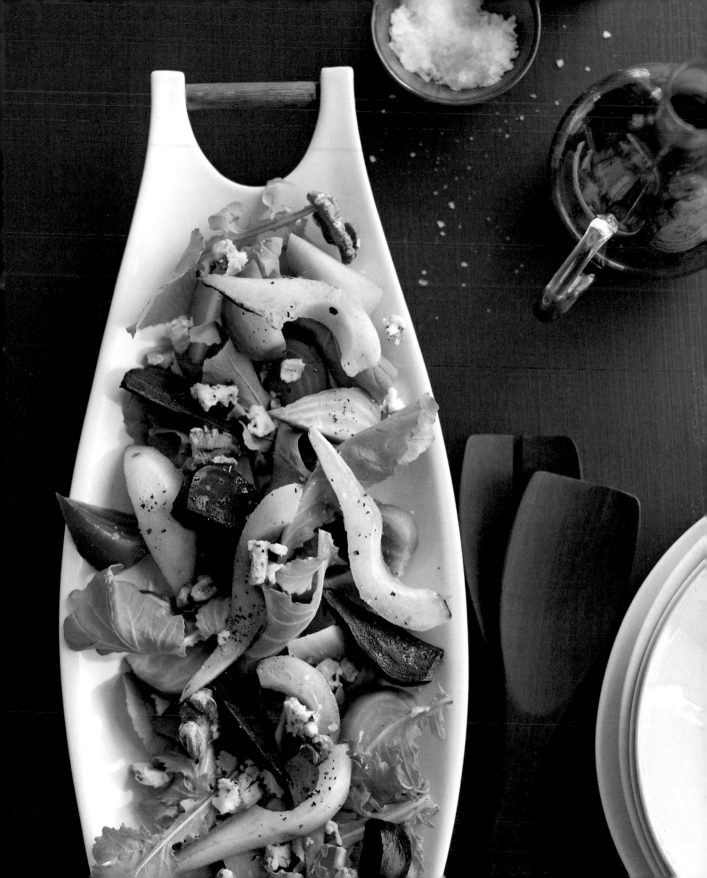

Fall Fruit Salad

4 SERVINGS / 182 CALORIES / MUFA: WALNUT OIL

Walnut oil's delicate bouquet is best enjoyed when it's not heated. It shines in this out-of-the-ordinary salad, which tastes divine with roast chicken.

5 MINUTES

¼ cup walnut oil

2 tablespoons orange juice

1 Gala apple, unpeeled

1 green Bartlett pear, unpeeled

2 tablespoons golden or regular raisins

Grated orange zest (optional)

Nutrition per serving

○ 182 calories

○ 0 g protein

○ 16 g carbohydrates

○ 14 g fat

○ 2 g saturated fat

○ 0 mg cholesterol

○ 0 mg sodium

○ 2 g fiber

1. Whisk the oil and juice in a small bowl.

2. Quarter and core the apple and pear. Cut into slices and arrange on 4 salad plates or a serving platter. Drizzle with the dressing. Scatter the raisins on top. Sprinkle with orange zest, if desired.

MAKE IT A FLAT BELLY DIET MEAL: Serve with 3 ounces precooked chicken breast (122) and 1 ounce whole grain French bread (90). **Total meal: 394 calories** To serve as part of another FBD meal, reduce the walnut oil to 2 tablespoons (122).

Green Bean and Pumpkin Seed Salad

4 SERVINGS (1 CUP EACH) / 140 CALORIES / MUFA: PUMPKIN SEEDS

The contrast between the tender beans and crunchy pumpkin seeds makes this salad especially appealing. Serve with grilled pork tenderloin.

10 MINUTES

2 teaspoons canola oil

½ teaspoon ground cumin

⅛ teaspoon salt

¾ pound green beans, broken into 2" lengths (about 3 cups)

½ cup shelled unsalted dry-roasted pumpkin seeds

½ small red onion, halved and thinly sliced

1 tablespoon fresh lime juice

Nutrition per serving

○ 140 calories
○ 5 g protein
○ 9 g carbohydrates
○ 10 g fat
○ 1.5 g saturated fat
○ 0 mg cholesterol
○ 75 mg sodium
○ 3 g fiber

1. Combine ¼ cup water, the oil, cumin, and salt in a large nonstick skillet. Cover and bring to a boil over high heat. Reduce the heat to medium. Add the beans and stir. Cook, tossing occasionally, for 5 minutes, or until the beans are tender and all the water is gone. Add the pumpkin seeds and cook, tossing, for about 2 minutes, or until the seeds are hot.

2. Transfer the mixture to a serving platter. Add the onion and lime juice and toss to combine.

MAKE IT A TEAM EFFORT Have the kids trim the beans; they can also squeeze the lime juice into a small bowl and help toss the salad just before serving.

MAKE IT A FLAT BELLY DIET MEAL: Serve with 3 ounces grilled or broiled pork tenderloin (99) and ¾ cup cooked brown rice (163). **Total meal: 402 calories**

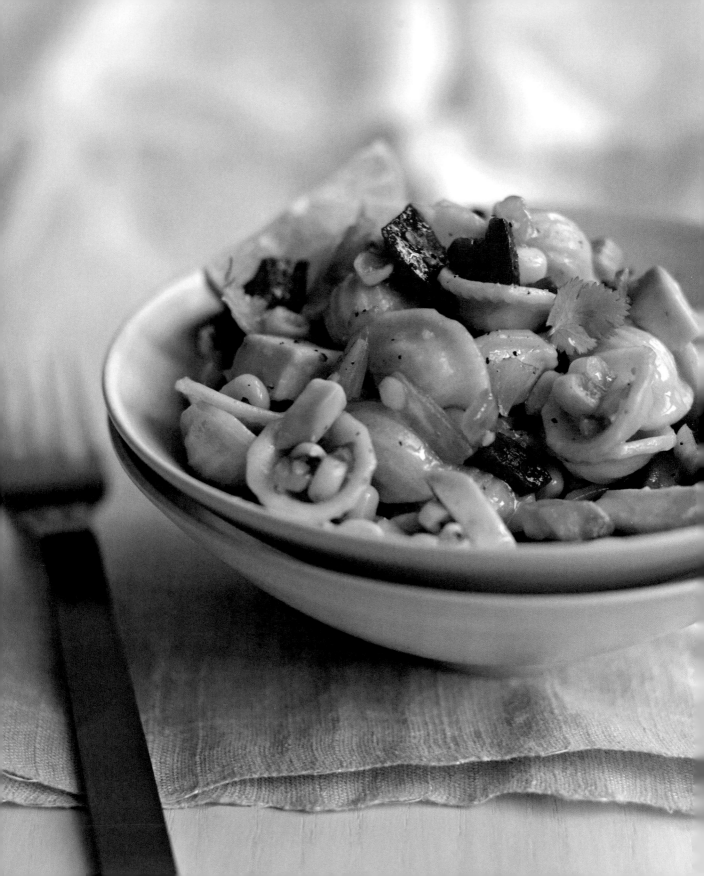

Roasted Pepper–Corn Pasta Salad

4 SERVINGS (1¼ CUPS EACH) / 344 CALORIES / MUFA: AVOCADO

The vegetables in this salad provide plenty of fiber, so here's one recipe where we don't call for multigrain pasta. Orecchiette are shaped roughly like small ears (*orecchiette* literally means "little ears" in Italian).

30 MINUTES

8 ounces orrechiette pasta
1 tablespoon olive oil
1 yellow onion, chopped
2 garlic cloves, minced
¾ cup corn kernels
1 roasted pepper, chopped (about ½ cup)
1 Hass avocado, chopped
3 tablespoons chopped fresh cilantro
2 tablespoons fresh lime juice
½ teaspoon salt
¼ teaspoon ground black pepper

Nutrition per serving
○ 344 calories
○ 10 g protein
○ 56 g carbohydrates
○ 10 g fat
○ 1.5 g saturated fat
○ 0 mg cholesterol
○ 380 mg sodium
○ 6 g fiber

1. Bring a large pot of water to a boil. Add the pasta and cook according to package directions. Drain.

2. Meanwhile, heat the oil in a large nonstick skillet over medium-high heat. Add the onion and garlic, and cook for 2 minutes. Stir in the corn and cook for 2 to 3 minutes, or until the onion begins to brown. Add the roasted pepper and cook for 1 minute. Transfer to a large bowl.

3. Add the pasta, avocado, cilantro, lime juice, salt, and black pepper to the bowl and toss gently but thoroughly.

MAKE IT A FLAT BELLY DIET MEAL: Serve with 6 dried apricot halves (51). Total meal: 395 calories

Pasta Salad with Caramelized Onions and Zucchini

4 SERVINGS (SCANT CUP EACH) / 258 CALORIES / MUFA: OLIVE OIL

The natural sweetness of caramelized onion combined with a touch of raisins should make this pasta salad a family favorite.

15 MINUTES

- 4 ounces multigrain penne pasta
- 4 tablespoons olive oil
- ½ red onion, halved and sliced
- ¼ teaspoon salt
- 1 small zucchini (4 ounces), cut into matchsticks
- 1 tablespoon raisins, finely chopped
- ¼ teaspoon dried oregano
- 2 tablespoons grated Parmesan cheese
- 2 teaspoons balsamic vinegar
- ⅛ teaspoon ground black pepper

Nutrition per serving

- 258 calories
- 5 g protein
- 26 g carbohydrates
- 15 g fat
- 2.5 g saturated fat
- 0 mg cholesterol
- 190 mg sodium
- 3 g fiber

1. Bring a large pot of water to a boil. Add the pasta and cook according to package directions. Drain, rinse under cold water, and drain again.

2. Meanwhile, heat 2 tablespoons of the oil in a large skillet over medium-high heat. Add the onion and salt and cook, stirring occasionally, for 6 minutes, or until very soft. Stir in the zucchini, raisins, and oregano. Cook, stirring occasionally, for 4 minutes, or until the zucchini is softened and the onion is caramelized. Remove from the heat.

3. Add the cheese, vinegar, pepper, pasta, and remaining 2 tablespoons oil to the skillet, and toss to combine. Serve warm or at room temperature.

MAKE IT A TEAM EFFORT Invite the kids to pick the pasta shape. It's fun and empowering for them to have a say in recipe choices. Elbows, penne, fusilli, rotini, or farfalle (bow tie) shapes all work well for this dish.

MAKE IT A FLAT BELLY DIET MEAL: Serve with 3 ounces cooked pork tenderloin (99) and 1 cup steamed spinach (41). Total meal: 398 calories

Broccoli Pasta Salad

4 SERVINGS (1½ CUPS EACH) / 248 CALORIES / MUFA: OLIVES

Rinsing pasta removes much of the starch that helps sauce cling to the noodles, so it's best avoided unless you're making a pasta salad like this one. Rinsing also stops the cooking process in its tracks so the vegetables retain their bright color.

30 MINUTES

4 ounces multigrain rotini pasta

2 cups broccoli florets

1 carrot, sliced

2 tablespoons olive oil

2 tablespoons cider vinegar

½ teaspoon dried oregano

½ teaspoon salt

¼ teaspoon ground black pepper

40 pitted black olives

1 red bell pepper, chopped

¼ red onion, sliced

Nutrition per serving

○ 248 calories
○ 7 g protein
○ 30 g carbohydrates
○ 12 g fat
○ 1.5 g saturated fat
○ 0 mg cholesterol
○ 710 mg sodium*
○ 6 g fiber

1. Bring a large pot of water to a boil. Add the pasta and cook according to package directions. Add the broccoli and carrot for the last 1 minute of cooking. Drain well. Run under cold water and drain again.

2. Meanwhile, whisk together the oil, vinegar, oregano, salt, and black pepper in a large bowl. Add the olives, bell pepper, and onion.

3. Add the drained pasta and vegetables to the bowl and toss to combine.

Limit saturated fat to no more than 10 percent of total calories—about 17 grams per day for most women or 21 grams for most men—and sodium intake to no more than 2,300 milligrams.

MAKE IT A FLAT BELLY DIET MEAL: Serve with 3 ounces water-packed chunk light tuna (105) and ½ cup sliced strawberries (27). **Total meal: 380 calories**

Sicilian Tuna Salad

4 SERVINGS (½ CUP EACH) / 160 CALORIES / MUFA: OLIVES

This seafood side dish also make a wonderful light lunch with some whole grain crackers.

5 MINUTES

2 cans (6 ounces each) low-sodium or no-salt-added water-packed solid white tuna, drained

40 pitted large green olives

1 celery rib, sliced

2 teaspoons red wine vinegar
Pinch of crushed red-pepper flakes

4 large red-leaf lettuce leaves

8 cherry tomatoes, halved or quartered

Toss together the tuna, olives, celery, vinegar, and red-pepper flakes in a bowl. Serve on a lettuce leaf, garnished with cherry tomatoes.

MAKE IT AHEAD Store the salad (without the lettuce or tomatoes) in an airtight container in the refrigerator for up to 3 days.

Nutrition per serving

- 160 calories
- 17 g protein
- 2 g carbohydrate
- 10 g fat
- 0.5 g saturated fat
- 30 mg cholesterol
- 470 mg sodium
- 1 g fiber

MAKE IT A FLAT BELLY DIET MEAL: Serve with 8 whole grain crackers (70) and 6 ounces fat-free vanilla yogurt (130) mixed with ½ cup blueberries (42). **Total meal: 402 calories**

Thai Peanut Slaw

4 SERVINGS (2 CUPS EACH) / 194 CALORIES / MUFA: PEANUTS

Just 1 serving of this slaw packs over 95 milligrams of vitamin C—even more than you'd get in a whole orange!

40 MINUTES

Combine the cabbage, carrot, pepper, peanuts, cilantro, lime juice, sugar, and fish sauce in a large bowl. Toss well and let stand for 30 minutes, stirring occasionally.

6 cups shredded green cabbage
1 carrot, grated
1 large red bell pepper, thinly sliced
½ cup unsalted dry-roasted peanuts
3 tablespoons chopped fresh cilantro
3 tablespoons fresh lime juice
3 tablespoons sugar
1 tablespoon fish sauce

MAKE IT FASTER If you have a food processor with a thin slicing blade, by all means use it for a dish like this. You'll easily cut your prep time in half.

Nutrition per serving
○ 194 calories
○ 7 g protein
○ 25 g carbohydrates
○ 9 g fat
○ 1.5 g saturated fat
○ 0 mg cholesterol
○ 380 mg sodium
○ 5 g fiber

MAKE IT A FLAT BELLY MEAL: Serve with 3 ounces grilled pork tenderloin (99) and ¾ cup sliced mango (80). Total meal: 373 calories

Spinach-Avocado Caesar Salad

4 SERVINGS (1 CUP EACH) / 177 CALORIES / MUFA: AVOCADO

Caesar salad seems to go with everything, and this version, which uses folate-rich spinach instead of the typical romaine is no exception.

15 MINUTES

- 2 slices crusty whole wheat bread (about 2 ounces)
- 1 tablespoon olive oil
- ¼ teaspoon Italian seasoning
- 1 hard-cooked egg
- 1 Hass avocado, coarsely chopped
- 2 tablespoons warm water
- 2 tablespoons grated Romano cheese
- 2 teaspoons red wine vinegar
- 1 teaspoon minced garlic
- ¼ teaspoon Dijon mustard
- ⅛ teaspoon salt
- ⅛ teaspoon ground black pepper
- 6 cups baby spinach

1. Toast the bread. Brush with the oil to coat. Sprinkle with the Italian seasoning. Cut into ½" cubes. Set aside.

2. Peel and halve the egg and place the yolk in a large bowl. Chop the white and set aside.

3. Add half the avocado to the yolk and smash against the side of the bowl with a fork until smooth. Stir in the water, cheese, vinegar, garlic, mustard, salt, and pepper to form a dressing. Add the spinach, remaining avocado, and reserved egg white and toss to coat. Serve individual salads with the croutons scattered on top.

Nutrition per serving
- 177 calories
- 5 g protein
- 15 g carbohydrates
- 12 g fat
- 2 g saturated fat
- 55 mg cholesterol
- 250 mg sodium
- 5 g fiber

MAKE IT A FLAT BELLY MEAL: Serve with 3 ounces grilled chicken breast (122) and 6 ounces fat-free plain Greek yogurt (90). **Total meal: 389 calories**

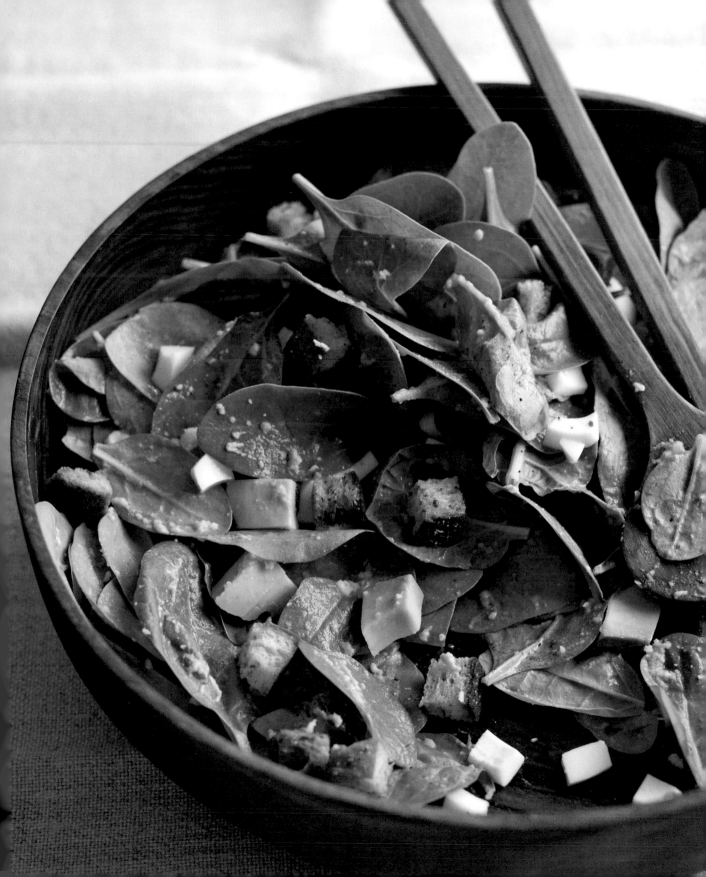

Creamy Sesame Greens

4 SERVINGS (½ CUP EACH) / 252 CALORIES / MUFA: TAHINI

Old-school creamed spinach is drenched in cream and butter. This MUFA-improved version uses kale instead of spinach and heart-healthy sesame paste to create a rich sauce to diminish the greens' bitter edge that so many kids find unpalatable.

15 MINUTES

½ pound kale or collard leaves, finely chopped

1 onion, chopped

1 teaspoon canola oil

½ cup tahini

2 tablespoons honey

¼ teaspoon salt

⅛ teaspoon ground red pepper

Nutrition per serving

○ 252 calories

○ 7 g protein

○ 22 g carbohydrates

○ 17 g fat

○ 2.5 g saturated fat

○ 0 mg cholesterol

○ 180 mg sodium

○ 3 g fiber

1. Bring a large covered pot of water to a boil over high heat. Add the greens. Stir. Cover the pot and boil for 5 minutes, or until wilted. Reserve ½ cup of the cooking water before draining the greens.

2. Meanwhile, combine the onion and oil in a large nonstick skillet. Cook over medium-low heat, stirring, for 5 minutes, or until the onion softens.

3. Combine the tahini, honey, salt, red pepper, and the reserved cooking water in a bowl. Whisk until smooth. Add the greens to the skillet and stir in the tahini mixture. Simmer over low heat for about 1 minute, or until the sauce is warm.

MAKE IT **FASTER**   Cooked kale and other greens can be refrigerated for several days, making this dish even faster to put together. Drain and rinse the cooked greens under cold running water. Drain again and pat dry. Store in an airtight plastic bag. For the sesame sauce, you can either save some of the greens, cooking water or use plain water.

MAKE IT A FLAT BELLY DIET MEAL: Serve with 3 ounces baked grouper (100) and ½ cup cooked whole wheat couscous (70). **Total meal: 422 calories**

Broccoli Rabe with Toasted Garlic

4 SERVINGS / 200 CALORIES / MUFA: OLIVE OIL

Broccoli rabe looks similar to small broccoli florets that are on long, thin stems. Its bitter but zesty flavor is rendered noticeably milder after cooking for a few minutes in boiling water.

10 MINUTES

2 **bunches broccoli rabe (about 2 pounds), tough stem ends removed**
¼ **cup extra-virgin olive oil**
6 **garlic cloves, thinly sliced**
¼ **teaspoon crushed red-pepper flakes**
½ **teaspoon salt**

Nutrition per serving
○ 200 calories
○ 8 g protein
○ 12 g carbohydrates
○ 14 g fat
○ 2 g saturated fat
○ 0 mg cholesterol
○ 360 mg sodium
○ 6 g fiber

1. Bring a large pot of lightly salted water to a boil. Add the broccoli rabe, return to a boil, and cook for 2 minutes. Drain and set aside.

2. Heat the oil in a large nonstick skillet over medium-high heat. Add the garlic and red-pepper flakes and cook for 1½ to 2 minutes, or until the garlic starts to brown. Add the reserved broccoli rabe and the salt. Cook, tossing, for 1 minute, or until hot.

MAKE IT A FLAT BELLY DIET MEAL: Serve with ½ cup unsweetened applesauce (52) and Chicken Cutlets Topped with Turkey Bacon and Avocado (page 150), but omit the avocado (152). **Total meal:** 404 calories

Haricots Verts

4 SERVINGS / 160 CALORIES / MUFA: ALMONDS

Haricots verts—that's French for "green beans"—are actually longer and thinner than most American varieties. They also have a more complex flavor, but if you can't find them, just look for the thinnest young green beans available.

20 MINUTES

1 pound haricots verts
½ cup sliced almonds
1 tablespoon unsalted butter
1 tablespoon extra-virgin olive oil
2 garlic cloves, minced
1 tablespoon fresh lemon juice
½ teaspoon salt
¼ teaspoon ground black pepper
1 teaspoon grated lemon zest

1. Bring a large pot of lightly salted water to a boil. Add the beans, return to a boil, and cook for 2 minutes. Drain.

2. Place the almonds in a large nonstick skillet and cook over medium-high heat, shaking the pan often, for 2 to 3 minutes, or until lightly toasted. Transfer to a plate.

3. Add the butter to the skillet and cook over medium-high heat for about 1 minute, or until it begins to brown slightly. Add the oil and garlic and cook for 15 seconds, or until fragrant. Add the lemon juice and cook for 10 seconds. Add the beans, salt, and pepper and cook, tossing, for 1 minute to heat through. Stir in the almonds and lemon zest.

Nutrition per serving
○ 160 calories
○ 5 g protein
○ 12 g carbohydrates
○ 12 g fat
○ 2.5 g saturated fat
○ 10 mg cholesterol
○ 300 mg sodium
○ 5 g fiber

MAKE IT A FLAT BELLY DIET MEAL: Serve with Tandoori Chicken Thighs (page 122), but omit the walnuts (263). Total meal: 423 calories. To serve as part of another FBD meal, omit the almonds (94).

Roasted Carrots and Hazelnuts

4 SERVINGS / 182 CALORIES / MUFA: HAZELNUTS

This autumnal dish is satisfying—and special enough with the addition of hazelnuts to grace the holiday table.

45 MINUTES

1 pound baby carrots
1 teaspoon canola oil
½ cup skinned hazelnuts
2 teaspoons honey
2 teaspoons balsamic vinegar
¼ teaspoon salt
1 tablespoon finely chopped parsley

Nutrition per serving
○ 182 calories
○ 4 g protein
○ 18 g carbohydrates
○ 11g fat
○ 1 g saturated fat
○ 0 mg cholesterol
○ 210 mg sodium
○ 4 g fiber

1. Preheat the oven to 375°F. Coat a rimmed baking sheet with cooking spray. Scatter the carrots on the baking sheet, drizzle with the oil, and toss to coat.

2. Roast the carrots for 20 minutes. Scatter the hazelnuts over the carrots and toss to combine. Bake for 20 minutes, or until the nuts are golden and the carrots are tender.

3. Whisk the honey, vinegar, and salt in a serving bowl. Add the carrots, hazelnuts, and parsley and toss to combine.

MAKE IT AHEAD This dish can be roasted and cooled, then refrigerated in an airtight container. Reheat on medium power in a microwaveable dish, covered with wax paper, for 3 to 4 minutes.

MAKE IT A FLAT BELLY DIET MEAL: Serve with ½ cup grapes (52) and Rosemary Pork and Rice Bake (page 192), but omit the pine nuts (146). **Total meal: 380 calories.** To serve as part of another FBD meal, omit the hazelnuts (72).

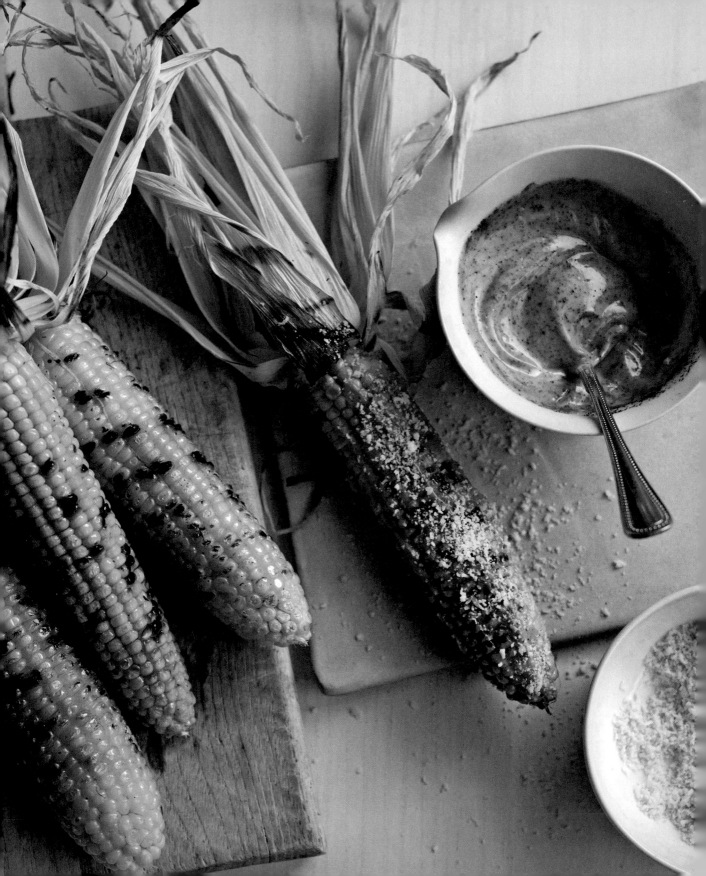

Mexican Grilled Corn on the Cob

4 SERVINGS / 199 CALORIES / MUFA: CANOLA OIL MAYONNAISE

This is such an easy dish to put together and throw on the grill. In fact, it might become one of your favorite ways to enjoy this summertime treat.

40 MINUTES

- 4 **ears corn**
- ¼ **cup canola oil mayonnaise**
- 1 **teaspoon fresh lime juice**
- 1 **teaspoon chili powder**
- 4 **teaspoons grated Parmesan cheese**

Nutrition per serving
- ○ 199 calories
- ○ 5 g protein
- ○ 18 g carbohydrates
- ○ 14 g fat
- ○ 1 g saturated fat
- ○ 5 mg cholesterol
- ○ 115 mg sodium
- ○ 2 g fiber

1. Preheat the grill to medium-high. Remove the outermost husks and silks, but leave the tender inner husks on the corn. Soak the ears in cold water for 15 minutes.

2. Combine the mayonnaise, lime juice, and chili powder in a small bowl. Set aside.

3. Grill the ears of corn over direct heat for 10 minutes, turning to prevent charring. Move to indirect heat and grill for 10 minutes longer, or until a kernel pops easily when pressed. If the corn appears dry, it's overcooked.

4. Peel back the husks and spread 1 tablespoon of the reserved mayonnaise mixture over each cob. Dust each with 1 teaspoon of cheese and serve hot.

MAKE IT FASTER If you're pressed for time, skip the soaking step and the grilling. Remove the outermost husks, leaving the tender inner husks and the silk in place. Microwave the corn on high (2 ears at a time) for 3 to 5 minutes, or just until the husk layer is hot. Let sit for 5 minutes, then remove the silk and inner husks. Serve spread with the mayonnaise mixture and sprinkled with the cheese.

MAKE IT A FLAT BELLY DIET MEAL: Serve with 3 ounces grilled chicken breast (122) and ½ mango, grilled (67). Total meal: 388 calories

Salt and Pepper Oven Fries

4 SERVINGS / 262 CALORIES / MUFA: CANOLA OIL

The tasters in our test kitchen couldn't believe how tossing the baked fries with a final coating of canola oil made them taste like they'd actually been fried!

40 MINUTES

1 pound russet (baking) potatoes, cut into 3½" x ½" sticks
¼ cup canola oil
3 garlic cloves, minced
¼ teaspoon salt
¼ teaspoon ground black pepper
1 tablespoon chopped parsley

Nutrition per serving
○ 262 calories
○ 4 g protein
○ 32 g carbohydrates
○ 14 g fat
○ 1 g saturated fat
○ 0 mg cholesterol
○ 150 mg sodium
○ 2 g fiber

1. Preheat the oven to 450°F. Coat a large baking sheet with cooking spray.

2. Combine the potatoes and 2 tablespoons of the oil in a large bowl, tossing to coat well. Arrange the potatoes in a single layer on the baking sheet. Bake for 30 minutes, turning the potatoes halfway through the cooking time, until golden brown and crisp. Remove from the oven and transfer to a large bowl.

3. Meanwhile, heat the remaining 2 tablespoons oil in a small skillet over medium heat. Add the garlic and cook until browned, about 4 minutes. Pour the oil and garlic over the potatoes. Add the salt, pepper, and parsley and toss well. Serve hot.

MAKE IT A FLAT BELLY DIET MEAL: Serve with 3 ounces baked cod (89) and 1 cup steamed broccoli (44). Total meal: 395 calories

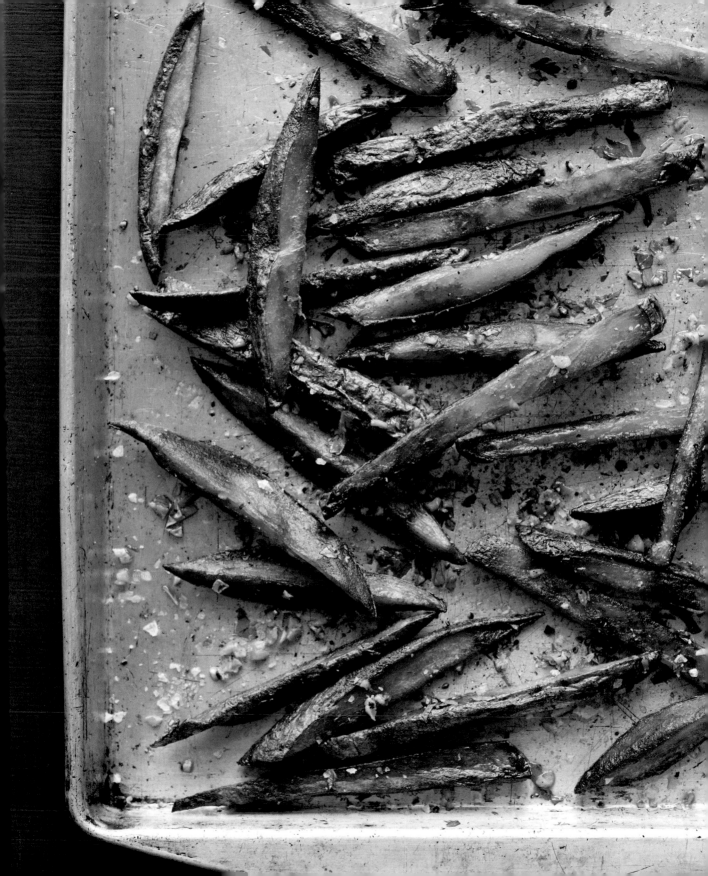

Garlic Mashed Potatoes

4 SERVINGS (¾ CUP EACH) / 257 CALORIES / MUFA: OLIVE OIL

If you want to retain even more fiber and nutrients in your dish, scrub your potatoes well but keep the skin on. Russet potatoes, also known as Idaho potatoes, are especially fluffy when cooked.

30 MINUTES

1½ pounds russet (baking) potatoes, cut into 1" to 2" pieces

¼ cup olive oil

2 teaspoons minced garlic

¾ teaspoon salt

Nutrition per serving

○ 257 calories
○ 3 g protein
○ 31 g carbohydrates
○ 14 g fat
○ 2 g saturated fat
○ 0 mg cholesterol
○ 440 mg sodium
○ 2 g fiber

1. Place the potatoes in a large pot and cover with 1" of water. Bring to a boil and cook for 20 minutes, or until the potatoes are easily pierced with a fork. Reserve ½ cup of the cooking liquid before draining the potatoes.

2. Add the oil and garlic to the potato cooking pot and cook over low heat, stirring, for 30 seconds, or until the garlic is fragrant. Remove from heat, return the potatoes to the pot, sprinkle with the salt, and mash until smooth. Add some or all of the reserved cooking liquid to achieve the desired consistency.

MAKE IT A FLAT BELLY DIET MEAL: Serve with a 4-ounce cooked center-cut pork chop (160). Total meal: 417 calories. To serve as part of another FBD meal, omit the oil from this recipe and add the garlic just before mashing the potatoes with 6 ounces fat-free plain Greek yogurt (160).

Golden Rice Pilaf

4 SERVINGS (¾ CUP EACH) / 275 CALORIES / MUFA: PISTACHIOS

Basmati rice, a long-grain rice with a distinct, nutty fragrance, is used in many Indian dishes. If you prefer to use brown basmati rice, increase the cooking time to 45 minutes and wait to add the peas until you let it stand, covered, for 10 minutes.

30 MINUTES

¾ cup basmati rice

½ cup frozen green peas

½ teaspoon cumin seeds

⅛ teaspoon saffron threads, lightly crushed

½ teaspoon salt

½ cup shelled unsalted roasted pistachios

1 tablespoon olive oil

2 large shallots, thinly sliced

Nutrition per serving
○ 275 calories
○ 8 g protein
○ 38 g carbohydrates
○ 11 g fat
○ 1.5 g saturated fat
○ 0 mg cholesterol
○ 310 mg sodium
○ 3 g fiber

1. Combine the rice, peas, cumin seeds, saffron, salt, and 1½ cups water in a medium saucepan. Bring to a boil over medium-high heat, stir once, reduce to a simmer, cover, and cook for 15 minutes, or until the liquid has been absorbed. Remove from the heat and let stand for 5 minutes. Stir in the pistachios.

2. Meanwhile, heat the oil in a small nonstick skillet over medium-high heat. Add the shallots and cook, stirring occasionally, for 5 to 6 minutes, or until golden.

3. Serve the rice topped with the shallots.

MAKE IT A FLAT BELLY DIET MEAL: Serve with 3 ounces cooked salmon fillet (156). Total meal: 431 calories. To serve as part of another FBD meal, omit the pistachios (187).

QUICK-FIX PANTRY RESCUES

"Fried" Corn
Warm 1 tablespoon **olive oil** (120) in a skillet over medium heat. Add ½ cup frozen corn kernels (72), 2 tablespoons chopped roasted pepper (8), and a dash of ground black pepper (0). Cook until warmed through and serve with 1 cup steamed cooked broccoli (44) and 3 ounces grilled chicken (122) topped with 1 tablespoon barbecue sauce (20). **Total Calories = 386**

Italian Orzo Salad
Toss ¾ cup cooked whole wheat orzo (195) with 2 tablespoons toasted **pine nuts** (113), 1 chopped plum tomato (11), 1 tablespoon chopped fresh parsley (1), 1 teaspoon olive oil (40), ½ teaspoon minced garlic (8), and ⅛ teaspoon salt (0). Sprinkle 1 tablespoon Parmesan cheese (22) over the top. **Total Calories = 390**

Bread Salad
Tear one 6″ whole wheat pita (120) into 1″ pieces and toss with 1 chopped tomato (22), 2 tablespoons crumbled feta cheese (50), 2 chopped scallions (10), 1 tablespoon olive oil (119), 1 tablespoon red wine vinegar (0), ¼ teaspoon dried oregano (1), and ground black pepper (0) to taste. Let sit for 5 to 10 minutes to allow the flavors to combine. Serve with 1 cup grapes (104). **Total Calories = 426**

Green Beans with Tapenade
Cook 1 cup frozen green beans (44) over medium heat and toss with 2 tablespoons **black olive tapenade** (88) and 1 cup grape tomatoes, halved (30). Serve with ½ cup cooked brown rice (109), 4 ounces broiled tilapia (145), and a wedge of lemon (1). **Total Calories = 417**

South-of-the-Border Baked Potato
Scrub a medium russet (baking) potato (168), prick the skin with a fork, and microwave on high for 5 to 8 minutes, or until cooked through. Split open and serve topped with ¼ cup shredded reduced-fat Cheddar cheese (80), 2 tablespoons salsa (10), ¼ cup mashed **Hass avocado** (96), and a dash of hot sauce (0), if desired. Serve with ½ cup sliced mango (54). **Total Calories = 408**

Menu for a Family-Style Buffet

Spinach-Avocado Caesar Salad (page 216)

Crunchy Crust Mac and Cheese (page 179)

Chicken Thighs with Green Beans (page 160)

Roasted Carrots and Hazelnuts (page 221)

Dark Chocolate Zucchini Bread (page 269)

NOTE: Double all the recipes except for the zucchini bread.

SERVES 8

⊙ **The night before:** Make Dark Chocolate Zucchini Bread. Grate the cheese for the macaroni. Make the croutons for the salad.

⊙ **About 90 minutes before serving:** Make Crunchy Crust Mac and Cheese and keep covered until ready to serve.

⊙ **About 45 minutes before serving:** Make Roasted Carrots and Hazelnuts. Keep covered until ready to serve.

⊙ **About 30 minutes before serving:** Make Chicken Thighs with Green Beans. Wash and rinse the spinach for the salad.

⊙ **About 10 minutes before serving:** Make Spinach-Avocado Caesar Salad.

MAKE IT A FLAT BELLY DIET MEAL: Enjoy *either* the mac and cheese (328) with the roasted carrots (omit the hazelnuts) (72) or the chicken thighs (269) with a half serving of the Caesar salad (89). **Total meal = 400 calories (macaroni and carrots) or 358 calories (chicken and salad).** Later in the day, enjoy a slice of zucchini bread (354) and $\frac{1}{2}$ cup grapes (52) as your FBD snack. **Total meal = 406 calories**

10

Snacks
FOR EVERYONE

- Mango-Avocado Salsa
- Pan-Roasted Sunflower Seeds with Dill
- Asian Snack Mix
- Tomato and Roasted Pepper Bruschetta
- Mashed Avocado Cakes
- Broccoli Florets with Thai Cashew Dip
- Easy Barbecue Pita Pizzas

- English Muffin Pizzas
- Pistachio Cheese Spread
- Apples with Honey-Yogurt Dip and Candied Walnuts
- Macadamia Coconut Clusters
- Marshmallow Cereal Bars
- Easy Peanut Brittle
- Sugar-Glazed Almond Trail Mix
- Chocolate-Covered Pretzels

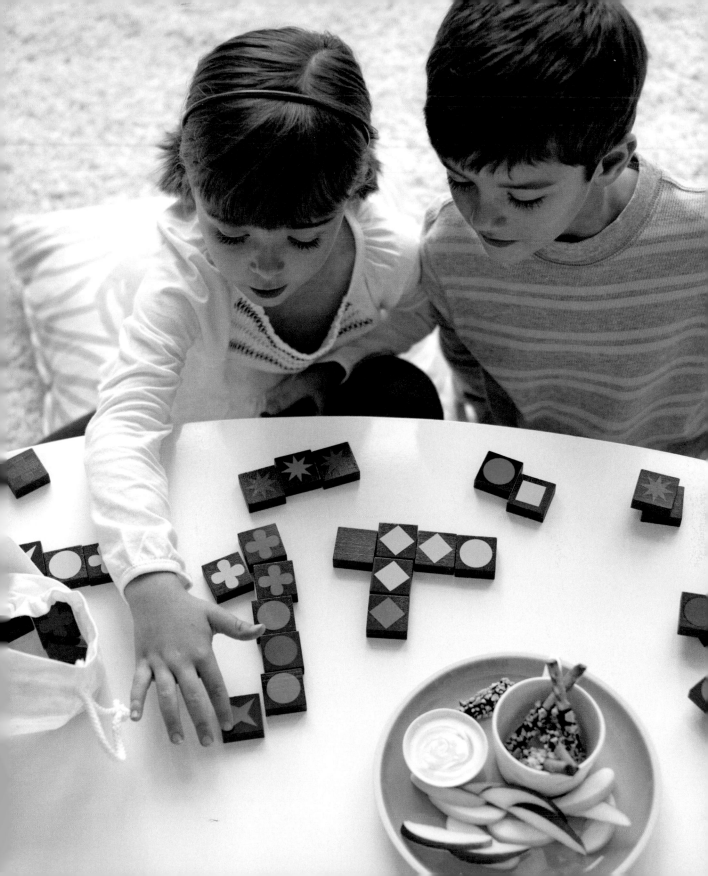

Mango-Avocado Salsa

4 SERVINGS (¾ CUP SALSA EACH) / 265 CALORIES / MUFA: AVOCADO

Mango and pineapple lends a sunny look—as well as lots of flavor—to this delicious salsa. If your family prefers a little spice, a few splashes of hot sauce will do the trick.

15 MINUTES

1 mango
1 Hass avocado
⅓ fresh pineapple
¼ red onion
2 tablespoons chopped fresh cilantro
1 tablespoon fresh lime juice
¼ teaspoon salt
4 ounces baked tortilla chips

Nutrition per serving
○ 265 calories
○ 10 g protein
○ 44 g carbohydrates
○ 10 g fat
○ 1.5 g saturated fat
○ 0 mg cholesterol
○ 430 mg sodium
○ 6 g fiber

1. Chop the mango into ¼″ to ½″ pieces. Chop the avocado into ½″ cubes. Chop the pineapple into ¼″ to ½″ pieces. Finely chop the onion.

2. Combine the mango, avocado, pineapple, onion, cilantro, lime juice, and salt in a bowl. Serve with the tortilla chips.

MAKE IT A FLAT BELLY DIET MEAL: Serve with 1 cup baby carrots (53) and 1 cup grapes (104).
Total meal: 422 calories

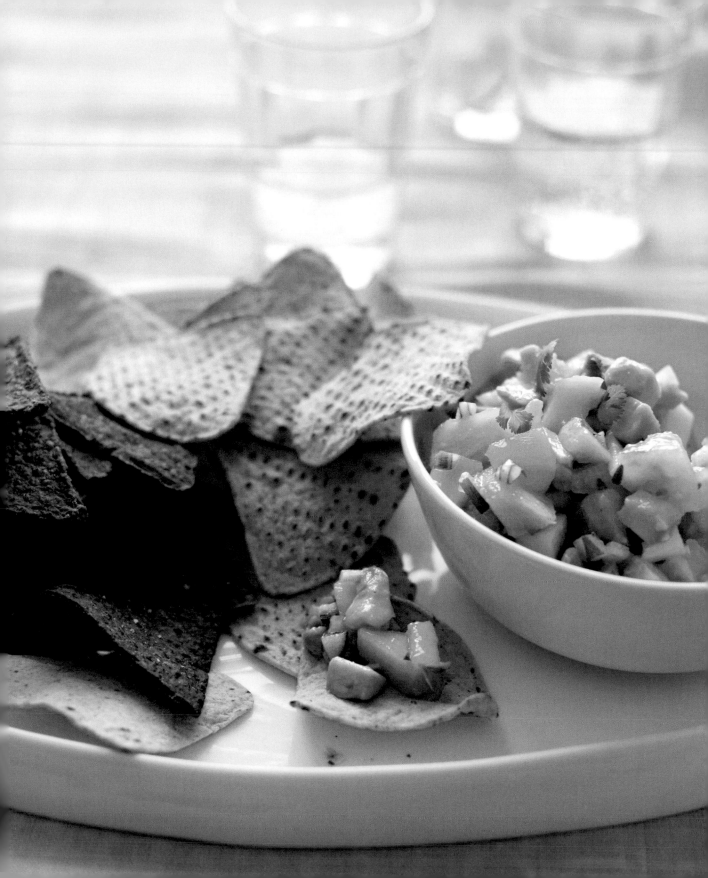

Pan-Roasted Sunflower Seeds with Dill

4 SERVINGS (2 TABLESPOONS EACH) / 100 CALORIES / MUFA: SUNFLOWER SEEDS

MUFA-rich ingredients should be as fresh as possible. Purchase seeds and nuts from a grocery or health food store that does a brisk business. And seek out stores that sell these items in bulk, which is less expensive than packaged.

5 MINUTES

½ teaspoon canola oil

½ cup shelled unsalted sunflower seeds

⅛ teaspoon garlic powder

¼ teaspoon dillweed

Pinch of salt

Nutrition per serving

○ 100 calories

○ 3 g protein

○ 4 g carbohydrates

○ 9 g fat

○ 1 g saturated fat

○ 0 mg cholesterol

○ 75 mg sodium

○ 2 g fiber

Heat the oil in a medium nonstick skillet over medium-high heat. Add the seeds and garlic powder. Cook, tossing occasionally, for 3 to 4 minutes, or until browned and fragrant. Stir in the dill and salt. Transfer to a plate to cool.

MAKE IT AHEAD For convenient grab-and-go snacks, divide the mixture into servings and put each serving in a zip-top sandwich bag. Store the bags in a cool cabinet for up to 2 weeks.

MAKE IT A FLAT BELLY DIET MEAL: Serve with one 6″ whole wheat pita (120), ¼ cup hummus (100), and 1 apple (77). Total meal: 397 calories

Asian Snack Mix

10 SERVINGS (½ CUP EACH) / 180 CALORIES / MUFA: PEANUTS

This snack mix can have a "wild" side if you make it with wasabi-coated peanuts. Just add 2½ cups wasabi-coated peanuts in place of the regular peanuts after the snack mix bakes. A ⅔-cup serving of the wild mix will have 227 calories.

20 MINUTES

2 tablespoons canola oil
2 teaspoons reduced-sodium soy sauce
¼ teaspoon garlic powder
¼ teaspoon ground ginger
2 cups toasted rice cereal squares
2 cups air-popped popcorn
1¼ cups unsalted dry-roasted peanuts

Nutrition per serving
○ 180 calories
○ 5 g protein
○ 10 g carbohydrates
○ 15 g fat
○ 1.5 g saturated fat
○ 0 mg cholesterol
○ 80 mg sodium
○ 2 g fiber

1. Preheat the oven to 325°F. Coat a large rimmed baking sheet with cooking spray.

2. Whisk together the oil, soy sauce, garlic powder, and ginger in a large bowl. Add the cereal, popcorn, and peanuts, tossing to coat evenly. Spread the mixture on the baking sheet. Bake for 15 minutes, stirring occasionally, until the cereal is very crisp. Watch carefully so the mixture does not burn.

3. Remove from the oven and let cool completely before storing in an airtight container.

MAKE IT **A TEAM EFFORT** Mixing ingredients is always a fun part of cooking. Let the kids toss the cereal, popcorn, and peanuts with their (freshly washed) hands.

MAKE IT A FLAT BELLY DIET MEAL: Serve with 1 piece reduced-fat mozzarella string cheese (70), 2 rye crispbread (62), and 8 dried apricot halves (67). **Total meal: 379 calories.** To serve as part of another FBD meal, omit the peanuts (110).

Tomato and Roasted Pepper Bruschetta

4 SERVINGS (4 PIECES EACH) / 329 CALORIES / MUFA: OLIVE OIL

How can you tell when a tomato is perfectly ripe? Your nose knows. A ripe tomato smells like a tomato; unripe ones have no aroma.

20 MINUTES

2 small baguettes (about 4 ounces each), cut on the diagonal into 16 slices total

¼ cup extra-virgin olive oil

1 small garlic clove

1 tomato, seeded and chopped

1 roasted pepper, patted dry and chopped (about ½ cup)

½ small red onion, finely chopped

2 tablespoons chopped fresh basil

1 tablespoon balsamic vinegar

⅛ teaspoon salt

¼ teaspoon ground black pepper

1. Preheat the oven to 400°F.

2. Arrange the baguette slices on a baking sheet in a single layer. Brush the tops with 2 tablespoons of the oil and bake for 7 to 8 minutes, or until crisp. Remove from the oven, let cool 1 minute, then rub the top of each slice with the garlic clove.

3. Meanwhile, combine the remaining 2 tablespoons oil, the tomato, roasted pepper, onion, basil, vinegar, salt, and black pepper in a bowl. Spoon the mixture over the toasts and serve.

Nutrition per serving
- 329 calories
- 8 g protein
- 40 g carbohydrates
- 15 g fat
- 2.5 g saturated fat
- 0 mg cholesterol
- 570 mg sodium
- 2 g fiber

MAKE IT A FLAT BELLY DIET MEAL: Serve with ½ cup red grapes (52). Total meal: 381 calories

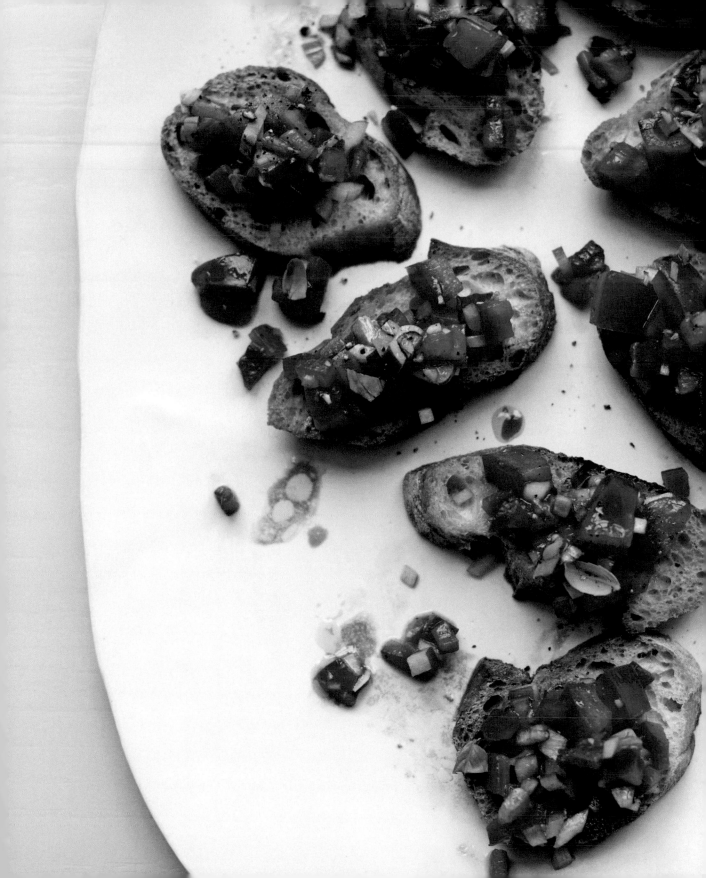

Mashed Avocado Cakes

4 SERVINGS / 188 CALORIES / MUFA: AVOCADO

Wonderful as guacamole is, when you're looking for an avocado change-up, this easy snack will fit the bill.

15 MINUTES

1 cup mashed Hass avocado
1 tablespoon stone-ground cornmeal
1 tablespoon finely chopped fresh cilantro
¼ teaspoon ground cumin
Pinch of salt
1 tablespoon olive oil
¼ cup mango chutney

1. Combine the avocado, cornmeal, cilantro, cumin, and salt in a shallow bowl. Stir with a fork to mix evenly.

2. Heat the oil in a large nonstick skillet over medium-high heat. Swirl to coat the pan bottom. When the oil is hot, drop 4 equal dollops of the avocado mixture onto the pan. Flatten slightly with the back of a spoon. Cook for 5 minutes, or until lightly browned on the bottom. Flip and cook for 2 to 3 minutes, or until set. Serve with the chutney.

🕐 **MAKE IT AHEAD** This snack can be refrigerated for up to 2 days and eaten at room temperature.

Nutrition per serving

○ 188 calories
○ 1 g protein
○ 19 g carbohydrates
○ 12 g fat
○ 1.5 g saturated fat
○ 0 mg cholesterol
○ 130 mg sodium
○ 4 g fiber

MAKE IT A FLAT BELLY DIET MEAL: Serve with 3 ounces deli roast turkey (92) and 1 ounce baked multigrain chips (118). Total meal: 398 calories

Broccoli Florets with Thai Cashew Dip

4 SERVINGS (1 CUP BROCCOLI PLUS 3 TABLESPOONS DIP EACH) / 212 CALORIES / MUFA: CASHEW BUTTER

If you don't have any cashew butter on hand, use whole cashews instead! Just toast lightly in a dry skillet over medium-high heat for 2 to 3 minutes, or until just fragrant. Then puree in a food processor with the other dip ingredients.

5 MINUTES

Combine the cashew butter, water, soy sauce, vinegar, and sugar in a bowl. Whisk until smooth. Stir in the scallions and red-pepper flakes (if using). Serve with the broccoli florets for dipping.

½ cup unsalted cashew butter
¼ cup warm water
1 tablespoon reduced-sodium soy sauce
2 teaspoons rice or white wine vinegar
½ teaspoon sugar
2 scallions, minced
¼ teaspoon crushed red-pepper flakes (optional)
4 cups broccoli florets

MAKE IT AHEAD The dip can be refrigerated in an airtight container for up to 1 week. Stir and allow to sit at room temperature for 10 minutes before serving.

Nutrition per serving
- 212 calories
- 8 g protein
- 13 g carbohydrates
- 16 g fat
- 3 g saturated fat
- 0 mg cholesterol
- 250 mg sodium
- 2 g fiber

MAKE IT A FLAT BELLY DIET MEAL: Serve with ½ ounce baked tortilla chips (59) and 1 pear (103). Total meal: 374 calories

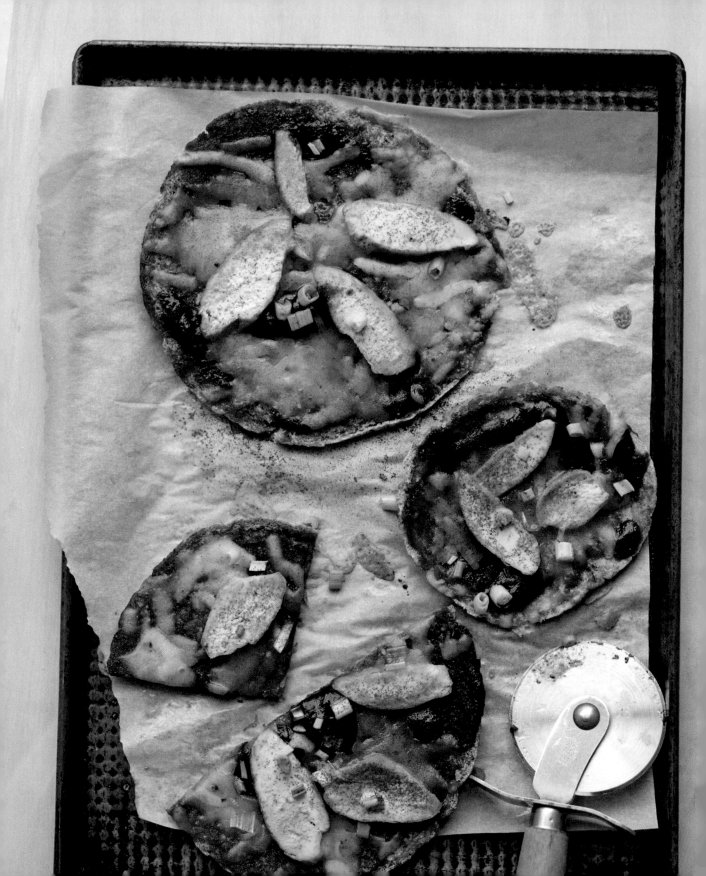

Easy Barbecue Pita Pizzas

2 SERVINGS / 410 CALORIES / MUFA: OLIVE OIL

When you need a pizza fix, this recipe will do the trick, especially if you love thin crusts. Adding a layer of olive oil between pita and sauce helps make the bread extra crispy.

15 MINUTES

2 whole wheat pitas (6"), split horizontally in half

2 tablespoons olive oil

4 tablespoons barbecue sauce

½ cup (2 ounces) shredded reduced-fat Cheddar cheese

4 ounces precooked chicken breast, sliced (see page 86)

2 scallions, thinly sliced
Chili powder (optional)

Nutrition per serving
○ 410 calories
○ 24 g protein
○ 39 g carbohydrates
○ 18 g fat
○ 3.5 g saturated fat*
○ 55 mg cholesterol
○ 730 mg sodium*
○ 4 g fiber

1. Preheat the oven to 375°F.

2. Arrange the pita halves rough side up on a baking sheet and drizzle 1½ teaspoons of the oil on each. Use the back of a spoon to spread the oil evenly to the edges. Top each with 1 tablespoon barbecue sauce, 2 tablespoons cheese, one-fourth of the chicken, and one-fourth of the scallions. Sprinkle with chili powder, if desired. Bake for 7 minutes, or until the cheese is melted.

* Limit saturated fat to no more than 10 percent of total calories—about 17 grams per day for most women or 21 grams for most men—and sodium intake to no more than 2,300 milligrams.

MAKE IT A FLAT BELLY DIET MEAL: A single serving of this recipe counts as a Flat Belly Diet Meal without any add-ons!

English Muffin Pizzas

4 SERVINGS / 311 CALORIES / MUFA: TAPENADE

To match the calorie count in this recipe, look for muffins that provide about 134 calories and 4 grams of fiber per serving.

15 MINUTES

4 whole wheat English muffins, split

$\frac{1}{2}$ cup black tapenade

1 tomato, cut into 8 slices

1 cup (4 ounces) shredded reduced-fat mozzarella cheese

4 teaspoons grated Parmesan cheese

8 fresh basil leaves

Nutrition per serving

○ 311 calories
○ 15 g protein
○ 29 g carbohydrates
○ 15 g fat
○ 4 g saturated fat*
○ 15 mg cholesterol
○ 700 mg sodium*
○ 5 g fiber

1. Preheat the oven to 400°F.

2. Toast the English muffins. Spread each muffin half with 1 tablespoon of the tapenade. Top each with 1 tomato slice, 2 tablespoons mozzarella, and $\frac{1}{2}$ teaspoon Parmesan. Place on a baking sheet and bake for 6 to 7 minutes, or until the cheese melts. Serve topped with a basil leaf.

Limit saturated fat to no more than 10 percent of total calories—about 17 grams per day for most women or 21 grams for most men—and sodium intake to no more than 2,300 milligrams.

MAKE IT A FLAT BELLY DIET MEAL: Serve with $\frac{1}{2}$ cup each carrot and celery sticks (35) and 1 orange (69). Total meal: 415 calories

Pistachio Cheese Spread

4 SERVINGS (ABOUT ¼ CUP EACH) / 280 CALORIES / MUFA: PISTACHIOS

Greek feta cheese adds tang to this spread. For a slightly less assertive spread, replace 1 ounce of the feta with 1 ounce fat-free cream cheese; the calories will be only slightly lower (273).

10 MINUTES

½ cup shelled unsalted roasted pistachios
2 ounces reduced-fat feta cheese, at room temperature
2 ounces fat-free cream cheese, at room temperature
1 tablespoon honey
1 tablespoon water
1 teaspoon salt-free lemon-pepper seasoning
2 whole grain pitas (6")

1. Place the pistachios in a food processor and pulse 6 to 8 times to coarsely chop. Add the feta, cream cheese, honey, water, and lemon-pepper seasoning. Pulse to incorporate.

2. Split the pitas horizontally in half and toast to desired crispness. Cut each pita into 8 wedges for a total of 32 and serve with the spread.

Nutrition per serving
○ 280 calories
○ 13 g protein
○ 26 g carbohydrates
○ 16 g fat
○ 3 g saturated fat
○ 5 mg cholesterol
○ 400 mg sodium
○ 5 g fiber

MAKE IT A FLAT BELLY DIET MEAL: Serve with ½ cup baby carrots (27) and ¼ cup dried cranberries (98). Total meal: 405 calories

Apples with Honey-Yogurt Dip and Candied Walnuts

1 SERVING / 273 CALORIES / MUFA: WALNUTS

Just a little sugar and water puts a whole new twist on a serving of walnuts.

5 MINUTES

1 teaspoon sugar
1 tablespoon warm water
2 tablespoons walnuts
⅓ cup fat-free plain Greek yogurt
1 tablespoon honey
1 apple, sliced

Nutrition per serving
○ 273 calories
○ 9 g protein
○ 46 g carbohydrates
○ 8 g fat
○ 1 g saturated fat
○ 0 mg cholesterol
○ 30 mg sodium
○ 3 fiber

1. Combine the sugar and water in a small bowl. Stir to dissolve the sugar.

2. Place the walnuts in a small skillet and cook over medium-high heat, shaking the pan often, for 3 to 5 minutes, until lightly toasted. Remove the skillet from the heat and stir in the sugar mixture, tossing to coat. Let cool.

3. Place the yogurt in a small bowl and cover with the honey and walnuts. Serve with apple slices for dipping.

MAKE IT A FLAT BELLY DIET MEAL: Serve with 1 cup whole strawberries (46) and 8 whole wheat crackers (70). Total meal: 389 calories

Macadamia Coconut Clusters

8 SERVINGS (2 CLUSTERS EACH) / 140 CALORIES / MUFA: MACADAMIA NUTS

Making these crunchy caramelized candies is easy but does require attention. Make sure there are pot holders and silicone or other heatproof utensils at hand. And never directly touch the sugar syrup with bare hands.

15 MINUTES

3 tablespoons sugar
1 tablespoon light corn syrup
1½ teaspoons coconut extract
1 cup unsalted macadamia nuts, quartered
2 tablespoons flaked coconut

Nutrition per serving
○ 140 calories
○ 1 g protein
○ 10 g carbohydrates
○ 10 g fat
○ 1 g saturated fat
○ 0 mg cholesterol
○ 10 mg sodium
○ 1 g fiber

1. Coat a baking sheet with cooking spray.

2. Place the sugar in a heavy 9″ skillet. Drizzle the corn syrup and coconut extract evenly over the sugar. Set over medium heat. Cook, without stirring, for 2 to 3 minutes, or until the sugar starts to melt. Tip the pan gently to help submerge any sugar that isn't dissolved. Scatter the nuts and coconut on top. Cook, stirring occasionally with a silicone spatula, for 6 to 7 minutes, or until the nuts turn a caramel color. Immediately scrape out onto the baking sheet. Use 2 spatulas to divide into 16 clusters, pressing the nuts together as you work. Do not touch the mixture while hot. Set aside to cool. Store in an airtight container at room temperature.

🕐 **MAKE IT AHEAD** Store the clusters, separated by wax or parchment paper, in an airtight container.

MAKE IT A FLAT BELLY DIET MEAL: Serve with 6 ounces fat-free vanilla yogurt (130) mixed with 1 cup sliced mango (108). Total meal: 378 calories

Marshmallow Cereal Bars

8 SERVINGS / 425 CALORIES / MUFA: CHOCOLATE

Remember the old-fashioned treats made with crisped rice cereal? Well, here that old favorite gets a bit of makeover with a different blend of cereals and a smooth layer of rich chocolate on top!

20 MINUTES

- 3 tablespoons trans-free margarine
- 1 bag (10 ounces) marshmallows
- 1 teaspoon vanilla extract
- $\frac{1}{4}$ teaspoon almond extract
- 4 cups cornflakes
- 2 cups Cheerios
- 2 cups semisweet chocolate baking chips

Nutrition per serving
- ○ 425 calories
- ○ 5 g protein
- ○ 73 g carbohydrates
- ○ 16 g fat
- ○ 8 g saturated fat*
- ○ 0 mg cholesterol
- ○ 230 mg sodium
- ○ 4 g fiber

1. Coat an 8" x 8" baking dish with cooking spray.

2. Melt the margarine in a large saucepan over medium-high heat. Add the marshmallows and vanilla and almond extracts. Cook, stirring, for 6 to 7 minutes, or until melted. Remove from the heat and stir in the cornflakes, Cheerios, and 1$\frac{1}{2}$ cups of the chocolate chips, stirring until well coated. Transfer the mixture to the baking dish. Set a piece of plastic wrap over the mixture and, with a pot holder, press down firmly with the palms of your hands to flatten the mixture into the pan. Remove the plastic wrap and let cool in the pan for 30 minutes. Remove from the pan and transfer to a wire rack.

3. Place the remaining $\frac{1}{2}$ cup chocolate chips in a small bowl set over a small saucepan of barely simmering water. Stir the chips often for 4 to 5 minutes, or until melted. Spread the melted chips evenly over the top of the cereal mixture with a small spatula. Allow to cool completely until the chocolate sets, about 45 minutes. Cut into 8 bars.

* Limit saturated fat to no more than 10 percent of total calories—about 17 grams per day for most women or 21 grams for most men—and sodium intake to no more than 2,300 milligrams.

MAKE IT A FLAT BELLY DIET MEAL: A single serving of this recipe counts as a Flat Belly Diet Meal without any add-ons!

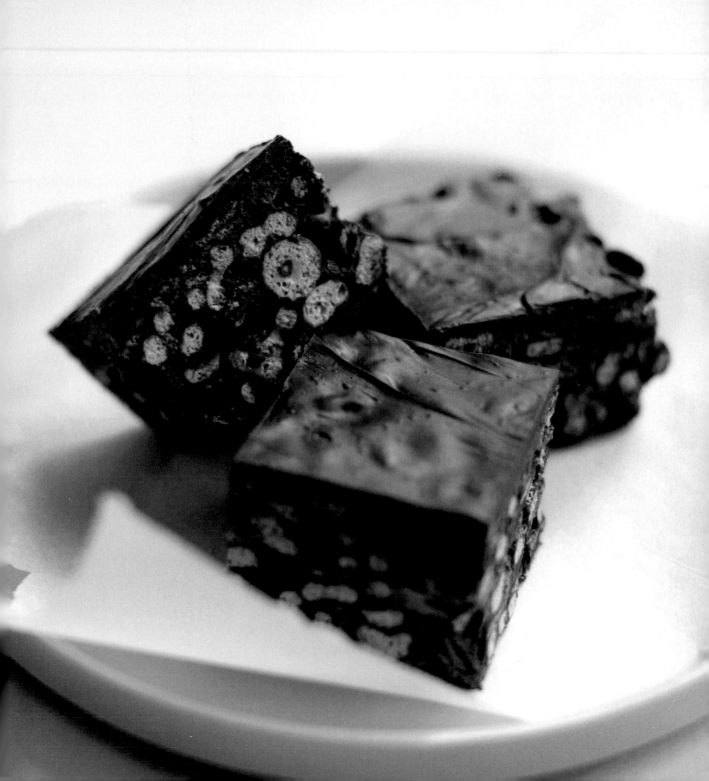

Easy Peanut Brittle

8 SERVINGS / 233 CALORIES / MUFA: PEANUTS

Peanut brittle comes together quickly, so make sure all your ingredients are measured ahead of time. And don't worry that you'll end up eating too much of it—this treat is sure to disappear fast if you have kids in the house!

15 MINUTES

¾ cup sugar
¼ cup light corn syrup
¼ teaspoon salt
 1 cup unsalted dry-roasted peanuts
 2 tablespoons trans-free margarine
 1 teaspoon vanilla extract
½ teaspoon baking soda

Nutrition per serving
○ 233 calories
○ 4 g protein
○ 31 g carbohydrates
○ 11 g fat
○ 1.5 g saturated fat
○ 0 mg cholesterol
○ 180 mg sodium
○ 1 g fiber

1. Coat a large baking sheet with cooking spray.

2. Combine the sugar, corn syrup, and salt in a medium saucepan. Bring to a boil over medium-high heat and cook, stirring occasionally, for 5 to 6 minutes, or until the sugar has dissolved and turned gold (or 275°F on a candy thermometer).

3. Stir in the peanuts, margarine, and vanilla extract and mix until the margarine is melted. Remove from the heat and quickly stir in the baking soda. Carefully pour the peanut mixture onto the baking sheet and spread with a wooden spoon or silicone spatula into a single layer. Do not touch the mixture until completely cool, about 1 hour. Break into smaller pieces to serve.

MAKE IT A FLAT BELLY DIET MEAL: Serve with 1 banana (105) and 1 piece reduced-fat mozzarella string cheese (70). **Total meal: 408 calories**

Sugar-Glazed Almond Trail Mix

8 SERVINGS / 263 CALORIES / MUFA: ALMONDS

No need to buy expensive snack mixes when you can put together this awesome treat instead. For even greater savings, look for dried fruits in the bulk bins at your grocery and buy only the amount you'll need.

1
HOUR
5 MIN

1 large egg white
1 cup unsalted natural (unblanched) whole almonds
⅓ cup sugar
¼ teaspoon ground cinnamon
½ teaspoon salt
1 cup low-fat granola
½ cup chopped dried pineapple
¼ cup golden raisins
¼ cup dried cranberries
¼ cup semisweet chocolate mini baking chips

Nutrition per serving
○ 263 calories
○ 6 g protein
○ 38 g carbohydrates
○ 11 g fat
○ 2 g saturated fat
○ 0 mg cholesterol
○ 190 mg sodium
○ 4 g fiber

1. Preheat the oven to 275°F.

2. Combine the egg white and 1 teaspoon water in a bowl and beat until frothy. Add the almonds and toss to coat. Transfer the almonds to a colander to drain for 10 minutes.

3. Meanwhile, combine the sugar, cinnamon, and salt in a large zip-top storage bag. Add the almonds and shake well to coat. Pour the almonds onto a large baking sheet. Bake for 15 minutes. Stir the almonds, return to the oven, and reduce the temperature to 250°F. Bake for 35 minutes longer, stirring occasionally. Remove from the oven, transfer to a bowl, and let cool for 15 minutes.

4. Stir in the granola, pineapple, raisins, cranberries, and chocolate chips. Store in an airtight container.

MAKE IT A FLAT BELLY DIET MEAL: Serve with 6 ounces fat-free vanilla yogurt (130).
Total meal: 393 calories

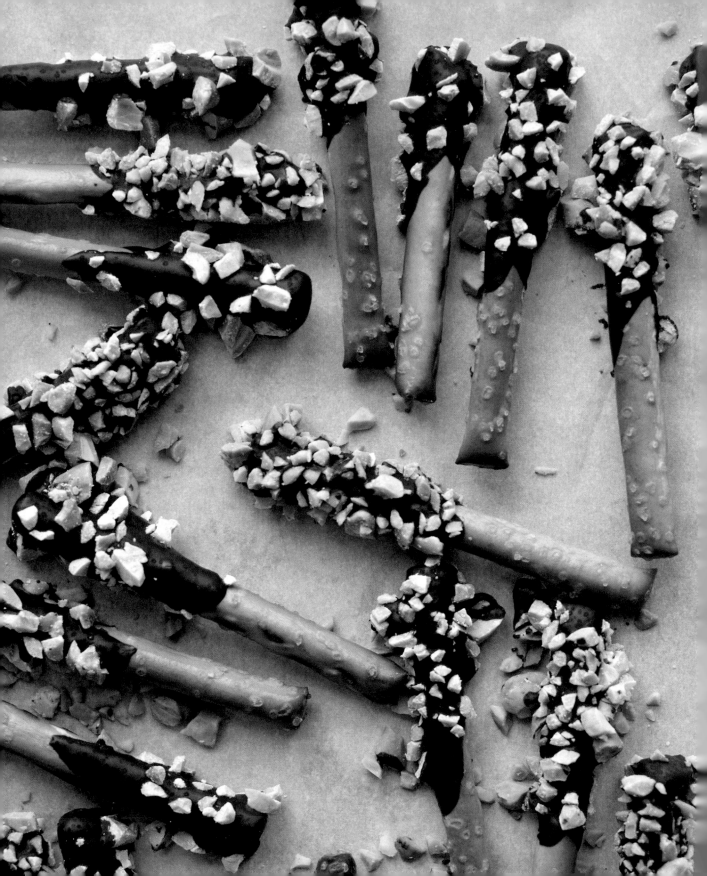

Chocolate-Covered Pretzels

1 SERVING / 309 CALORIES / MUFA: CASHEWS

This quick and easy snack takes the sweet-and-salty combination to new heights, and rolling the pretzel rods in nuts is a lot of fun for young helpers.

5 MINUTES

- 2 tablespoons semisweet chocolate baking chips
- 2 tablespoons cashews, chopped
- 3 pretzel rods

Nutrition per serving
- 309 calories
- 7 g protein
- 41 g carbohydrates
- 15 g fat
- 5 g saturated fat*
- 0 mg cholesterol
- 620 mg sodium*
- 3 g fiber

Place the chocolate chips in a large flat microwaveable bowl or plate and microwave until melted (oven power varies, so microwave in 20-second increments). Place the cashews on a second plate. Roll one end of each pretzel rod in chocolate followed by cashews. Let cool until firm.

Limit saturated fat to no more than 10 percent of total calories—about 17 grams per day for most women or 21 grams for most men—and sodium intake to no more than 2,300 milligrams.

MAKE IT A FLAT BELLY DIET MEAL: Serve with 8 ounces cappuccino made with 1 cup fat-free milk (83). Total meal: 392 calories

QUICK-FIX PANTRY RESCUES

Superfast Chips and Dip

Heat 1 tablespoon **olive oil** (119) in a skillet over medium-high heat. Cook one 8″ whole wheat tortilla (106) for 1 to 2 minutes per side until browned. Transfer to a cutting board and slice into chip-size wedges when cool. Then, without wiping skillet, add ½ cup rinsed and drained canned black beans, (100). Mash gently with the back of a spoon until heated through. Stir in ¼ cup shredded reduced-fat Cheddar cheese (80) and hot-pepper sauce to taste. **Total Calories = 405**

Cheese Plate

Arrange a 1-ounce wedge of room-temperature Brie (95) on a plate along with 8 small whole wheat crackers (70), 1 cup grapes (104), and 2 tablespoons unsalted dry-roasted **cashews** (100). **Total Calories = 369**

PB and Pineapple Snack Sandwich

Spread 2 tablespoons **peanut butter** (188) on 2 slices whole wheat bread (140). Top with ½ cup pineapple tidbits (59). **Total Calories = 387**

Emergency Fondue

Combine ¼ cup **semisweet chocolate chips** (207), 2 tablespoons fat-free evaporated milk (25), and 2 teaspoons honey (43) in a microwaveable bowl. Heat in the microwave in 20-second increments, stirring after each, until smooth and warmed through. Serve with 1 cup juice-packed canned pineapple chunks (104). **Total Calories = 379**

Caramel-Pecan Sundae

Top 1 cup slow-churned vanilla ice cream (200) with 2 tablespoons fat-free caramel topping (110) and 2 tablespoons toasted **pecans** (90). **Total Calories = 400**

Menu for an Impromptu Party

Asian Snack Mix (page 235)
Broccoli Florets with Thai Cashew Dip (page 239)
Steamed edamame (below)
Shrimp and Broccoli with Peanut BBQ Sauce

SERVES 4

🕐 **Up to 2 days before:** Make Asian Snack Mix. Store in a tightly covered container.

🕐 **About 1 hour before serving:** Thaw the shrimp (if frozen) and make Peanut BBQ Sauce. Make Thai Cashew Dip.

🕐 **About 30 minutes before serving:** Prepare the broccoli florets for both dishes.

🕐 **About 10 minutes before serving:** Cook the shrimp. Steam the edamame in the microwave according to package directions. Sprinkle with ¼ to ½ teaspoon salt and fresh lemon juice to taste just before serving.

MAKE IT A FLAT BELLY DIET MEAL: Enjoy *either* the snack mix (180) and broccoli with dip (212), or the shrimp and broccoli with Peanut BBQ Sauce (420), or the broccoli with dip (212) and ¾ cup shelled edamame (183). **Total meal: 392 calories (snack mix and dip) or 420 calories (shrimp) or 395 calories (dip and edamame)**

11

Delicious DESSERTS

- Tropical Fruit Salad
- Citrus-Avocado Gelatin Mold
- Crunchy Peanut Butter Cookies
- Dark Chocolate Swirled Meringues
- Pistachio Biscotti
- Fudgy Dark Chocolate–Raspberry Brownies
- Oatmeal Cookie Bars
- Pecan Bars
- Carrot Cake Cupcakes with Orange Icing
- Chocolate-Orange Snack Cakes
- Dark Chocolate Zucchini Bread
- Lemon Bundt Cake
- Banana-Walnut Cake
- Almond-Apple Crumble
- Strawberry Sponge Shortcake
- Blueberry Pie
- Mango Tart with Macadamia Crust
- Bananas Imposter
- Avocado Ice Cream
- Peanut Butter and Banana Malted Milk

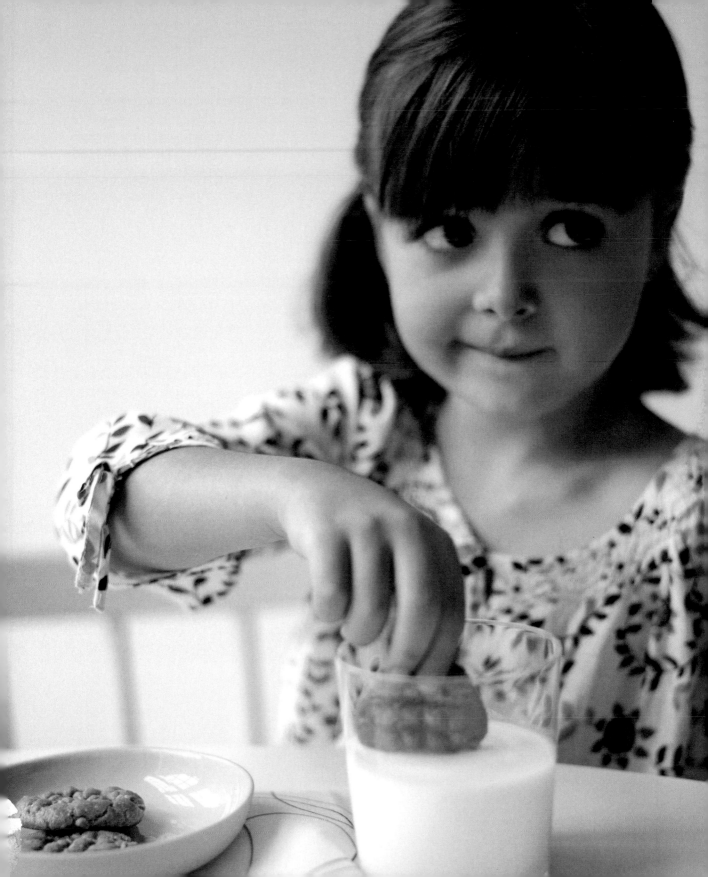

Tropical Fruit Salad

4 SERVINGS (1½ CUPS EACH) / 235 CALORIES / MUFA: AVOCADO

Though available year-round, pineapple season peaks from March through the end of July. For best results, store fresh pineapple in the refrigerator up to 5 days.

45 MINUTES

Combine the mango, pineapple, bananas, avocado, lime juice, honey, and cilantro in a bowl. Toss well. Let stand for 30 minutes before serving.

1 mango, cut into ½" pieces

½ pineapple, cut into ½" chunks (about 3 cups)

2 bananas, halved lengthwise and cut crosswise into 1"-thick slices

1 Hass avocado, cut into 1" cubes

2 tablespoons fresh lime juice

2 tablespoons honey

1 tablespoon chopped fresh cilantro

MAKE IT A TEAM EFFORT

If you're not concerned about having uniform pieces in your salad, give your younger helpers some large slices of the softer fruits to chop into smaller pieces using a table knife. They'll be inclined to try more than a polite bite.

Nutrition per serving

○ 235 calories
○ 2 g protein
○ 50 g carbohydrates
○ 6 g fat
○ 1 g saturated fat
○ 0 mg cholesterol
○ 5 mg sodium
○ 7 g fiber

MAKE IT A FLAT BELLY DIET MEAL: Serve with ½ cup low-fat cottage cheese (81) and 8 small wheat crackers (70). **Total meal: 386 calories.** To make it part of another FBD meal, omit the avocado (177).

Citrus-Avocado Gelatin Mold

6 SERVINGS / 237 CALORIES / MUFA: AVOCADO

Avocado, a true culinary chameleon, lends itself to a creamy citrus layer in this delicious molded dessert.

10 MINUTES + CHILLING

2½ tablespoons unflavored gelatin

2 cups cold unsweetened apple juice

1 can (11 ounces) juice-packed mandarin oranges, drained (reserve ½ cup juice) and patted dry

3 tablespoons honey

¼ cup cold water

1½ cups Hass avocado chunks

¼ cup confectioners' sugar
Grated zest of 1 lime

2 tablespoons fresh lime juice

2 cups mini marshmallows

Nutrition per serving
○ 237 calories
○ 4 g protein
○ 46 g carbohydrates
○ 6 g fat
○ 1 g saturated fat
○ 0 mg cholesterol
○ 50 mg sodium
○ 3 g fiber

1. Sprinkle 1½ tablespoons of the gelatin over 1 cup of the apple juice and the reserved mandarin orange juice in a bowl. Set aside for 1 minute.

2. Microwave the remaining 1 cup apple juice and the honey in a microwaveable measuring cup on high power for 2 minutes, or until it just comes to a boil. Whisk to completely dissolve the honey. Add to the gelatin mixture, whisking constantly, until no beads of gelatin remain. Refrigerate the apple-orange gelatin for 1 to 1½ hours, or until just beginning to set, with a consistency similar to raw egg whites.

3. Meanwhile, combine the remaining 1 tablespoon gelatin and the water in a small microwaveable dish. Set aside for 1 minute, or until the gelatin is softened. Microwave on high for 25 seconds, or until dissolved.

4. Combine the avocado, sugar, and lime zest and juice in a food processor and process for 2 to 3 minutes, or until the mixture is very smooth. With the machine running, add the gelatin-water mixture through the feed tube. Process until combined. Transfer to a bowl and fold in the marshmallows. Cover with plastic wrap, pressing the wrap firmly against the avocado mixture. Set aside.

5. Coat a 6-cup ring mold with cooking spray. When the apple-orange gelatin has reached the consistency of raw egg whites, pour half of it into the mold. Spread the avocado mixture evenly over it, then pour the remaining apple-orange gelatin on top. Press the drained mandarin oranges into the top layer. Refrigerate for about 1½ hours, or until completely set. (The dessert may be refrigerated for up to 24 hours, if desired.)

MAKE IT A FLAT BELLY DIET MEAL: Serve with 1 cup 1% milk (102) and 1 cup sliced strawberries (54).
Total meal: 393 calories

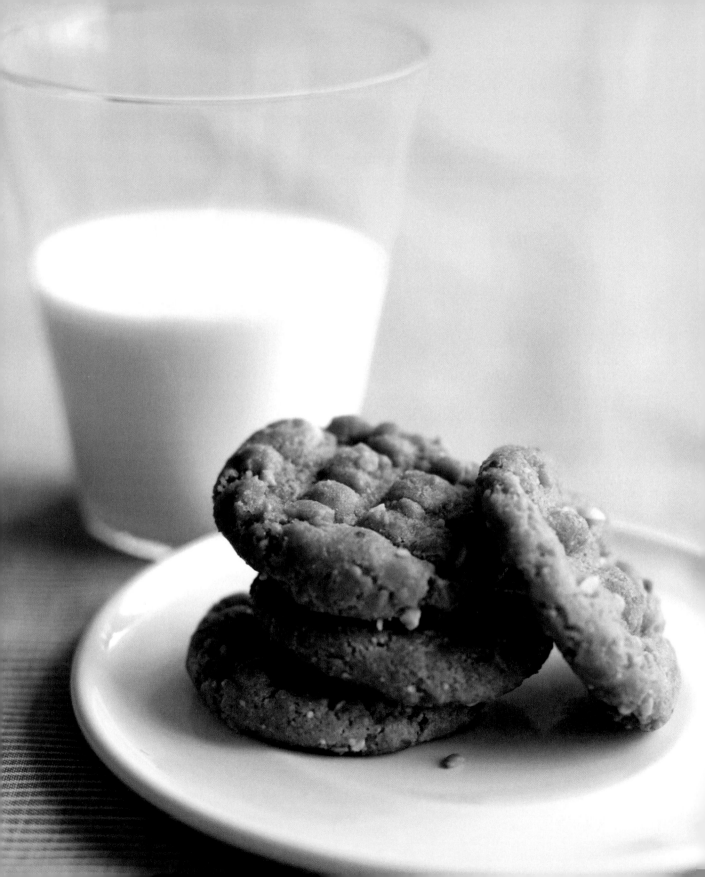

Crunchy Peanut Butter Cookies

8 SERVINGS (3 COOKIES EACH) / 315 CALORIES / MUFA: PEANUT BUTTER

Definitely dunkers! Have a cold glass of milk at the ready to submerge these treats.

35 MINUTES

1 cup natural unsalted crunchy peanut butter
1 cup packed light brown sugar
½ teaspoon baking soda
¼ teaspoon salt
1 large egg, lightly beaten
1 teaspoon vanilla extract
All-purpose flour for shaping cookies

1. Preheat the oven to 350°F. Coat several large baking sheets with cooking spray.

2. Combine the peanut butter, brown sugar, baking soda, and salt in a bowl. Add the egg and vanilla extract and beat until smooth.

3. Shape the dough into 24 balls and arrange on the sheets. Dip the tines of a fork into flour and gently press a crisscross pattern into the top of each cookie.

4. Bake for 10 to 12 minutes, or until lightly browned on the bottom. Transfer to a rack to cool. Store in an airtight container at room temperature.

Nutrition per serving
- 315 calories
- 8 g protein
- 34 g carbohydrates
- 17 g fat
- 2 g saturated fat
- 25 mg cholesterol
- 170 mg sodium
- 2 g fiber

MAKE IT A FLAT BELLY DIET MEAL: Serve with 1 cup fat-free milk (83). Total meal: 398 calories

Dark Chocolate Swirled Meringues

4 SERVINGS (8 COOKIES EACH) / 255 CALORIES / MUFA: CHOCOLATE

As an alternative to drizzling the chocolate, try dipping the flat side of each cookie into the melted chocolate. Arrange the meringues on parchment paper and let sit until the chocolate sets completely.

3 HOURS 20 MIN

- 3 large egg whites, at room temperature
- ¼ teaspoon cream of tartar
- ⅛ teaspoon ground cinnamon
- ½ cup sugar
- 1 teaspoon vanilla extract
- 4 ounces semisweet chocolate, chopped
- 1 tablespoon trans-free margarine

Nutrition per serving
- ○ 255 calories
- ○ 5 g protein
- ○ 42 g carbohydrates
- ○ 9 g fat
- ○ 5 g saturated fat*
- ○ 0 mg cholesterol
- ○ 40 mg sodium
- ○ 2 g fiber

1. Preheat the oven to 350°F. Line a large baking sheet with parchment paper.

2. Combine the egg whites, cream of tartar, and cinnamon in a medium bowl. Beat with an electric mixer on high speed until soft peaks form. With the mixer running, slowly add the sugar in a steady stream, beating until the mixture is glossy and stiff peaks form. Beat in the vanilla extract until well combined.

3. Transfer the mixture to a large plastic bag with 1 corner snipped off. Gently squeezing the bag, pipe 32 mounds about 1½" in diameter and ¾" apart onto the parchment-covered baking sheet. Place the baking sheet in the oven and reduce the heat to 250°F. Bake for 1 hour, or until the meringues are very lightly colored. Turn off the heat and leave in the oven for 1 hour. Transfer the meringues to a wire rack.

4. Combine the chocolate and margarine in a small bowl set over a saucepan of barely simmering water. Stir the chocolate mixture for 3 to 4 minutes, or until melted. Transfer the mixture to a small plastic bag with 1 corner snipped off. Place paper towels or parchment paper under the racks with the meringues. Working with one meringue at a time, gently squeeze the bag in a back-and-forth motion to make thin lines of chocolate. Then repeat over the same meringue in lines perpendicular to the first lines to create a crisscross pattern. Set the meringues in a cool place and let sit for 1 hour, or until the chocolate sets.

Limit saturated fat to no more than 10 percent of total calories—about 17 grams per day for most women or 21 grams for most men—and sodium intake to no more than 2,300 milligrams.

MAKE IT A FLAT BELLY DIET MEAL: Serve with 1 cup fat-free milk (83) and 1 cup sliced strawberries (54). Total meal: 392 calories

Pistachio Biscotti

8 SERVINGS (3 COOKIES EACH) / 254 CALORIES / MUFA: PISTACHIOS

If you prefer to remove the brownish skin from pistachios before using them in this recipe, blanch the nuts first in boiling water for about 2 minutes. Drain and cool slightly, then rub off the skins while still warm.

1 HOUR 10 MIN

½ cup sugar

2 tablespoons unsalted butter, at room temperature

1 large egg

1 tablespoon vanilla extract

1½ cups all-purpose flour

1 teaspoon baking powder

⅛ teaspoon salt

1 cup shelled unsalted pistachios

Nutrition per serving

○ 254 calories

○ 6 g protein

○ 34 g carbohydrates

○ 11 g fat

○ 3 g saturated fat

○ 35 mg cholesterol

○ 110 mg sodium

○ 2 g fiber

1. Preheat the oven to 350°F. Line a large baking sheet with parchment paper.

2. Combine the sugar, butter, egg, and vanilla extract in the bowl of an electric mixer. Beat on high speed until well combined. Meanwhile, combine the flour, baking powder, and salt in a bowl. With the mixer on low, beat in the flour mixture until moistened and a dough forms. Add the pistachios and mix for 15 seconds.

3. Shape the dough into 2 logs, each about 6" long x 2½" wide x ¾" high. Place on the baking sheet and bake for 24 to 25 minutes, or until slightly firm. Remove from the oven and let cool for 10 minutes. Trim the ends and slice each log with a serrated knife into 12 (½"-thick) cookies (24 total). Set the cookies upright on the baking sheet. Reduce the oven temperature to 300°F and return to the oven. Bake the cookies for 25 minutes. Transfer to a wire rack to cool. Cookies will crisp as they cool.

MAKE IT A FLAT BELLY DIET MEAL: Serve with 8 ounces cappuccino made with ½ cup fat-free milk (42) and ¼ cup dried cranberries (98). **Total meal: 394 calories**

Fudgy Dark Chocolate–Raspberry Brownies

8 SERVINGS (2 BROWNIES EACH) / 347 CALORIES / MUFA: CHOCOLATE

Baking brownies in parchment paper lets you lift them out of the pan when they're cool and makes dividing them into picture-perfect squares a snap. For a more precise cut, refrigerate beforehand.

1 HOUR

- 8 **ounces semisweet chocolate, chopped**
- 5 **tablespoons trans-free margarine**
- 2 **large eggs**
- 1 **large egg white**
- 1 **cup granulated sugar**
- 1 **teaspoon vanilla extract**
- ½ **cup all-purpose flour**
- ½ **teaspoon baking powder**
- ⅛ **teaspoon salt**
- 1 **cup raspberries**
- 1 **tablespoon confectioners' sugar (optional)**

Nutrition per serving
- 347 calories
- 5 g protein
- 50 g carbohydrates
- 15 g fat
- 6 g saturated fat*
- 55 mg cholesterol
- 140 mg sodium
- 3 g fiber

1. Preheat the oven to 325°F. Press parchment paper into the bottom of a 9" x 9" baking pan, making sure there is enough paper to overhang two opposite edges. Coat generously with cooking spray and dust lightly with flour.

2. Combine the chocolate and margarine in a bowl set over a saucepan of barely simmering water. Cook, stirring occasionally, until the mixture is melted and smooth. Remove from the heat and let cool 2 minutes.

3. Meanwhile, combine the whole eggs, egg white, granulated sugar, and vanilla extract in a bowl. Combine the flour, baking powder, and salt in a separate bowl. Whisk the slightly cooled chocolate mixture into the egg mixture until smooth. Add the flour mixture, stirring until combined. Gently fold in the raspberries. Pour the batter into the pan.

4. Bake for 48 to 50 minutes, or until a toothpick inserted in the center comes out with moist crumbs. Cool in the pan for 10 minutes. Carefully lift the foil from the pan and cool completely on a rack. Cut into 16 squares and sprinkle with confectioners' sugar, if desired, before serving.

* Limit saturated fat to no more than 10 percent of total calories—about 17 grams per day for most women or 21 grams for most men—and sodium intake to no more than 2,300 milligrams.

MAKE IT A FLAT BELLY DIET MEAL: Serve with ½ cup of soy chai, warm or iced (65).
Total meal: 412 calories

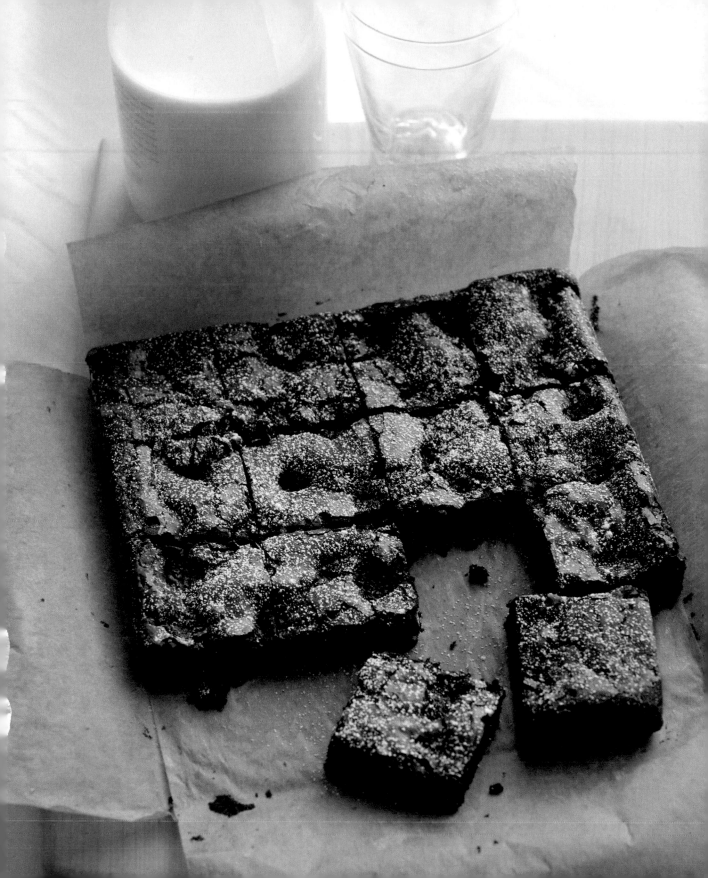

Oatmeal Cookie Bars

6 SERVINGS (2 BARS EACH) / 275 CALORIES / MUFA: CHOCOLATE

Eating oatmeal has never been more enticing than with these yummy chocolate-crowned confections. Tuck one into a lunch box and you're sure to get rave reviews.

25 MINUTES

½ cup old-fashioned rolled oats

¼ cup whole wheat pastry flour

½ teaspoon baking powder

½ teaspoon ground cinnamon

⅛ teaspoon baking soda

1 large egg

3 tablespoons honey

5 tablespoons fat-free milk

2 tablespoons canola oil

6 ounces semisweet chocolate, chopped

1 teaspoon vanilla extract

Nutrition per serving
○ 275 calories
○ 4 g protein
○ 36 g carbohydrates
○ 15 g fat
○ 6 g saturated fat*
○ 35 mg cholesterol
○ 90 mg sodium
○ 3 g fiber

1. Preheat the oven to 350°F. Coat an 8" x 8" baking pan with cooking spray.

2. Process the oats in a food processor until finely ground. Add the flour, baking powder, cinnamon, and baking soda. Pulse to mix.

3. Beat the egg in a small bowl. Stir in the honey, 2 tablespoons of the milk, and 1 tablespoon of the oil. Add the egg mixture to the oat mixture, pulsing to blend.

4. Spread the batter in the baking pan. Bake for 10 to 12 minutes, or until browned and slightly puffed.

5. Meanwhile, combine the chocolate, the remaining 3 tablespoons milk, and remaining 1 tablespoon oil in a microwaveable bowl. Cook on high power for 1 minute. Stir until smooth. If necessary, return to the microwave and cook in 10-second increments until the chocolate is completely melted. Add the vanilla extract and stir until the mixture is smooth and glossy. Spread the chocolate topping over the warm cookie base. Allow to cool before cutting into 12 bars.

Limit saturated fat to no more than 10 percent of total calories—about 17 grams per day for most women or 21 grams for most men—and sodium intake to no more than 2,300 milligrams.

MAKE IT A FLAT BELLY DIET MEAL: Serve with 6 ounces fat-free vanilla yogurt (130).
Total meal: 405 calories

Pecan Bars

8 SERVINGS / 375 CALORIES / MUFA: PECANS

Nothing beats the real maple flavor in these nutty bars. Unlike traditional recipes with a shortbread crust, this one includes syrup to render a softer bottom in these wholesome treats.

50 MINUTES

1½ cups all-purpose flour
½ cup packed light brown sugar
½ teaspoon salt
½ cup trans-free margarine
1 cup pecans
½ cup maple syrup
2 large eggs, lightly beaten
1 tablespoon vanilla extract

Nutrition per serving
○ 375 calories
○ 5 g protein
○ 46 g carbohydrates
○ 19 g fat
○ 2 g saturated fat
○ 55 mg cholesterol
○ 180 mg sodium
○ 2 g fiber

1. Preheat the oven to 350°F.

2. Combine the flour, brown sugar, and salt in a food processor. Add the margarine and pulse for about 30 seconds, or until the mixture has the consistency of sand. Press the mixture into the bottom of an 8″ x 8″ baking pan. Bake for 10 minutes.

3. Meanwhile, combine the pecans, maple syrup, eggs, and vanilla extract in a bowl.

4. Remove the pan from the oven and top with the pecan mixture. Spread the nuts with a fork to ensure as even a layer as possible. Bake for 30 minutes, or until the topping is set. Let cool completely before cutting into 8 bars.

MAKE IT A FLAT BELLY DIET MEAL: Serve with 6 dried apricot halves (51). Total meal: 426 calories

Carrot Cake Cupcakes with Orange Icing

12 SERVINGS / 386 CALORIES / MUFA: CANOLA OIL

These delicious cupcakes are a snap to put together and taste like a lighter version of regular carrot cake, each perfectly portioned into a single serving.

50 MINUTES

1¼ cups granulated sugar
¾ cup canola oil
⅓ cup low-fat buttermilk
2 large eggs
1 teaspoon vanilla extract
2 cups all-purpose flour
1½ teaspoons baking powder
1 teaspoon ground allspice
½ teaspoon baking soda
½ teaspoon salt
2 carrots, grated
½ cup golden raisins
1½ cups confectioners' sugar
2 tablespoons orange juice
2 teaspoons grated orange zest

1. Preheat the oven to 350°F. Line a 12-cup muffin pan with paper liners.

2. Combine the granulated sugar, oil, buttermilk, eggs, and vanilla extract in a bowl. Combine the flour, baking powder, allspice, baking soda, and salt in a separate bowl. Add the flour mixture to the oil mixture and stir until smooth. Fold in the carrots and raisins.

3. Spoon the batter into the muffin cups and bake for 19 to 20 minutes, or until golden and the cupcakes are slightly springy when touched. Cool the cupcakes in the pan for 5 minutes, then transfer to a rack to cool completely.

4. Combine the confectioners' sugar and orange juice and zest in a bowl, stirring until smooth. Spread some of the icing over each cupcake with a small spatula and let stand for 15 minutes before serving.

Nutrition per serving
- 386 calories
- 4 g protein
- 62 g carbohydrates
- 15 g fat
- 1.5 g saturated fat
- 36 mg cholesterol
- 239 mg sodium
- 1 g fiber

MAKE IT A FLAT BELLY DIET MEAL: Serve with ½ cup fat-free milk (42). Total meal: 428 calories

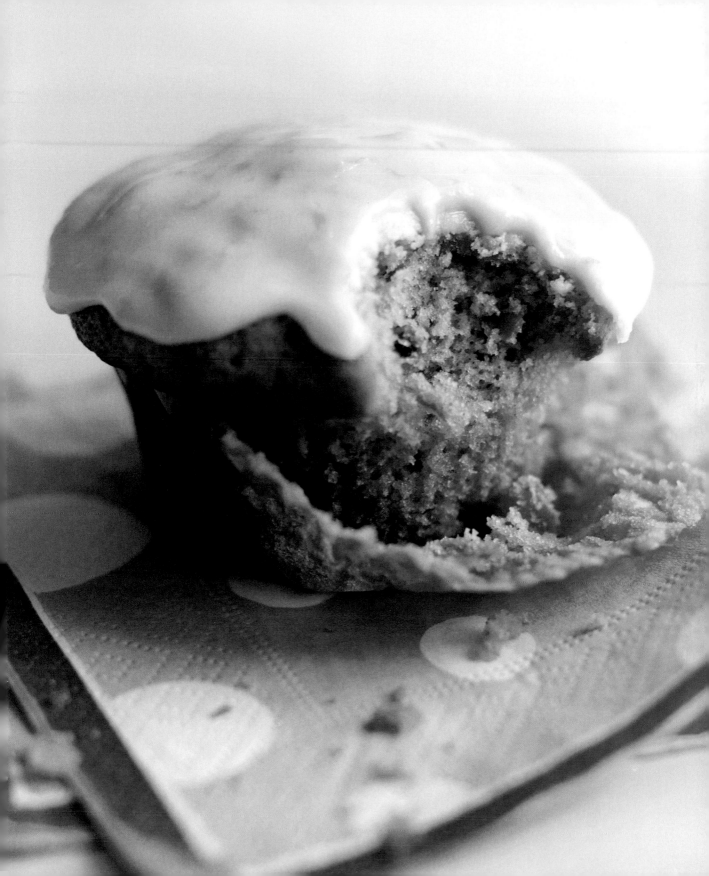

Chocolate-Orange Snack Cakes

4 SERVINGS (3 CAKES EACH) / 257 CALORIES / MUFA: CHOCOLATE

These bite-size treats provide a sophisticated pairing of chocolate and orange, so consider making a double batch and freezing one for when you need a quick dessert.

25 MINUTES

4 ounces bittersweet or semisweet chocolate, finely chopped

6 tablespoons all-purpose flour

¼ teaspoon baking powder

⅛ teaspoon baking soda

Pinch of salt

1 large egg white

3 tablespoons light brown sugar

3 tablespoons unsweetened applesauce

2 teaspoons canola oil

¾ teaspoon orange extract

1½ teaspoons whole milk

Nutrition per serving
- 257 calories
- 4 g protein
- 35 g carbohydrates
- 15 g fat
- 6 g saturated fat*
- 0 mg cholesterol
- 105 mg sodium
- 2 g fiber

1. Preheat the oven to 350°F. Coat a 12-cup mini-muffin pan with cooking spray.

2. Place 2½ ounces of the chocolate in a microwaveable bowl. Microwave on high power for 60 seconds, or until melted. Cook in 10-second increments, if needed, to melt completely. Stir until smooth.

3. Combine the flour, baking powder, baking soda, and salt on a sheet of wax paper.

4. Beat the egg white with a fork in a mixing bowl. Add the brown sugar, applesauce, 1½ teaspoons of the oil, the orange extract, and melted chocolate. Stir until smooth. Stir the flour mixture into the wet ingredients just until no flour is visible. Dollop into the muffin cups.

5. Bake for 10 minutes, or until the tops are set but yield slightly when pressed. (Do not overbake.) Cool in the pan on a rack for 3 minutes, then remove from the pan to cool completely.

6. Meanwhile, combine the remaining 1½ ounces chocolate, the milk, and the remaining ½ teaspoon oil in a microwaveable bowl. Microwave on high power for 30 seconds, or until melted. Stir until smooth. Spread glaze over each cake.

* Limit saturated fat to no more than 10 percent of total calories—about 17 grams per day for most women or 21 grams for most men—and sodium intake to no more than 2,300 milligrams.

MAKE IT A FLAT BELLY DIET MEAL: Serve with 1 banana (105) and ½ cup fat-free milk (42). Total meal: 404 calories

Dark Chocolate Zucchini Bread

16 SERVINGS (1 SLICE EACH) / 354 CALORIES / MUFA: CANOLA OIL

While smaller zucchini have the most flavor, this recipe provides an ideal way to handle those jumbo squash that always appear with the late-summer bumper crop. Plus, they're a good source of vitamin B$_6$!

1 HOUR 30 MIN

2$\frac{1}{2}$ cups all-purpose flour
1$\frac{1}{2}$ cups semisweet chocolate
mini baking chips
$\frac{1}{4}$ cup unsweetened cocoa
powder (not Dutch process)
1 teaspoon baking soda
1 teaspoon ground cinnamon
1 teaspoon salt
1$\frac{1}{2}$ cups sugar
1 cup canola oil
2 large eggs, lightly beaten
1 teaspoon vanilla extract
2 cups shredded zucchini
(about $\frac{3}{4}$ pound)
$\frac{1}{4}$ cup fat-free plain Greek
yogurt

Nutrition per serving
○ 354 calories
○ 4 g protein
○ 44 g carbohydrates
○ 20 g fat
○ 4 g saturated fat*
○ 25 mg cholesterol
○ 240 mg sodium
○ 2 g fiber

1. Preheat the oven to 350°F. Coat two 9" x 5" loaf pans with cooking spray.

2. Combine the flour, 1 cup of the chocolate chips, the cocoa, baking soda, cinnamon, and salt in a large bowl.

3. Place the remaining $\frac{1}{2}$ cup chocolate chips in a small microwaveable cup or bowl and melt in the microwave. (Oven power can vary, so microwave in 10-second increments until the chocolate is easy to stir.)

4. Stir together the melted chocolate, sugar, oil, eggs, and vanilla extract in another large bowl. Add the flour mixture and stir until thoroughly combined. Add the zucchini and yogurt in alternating batches, stirring well after each addition. (The batter will be very thick.)

5. Divide the batter between the 2 loaf pans and bake for 1 hour, or until a cake tester inserted in the center comes out clean. Cool in the pans on a rack for 10 minutes, then turn out of the pans onto the rack to cool completely. Cut each loaf into 8 slices.

* Limit saturated fat to no more than 10 percent of total calories—about 17 grams per day for most women or 21 grams for most men—and sodium intake to no more than 2,300 milligrams.

MAKE IT A FLAT BELLY DIET MEAL: Serve with 1 apple (77). Total meal: 431 calories

Lemon Bundt Cake

16 SERVINGS / 317 CALORIES / MUFA: SAFFLOWER OIL

To extract the most juice from a lemon, warm it to room temperature by running it under hot water, and then roll it under the palm of your hand on a flat surface before cutting and squeezing.

1 HOUR 45 MIN

- 3 cups all-purpose flour
- 1½ cups granulated sugar
- 2 teaspoons baking powder
- ½ teaspoon baking soda
- ¼ teaspoon salt
- 1 cup safflower oil
- ¾ cup + 2 tablespoons low-fat buttermilk
- 3 large eggs
- ¼ cup fresh lemon juice
- 1 teaspoon lemon extract
- 1 cup confectioners' sugar

Nutrition per serving
- 317 calories
- 4 g protein
- 44 g carbohydrates
- 15 g fat
- 1.5 g saturated fat
- 40 mg cholesterol
- 160 mg sodium
- 0 g fiber

1. Preheat the oven to 350°F. Spray a 12-cup Bundt pan with cooking spray and lightly coat with flour.

2. Combine the flour, granulated sugar, baking powder, baking soda, and salt in a large bowl. Combine the oil, ¾ cup of the buttermilk, the eggs, lemon juice, and lemon extract in a separate bowl. Add the oil mixture to the flour mixture and stir until well combined. Pour the batter into the Bundt pan.

3. Bake for 43 to 45 minutes, or until a toothpick inserted halfway between the tube and sides comes out clean. Cool in the pan for 15 minutes. Turn out of the pan onto a rack to cool for 30 minutes.

4. Meanwhile, combine the remaining 2 tablespoons buttermilk and confectioners' sugar in a bowl, stirring until smooth. Drizzle the mixture over the cake and wait at least 10 minutes before slicing into 16 pieces.

MAKE IT A FLAT BELLY DIET MEAL: Serve with 1 cup raspberries (64). Total meal: 381 calories

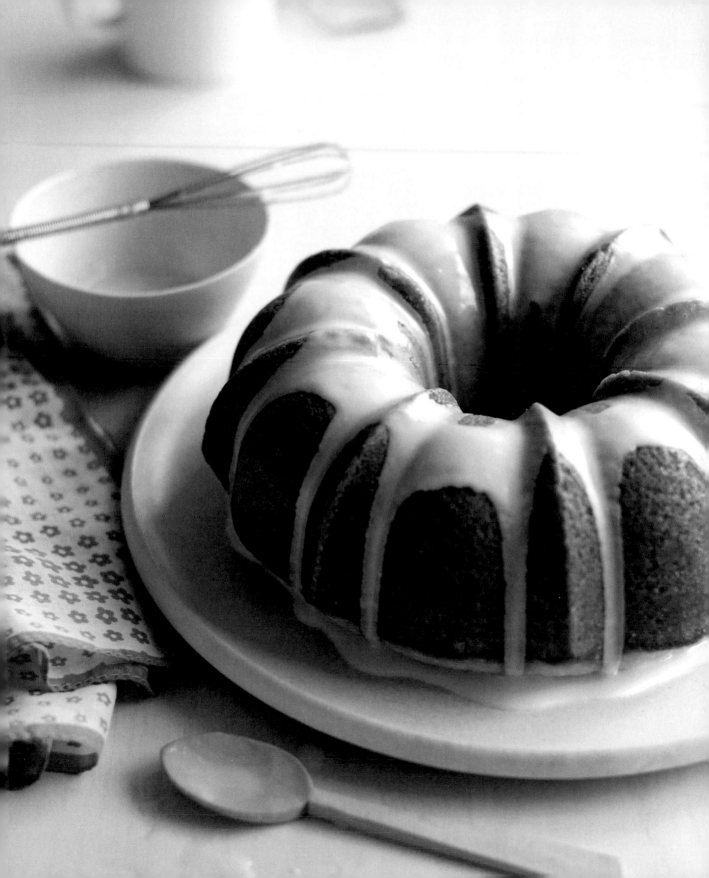

Banana-Walnut Cake

12 SERVINGS / 301 CALORIES / MUFA: WALNUTS

This extra-nutty cake would be perfect served with a hot cup of tea.

50 MINUTES

⅔ cup granulated sugar
2 ripe bananas, mashed
2 large eggs
½ cup + 1 tablespoon 1% milk
¼ cup canola oil
2 teaspoons vanilla extract
1¾ cups all-purpose flour
2 teaspoons baking powder
1 teaspoon ground cinnamon
¼ teaspoon salt
1½ cups walnuts
1 cup confectioners' sugar

Nutrition per serving

○ 301 calories
○ 5 g protein
○ 41 g carbohydrates
○ 14 g fat
○ 1.5 g saturated fat
○ 35 mg cholesterol
○ 150 mg sodium
○ 2 g fiber

1. Preheat the oven to 350°F. Coat a 9" x 9" baking pan with cooking spray and lightly coat with flour.

2. Combine the granulated sugar, bananas, eggs, ½ cup of the milk, the oil, and 1 teaspoon of the vanilla extract in a bowl, mixing well. Combine the flour, baking powder, cinnamon, and salt in a separate bowl. Add the flour mixture to the banana mixture and stir until just combined. Fold in the walnuts. Pour the batter into the baking pan.

3. Bake for 28 to 30 minutes, or until a toothpick inserted in the center comes out clean. Cool in the pan for 10 minutes. Turn out of the pan onto a rack to cool completely.

4. Meanwhile, combine the confectioners' sugar, remaining 1 tablespoon milk, and remaining 1 teaspoon vanilla extract in a small bowl. Spread the glaze over the banana cake with a small spatula. Cut into 12 squares.

MAKE IT A FLAT BELLY DIET MEAL: Serve with 1 apple (77) and 1 cup of hot tea (0).
Total meal: 378 calories

Almond-Apple Crumble

6 SERVINGS / 325 CALORIES / MUFA: ALMONDS

The old-time goodness of a baked fruit crumble makes an ideal cool-weather dessert, filling the kitchen with delicious aromas.

1 HOUR 15 MIN

- ¼ cup unsweetened applesauce
- 2 tablespoons honey
- 1 tablespoon cornstarch
- 1 pound baking apples, sliced
- ¼ cup dried cranberries
- ¾ cup old-fashioned rolled oats
- ¾ cup slivered almonds
- ¼ cup whole wheat pastry flour
- ¼ cup packed light brown sugar
- ¼ teaspoon ground cinnamon
  Pinch of salt
- 3 tablespoons cold trans-free margarine, cut into small pieces

Nutrition per serving

- ○ 325 calories
- ○ 6 g protein
- ○ 46 g carbohydrates
- ○ 14 g fat
- ○ 2 g saturated fat
- ○ 0 mg cholesterol
- ○ 75 mg sodium
- ○ 5 g fiber

1. Preheat the oven to 350°F. Coat an 8″ x 8″ baking dish with cooking spray.

2. Combine the applesauce, honey, and cornstarch in a large bowl. Blend until smooth. Stir in the apples and dried cranberries. Transfer to the baking dish. Wipe out the bowl with a paper towel.

3. Place the oats, almonds, flour, brown sugar, cinnamon, and salt in the bowl. Toss with a fork. Add the margarine and blend into the dry ingredients with a fork or pastry blender. Sprinkle over the fruit.

4. Bake for 45 minutes, or until the top is browned and fruit is bubbling. Let rest for 15 minutes before serving.

MAKE IT A FLAT BELLY DIET MEAL: Serve with ½ cup slow-churned reduced-fat vanilla ice cream (100). Total meal: 425 calories

Strawberry Sponge Shortcake

8 SERVINGS / 286 CALORIES / MUFA: CANOLA OIL

When a dessert is prepared with healthy monounsaturated canola oil and fresh berries, you can feel good about serving it to your family.

40 MINUTES

1 cup all-purpose flour
1 teaspoon baking powder
1/8 teaspoon baking soda
1/2 cup + 2 tablespoons sugar
3 large egg whites
Pinch of salt
1/2 cup canola oil
1/4 cup fat-free milk
1 1/2 teaspoons vanilla extract
1 quart strawberries, sliced
8 tablespoons fat-free whipped topping

Nutrition per serving
○ 286 calories
○ 4 g protein
○ 36 g carbohydrates
○ 15 g fat
○ 1.5 g saturated fat
○ 0 mg cholesterol
○ 130 mg sodium
○ 2 g fiber

1. Preheat the oven to 350°F. Coat a 9" round cake pan with cooking spray.

2. Whisk together the flour, baking powder, baking soda, and 1/4 cup of the sugar in a bowl.

3. Place the egg whites and salt in a bowl and, with an electric mixer, beat on medium speed until the whites start to turn opaque. Increase the speed to high. Continue beating, gradually adding the remaining 1/4 cup of the sugar until soft peaks form.

4. Whisk the oil, milk, and vanilla extract into the flour mixture until smooth. Dollop one-third of the beaten egg whites onto the batter and gently whisk in. Dollop on the remaining whites and gently fold into the batter. Pour into the cake pan and smooth the top.

5. Bake for 25 minutes, or until the top is browned and the cake springs back when pressed with a fingertip. Cool in the pan on a rack.

6. Meanwhile, combine the strawberries and the remaining 2 tablespoons sugar in a bowl. Refrigerate until serving.

7. Cut the cake into 8 wedges. Cut each wedge horizontally in half. Place the bottom halves on 8 dessert plates. Dividing evenly, top the wedges with half the strawberry mixture. Cover with the cake tops. Spoon on the remaining strawberry mixture and 1 tablespoon of whipped topping. Serve right away.

MAKE IT A FLAT BELLY DIET MEAL: Serve with 1 cup rice milk (120). Total meal: 406 calories

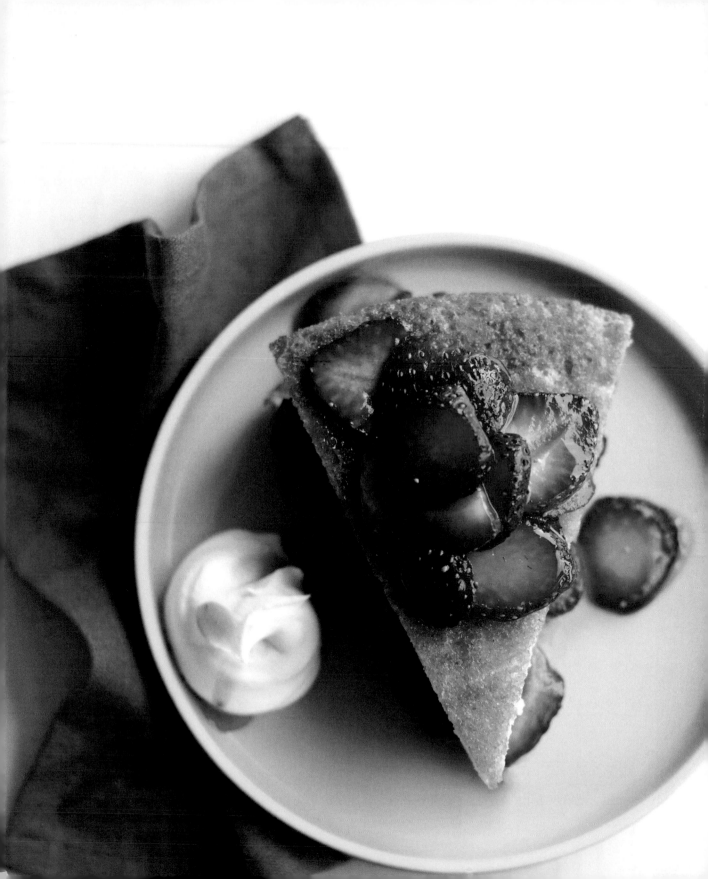

Blueberry Pie

8 SERVINGS / 435 CALORIES / MUFA: CANOLA OIL

Fruit pies are always a summertime favorite. And with this easy canola-oil crust, you don't have to resort to prepared crusts, which may contain less healthful types of fat.

1 HOUR 5 MIN

2½ cups all-purpose flour

½ teaspoon salt

½ cup canola oil

6 to 8 tablespoons cold 1% milk

4 cups blueberries

¼ cup cornstarch

½ cup granulated sugar

1 tablespoon fresh lemon juice

2 teaspoons grated lemon zest

⅓ cup old-fashioned rolled oats

¼ cup packed light brown sugar

2 tablespoons trans-free margarine, melted

1 teaspoon ground cinnamon

Nutrition per serving

○ 435 calories

○ 6 g protein

○ 67 g carbohydrates

○ 17 g fat

○ 2 g saturated fat

○ 0 mg cholesterol

○ 178 mg sodium

○ 3 g fiber

1. Preheat the oven to 375°F.

2. Place the flour and salt in a food processor. With the processor running, add the oil. Add the milk 1 tablespoon at a time until the mixture comes together and can be formed into a ball. On a lightly floured surface, press the mixture into a 12″ disk. Transfer the dough to a 9″ deep-dish pie plate and press into the bottom and up the sides of the pan. Form a decorative edge, if desired. Prick the bottom of the crust with a fork and bake for 10 minutes. Remove from the oven and reduce the temperature to 350°F.

3. Combine the blueberries, cornstarch, granulated sugar, lemon juice, and lemon zest in a large bowl. Toss gently and scrape the mixture into the pie shell.

4. Combine the oats, brown sugar, margarine, and cinnamon in a small bowl. Drop small pieces of the mixture on top of the blueberries to cover (the mixture will be loose).

5. Bake for 45 to 50 minutes, or until the blueberries are bubbling. Cool completely before cutting into 8 wedges.

MAKE IT A FLAT BELLY DIET MEAL: A single serving of this recipe counts as a Flat Belly Diet Meal without any add-ons!

Mango Tart with Macadamia Crust

8 SERVINGS / 336 CALORIES / MUFA: MACADAMIA NUTS

Apricot nectar is usually sold with other tropical juices in the Latin food section of your grocery store and sometimes in the produce section of a health food store.

1
HOUR
30 MIN

1 cup unsalted macadamia
   nuts
1 cup whole wheat pastry flour
   Grated zest and juice of 1 lime
½ teaspoon salt
4 tablespoons cold trans-free
   margarine, cut into pieces
1 large egg white, beaten
¼ cup apricot nectar
3 tablespoons mango chutney
3 tablespoons light brown
   sugar
2 tablespoons cornstarch
2½ pounds firm-ripe mango,
   sliced (about 4 cups)
8 tablespoons fat-free
   whipped topping

Nutrition per serving
○ 336 calories
○ 4 g protein
○ 42 g carbohydrates
○ 18 g fat
○ 3.5 g saturated fat
○ 0 mg cholesterol
○ 250 mg sodium
○ 4 g fiber

1. Preheat the oven to 375°F. Coat a 9″ fluted tart pan with a removable bottom or a springform pan with cooking spray.

2. Reserve 4 nuts. Place the remaining nuts in a food processor and process until finely ground. Add the flour, lime zest, and salt. Process briefly to blend. Scatter the margarine pieces over the mixture and pulse until incorporated. Combine the egg white and 1 tablespoon of the lime juice in a measuring cup. With the machine running, drizzle in the egg-white mixture, adding up to 1 tablespoon more lime juice (or water if not enough juice) so the dough starts to mass together.

3. Turn the mixture onto a lightly floured work surface. (Do not wash the food processor bowl.) Pat the dough into an 8″ disk (the mixture will be soft). Transfer to the bottom of the tart or spring-form pan. Press into the bottom and ½″ up the sides. Refrigerate for 15 minutes.

4. Meanwhile, combine the apricot nectar, chutney, brown sugar, and cornstarch in the food processor bowl and process until smooth. Transfer to a bowl. Add the mango slices and toss gently to mix. Spoon into the prepared crust. Bake for 1 hour, or until the juices are bubbling. Transfer to a rack to cool completely. Crush the 4 reserved nuts and sprinkle over the tart.

5. Unmold and cut into 8 wedges. Dollop 1 tablespoon whipped topping on each wedge just before serving.

MAKE IT A FLAT BELLY DIET MEAL:
Serve with a large (12 ounces) cappuccino made with ¾ cup fat-free milk (63). **Total meal: 398 calories**

Bananas Imposter

4 SERVINGS / 402 CALORIES / MUFA: CANOLA OIL

This alcohol-free, family-friendly version of the Crescent City classic comes together in minutes. It is a delightful closing for a weekend brunch.

10 MINUTES

- 3 **tablespoons confectioners' sugar**
- ½ **teaspoon ground cinnamon**
- 4 **firm-ripe bananas, sliced crosswise into 1″ pieces**
- ¼ **cup canola oil**
- 3 **tablespoons honey**
- 1 **teaspoon vanilla extract**
- 2 **cups slow-churned reduced- fat vanilla ice cream**

Nutrition per serving
○ 402 calories
○ 4 g protein
○ 61 g carbohydrates
○ 18 g fat
○ 3 g saturated fat
○ 20 mg cholesterol
○ 45 mg sodium
○ 3 g fiber

1. Mix together the confectioners' sugar and ¼ teaspoon of the cinnamon on a small plate. Dip the cut sides of the bananas in the sugar mixture and set aside.

2. Heat the oil in a large skillet over medium-high heat. Working in batches, place the bananas cut side down in the skillet. Cook for 2 minutes, or until browned on the bottom. Use tongs to carefully flip the pieces and cook for 1 minute longer. As they finish cooking, divide the banana pieces among 4 dessert plates.

3. Remove the skillet from the heat. Carefully stir in the honey, vanilla extract, and remaining ¼ teaspoon cinnamon. Spoon the sauce over the bananas. Top each serving with ½ cup ice cream.

MAKE IT A FLAT BELLY DIET MEAL: A single serving of this recipe counts as a Flat Belly Diet Meal without any add-ons!

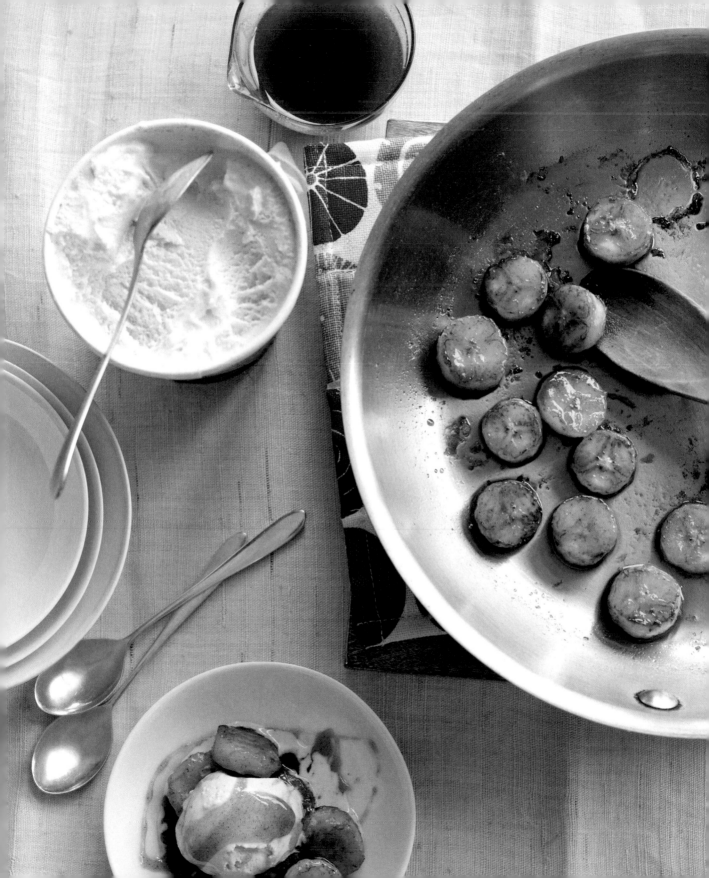

Flat Belly Diet! Family Cookbook

Avocado Ice Cream

4 SERVINGS (1 CUP EACH) / 348 CALORIES / MUFA: AVOCADO

Here's a recipe that could convert even the most diehard avocado skeptics. The vanilla and almond extracts actually make this homemade treat taste more like pistachio.

20 MINUTES + CHILLING

  3 Hass avocados, scooped out
1½ cups 1% milk
  1 cup fat-free plain Greek yogurt
  ½ cup sugar
  1 tablespoon vanilla extract
  1 teaspoon almond extract

Nutrition per serving
○ 348 calories
○ 7 g protein
○ 41 g carbohydrates
○ 17 g fat
○ 2.5 g saturated fat
○ 5 mg cholesterol
○ 70 mg sodium
○ 7 g fiber

1. Combine the avocados, milk, yogurt, sugar, and vanilla and almond extracts in a food processor. Process for 2 to 3 minutes, or until completely smooth.

2. Transfer the mixture to a bowl, cover, and refrigerate for 4 to 6 hours, or until thoroughly chilled.

3. Process the mixture in an ice-cream maker according to the manufacturer's instructions. For soft-serve ice cream, serve at once. If a firmer texture is desired, freeze overnight. Let sit at room temperature for about 15 minutes before serving.

MAKE IT A FLAT BELLY DIET MEAL: Serve topped with ½ cup sliced strawberries (27) and 1 tablespoon fat-free chocolate syrup (50). **Total meal: 425 calories**

Peanut Butter and Banana Malted Milk

2 SERVINGS / 404 CALORIES / MUFA: PEANUT BUTTER

Smooth, cold, and perfectly refreshing—what a delicious way to end the day!

5 MINUTES

Combine the peanut butter, banana, malted milk powder, milk, and ice cream in a blender. Blend until smooth and creamy.

¼ cup natural unsalted creamy peanut butter

1 ripe banana, frozen

4 tablespoons natural flavor malted milk powder

1 cup fat-free milk

½ cup 98% fat-free vanilla ice cream

Nutrition per serving

○ 404 calories
○ 15 g protein
○ 47 g carbohydrates
○ 18 g fat
○ 3 g saturated fat
○ 10 mg cholesterol
○ 160 mg sodium
○ 5 g fiber

MAKE IT A FLAT BELLY DIET MEAL: A single serving of this recipe counts as a Flat Belly Diet Meal without any add-ons!

Your MUFA Serving Chart

Food	Serving	Calories
OILS		
Canola oil	1 Tbsp	124
Canola oil mayonnaise	1 Tbsp	100
Flaxseed oil (cold-pressed organic)	1 Tbsp	120
Olive oil	1 Tbsp	119
Peanut oil	1 Tbsp	119
Pesto sauce	1 Tbsp	80
Safflower oil (high oleic)	1 Tbsp	120
Sesame (cold-pressed) or soybean oil	1 Tbsp	120
Sunflower oil (high oleic)	1 Tbsp	120
Walnut oil	1 Tbsp	120
NUTS, LEGUMES, AND SEEDS		
Almonds	2 Tbsp	109
Almond butter	2 Tbsp	200
Brazil nuts	2 Tbsp	110
Cashews	2 Tbsp	100
Cashew butter	2 Tbsp	190
Hazelnuts	2 Tbsp	110
Macadamia nuts	2 Tbsp	120
Natural peanut butter, crunchy	2 Tbsp	188
Natural peanut butter, smooth	2 Tbsp	188
Peanuts	2 Tbsp	110
Pecans	2 Tbsp	90
Pine nuts	2 Tbsp	113
Pistachios	2 Tbsp	88
Pumpkin seeds (without the shell)	2 Tbsp	148
Sesame seeds (without the shell)	2 Tbsp	91
Soybeans (edamame), shelled and boiled	1 cup	244
Sunflower seeds (without the shell)	2 Tbsp	90
Sunflower seed butter	2 Tbsp	190
Tahini (sesame seed paste)	2 Tbsp	178
Walnuts	2 Tbsp	82
AVOCADOS		
Avocado, California (Hass)	¼ cup	96
Avocado, Florida	¼ cup	69
OLIVES		
Black olive tapenade	2 Tbsp	88
Green olive tapenade	2 Tbsp	54
Green or black olives	10 large	50
Kalamata olives	10 large	105
DARK CHOCOLATE		
Semisweet chocolate chips	¼ cup	207

Family Snack Pack Guide

Building your own Flat Belly Diet snack is easy
when you follow these three simple steps.

Step 1:
Pick a MUFA from the list in Appendix A.

Step 2:
Choose from any of the following selections.

Step 3:
Keep your calorie count under 400.

GRAINS

○ **100% whole wheat bread** (1 slice), 70 calories

○ **100% light whole wheat bread** (1 slice), 40 calories

○ **Whole wheat tortilla** (one 8"), 105 calories

○ **Whole wheat pita** (one 6"), 120 calories

○ **Whole wheat bagel** (2 ounces), 120 calories

○ **Whole grain crackers,** such as Triscuit Thin Crisps (8), 70 calories

○ **Whole grain crispbread,** such as Wasa Multi Grain (2), 80 calories

○ **Whole wheat English muffin** (1 whole), 135 calories

○ **Baked multigrain tortilla chips** ($\frac{1}{2}$ ounce), 60 calories

○ **Popcorn** (4 cups light microwave), 100 calories

○ **Whole grain cereal** with at least 3 grams of fiber per serving, such as bran flakes, shredded wheat, or Kashi GoLean (1 cup), 150 calories

○ **Whole grain waffle** (1 waffle), 80 calories

○ **Oatmeal, instant,** plain (1 packet), 100 calories

DAIRY

○ **Reduced-fat mozzarella string cheese** (1-ounce piece), 80 calories

○ **Low-fat cottage cheese** ($\frac{1}{2}$ cup), 80 calories

○ **Reduced-fat Cheddar cheese** ($\frac{1}{4}$ cup shredded), 80 calories

○ **Greek yogurt,** fat-free plain, such as Fage 0% (6 ounces), 90 calories

○ **Fat-free vanilla yogurt,** such as Stonyfield Farm (6 ounces), 130 calories

○ **Trans-free margarine** (2 teaspoons), 55 calories

○ **Fat-free milk** (1 cup), 83 calories

○ **Low-fat soy milk** (1 cup), 70 calories

FRUITS

- **Apple** (1 medium/size of tennis ball), 77 calories
- **Applesauce,** unsweetened (½ cup), 55 calories
- **Banana** (1 medium/7" to 8"), 105 calories
- **Blueberries** (1 cup), 84 calories
- **Grapefruit** (½ medium), 60 calories
- **Grapes,** red or green (1 cup), 104 calories
- **Juice, apple or orange** (½ cup), 60 calories
- **Orange** (1 medium), 69 calories
- **Pear** (1 medium), 105 calories
- **Pineapple,** juice-packed tidbits, drained (4 ounces or ½ cup), 59 calories
- **Raisins** (¼ cup), 123 calories
- **Strawberries** (1 cup sliced), 54 calories

VEGETABLES

- **Baby carrots** (1 cup), 53 calories
- **Bell pepper** (1 cup sliced), 30 calories
- **Broccoli florets** (1 cup), 20 calories
- **Cauliflower florets** (1 cup), 30 calories
- **Celery** (1 medium rib), 8 calories
- **Cherry or grape tomatoes** (1 cup), 30 calories
- **Cucumber** (1 cup chopped), 16 calories
- **Mixed salad greens** (2 cups), 20 calories
- **Salsa** (¼ cup), 20 calories

PROTEIN

- **Turkey deli meat** (2 ounces), 61 calories
- **Chicken breast,** precooked (3 ounces), 122 calories
- **Ground beef,** 95% extra-lean, cooked (4 ounces), 193 calories
- **Chunk light tuna,** water-packed (3 ounces), 105 calories
- **Canned salmon** (3 ounces), 155 calories
- **Hard-cooked egg** (1 large), 78 calories
- **Fat-free refried beans** (½ cup), 100 calories
- **Hummus** (¼ cup), 100 calories

14-Day Meal Plan

This meal plan is designed for a woman who wants to lose weight. (Men who are trying to drop pounds should add one additional 400-calorie snack to each day.) All of these foods are appropriate for your kids, too—but you shouldn't count calories where they're concerned.

DAY 1

Breakfast

- ○ Apricot-Peach Smoothie (page 60)
- ○ 1 piece reduced-fat mozzarella string cheese
- ○ ½ cup blueberries

Lunch

- ○ Salad prepared with 2 cups mixed baby greens and 3 ounces water-packed chunk-light tuna topped with 2 tablespoons sunflower seeds and 2 tablespoons reduced-calorie balsamic vinaigrette dressing
- ○ 1 whole wheat pita (6")
- ○ ½ cup unsweetened applesauce

Dinner

- ○ Chicken and Almond Dumplings (page 186)

Snack

- ○ ½ cup fat-free vanilla yogurt mixed with 1 cup sliced strawberries and ¼ cup semisweet chocolate baking chips

Nutrition for Total Day:
1,594 calories
84 g protein
199 g carbohydrate
6 g fat
16 g sat fat
136 mg cholesterol
2,150 mg sodium
23 g fiber

DAY 2

Breakfast

- ○ 1 whole grain waffle topped with 2 tablespoons peanut butter
- ○ 1 cup blueberries

Lunch

- ○ Penne Pasta Salad (page 95)

Dinner

- ○ One 3-ounce turkey burger topped with 1 slice tomato, 1 large romaine leaf, and ¼ cup sliced avocado on a whole grain hamburger bun
- ○ ½ cup steamed broccoli florets

Snack

- ○ Almond-Apple Crumble (page 273)
- ○ ½ cup slow-churned reduced-fat vanilla ice cream

Nutrition for Total Day:
1,600 calories
84 g protein
169 g carbohydrate
70 g fat
13 g sat fat
185 mg cholesterol
1,040 mg sodium
26 g fiber

DAY 3

Breakfast

- o Chocolate-Stuffed French Toast (page 71)

Lunch

- o Chicken Salad with Wheat Crackers (page 91)
- o 1 pear
- o $\frac{1}{2}$ cup baby carrots

Dinner

- o 3 ounces roasted pork tenderloin
- o Garlic Mashed Potatoes (page 226)

Snack

- o 3 cups light microwave popcorn mixed with 2 tablespoons dry-roasted peanuts and $\frac{1}{4}$ cup raisins
- o 1 cup fat-free milk

Nutrition for Total Day:
1,650 calories
69 g protein
206 g carbohydrate
67 g fat
16 g sat fat
210 mg cholesterol
1,700 mg sodium
25 g fiber

DAY 4

Breakfast

- o 1 packet plain instant oatmeal cooked in $\frac{1}{2}$ cup fat-free milk and topped with 1 cup frozen raspberries, 2 tablespoons almonds, and 2 teaspoons honey
- o $\frac{1}{2}$ medium banana

Lunch

- o English Muffin Pizza (page 242)
- o 1 cup celery sticks
- o 1 cup red or green grapes

Dinner

- o Fish Nuggets with Tartar Sauce (page 177)
- o $\frac{1}{4}$ pound asparagus spears, steamed

Snack

- o 1 Carrot Cake Cupcake with Orange Icing (page 266)
- o $\frac{1}{2}$ cup fat-free milk

Nutrition for Total Day:
1,610 calories
78 g protein
210 g carbohydrate
56 g fat
8 g sat fat
240 mg cholesterol
1,840 mg sodium
26 g fiber

DAY 5

Breakfast

- O 2 Lemon-Blueberry Buttermilk Muffins (page 74)
- O 1 cup fat-free milk

Lunch

- O 1 whole wheat pita (6") filled with 2 ounces deli turkey, 1 slice low-sodium Swiss cheese, and ¼ cup sliced avocado
- O 1 cup cherry tomatoes

Dinner

- O Florentine Baked Beans (page 176)
- O ½ cup cooked brown rice
- O 1 cup cooked kale tossed with 1 teaspoon trans-free margarine

Snack

- O Sugar-Glazed Almond Trail Mix (page 249)
- O ½ cup fat-free plain Greek yogurt

Nutrition for Total Day:
1,580 calories
69 g protein
198 g carbohydrate
61 g fat
12 g sat fat
120 mg cholesterol
1,540 mg sodium
22 g fiber

DAY 6

Breakfast

- O 2 slices light whole grain toast spread with 2 tablespoons peanut butter
- O 1 cup canned juice-packed pineapple chunks, drained

Lunch

- O Orange, Apple, and Jicama Slaw with Shrimp (page 101)

Dinner

- O Crunchy Crust Mac and Cheese (page 179)
- O 1 cup cooked carrots tossed with 1 teaspoon trans-free margarine

Snack

- O 1 whole wheat tortilla (8") spread with 1 tablespoon pesto sauce and sprinkled with ¼ cup shredded reduced-fat mozzarella cheese (warm in toaster oven or broiler and roll up)
- O ½ cup fat-free milk
- O 1 cup green or red grapes

Nutrition for Total Day:
1,570 calories
68 g protein
193 g carbohydrate
64 g fat
13 g sat fat
165 mg cholesterol
1,870 mg sodium
35 g fiber

DAY 7

Breakfast

- ○ Almond, Oat, and Dried Cranberry-Cherry Granola (page 62)
- ○ 1 cup fat-free milk

Lunch

- ○ Avocado-Orange Salad (page 100)
- ○ 3 ounces precooked chicken breast
- ○ 1-ounce whole wheat roll
- ○ 1 apple

Dinner

- ○ 3 ounces broiled flank steak
- ○ ½ cup cooked brown rice
- ○ Haricots Verts (page 220)

Snack

- ○ 10 large black olives
- ○ ¼ cup hummus with 1 whole wheat pita (6″) and 1 cup baby carrots

Nutrition for Total Day:
1,550 calories
89 g protein
187 g carbohydrate
54 g fat
10 g sat fat
125 mg cholesterol
1,780 mg sodium
33 g fiber

DAY 8

Breakfast

- ○ 1 Maple-Pecan Cinnamon Roll (page 76)
- ○ ½ cup fat-free milk

Lunch

- ○ Pasta salad made with ½ cup cooked whole wheat pasta tossed with 3 ounces precooked chicken, ½ cup chopped baby carrots, ½ cup grape tomatoes, 2 tablespoons pine nuts, and 1 tablespoon reduced-calorie balsamic vinaigrette

Dinner

- ○ Shrimp and Ham Jambalaya (page 183)
- ○ Half wedge of Cornbread (page 199)
- ○ ½ cup steamed green beans

Snack

- ○ Tropical Fruit Salad (page 254)
- ○ ½ cup low-fat cottage cheese
- ○ 2 whole grain crispbreads

Nutrition for Total Day:
1,550 calories
90 g protein
195 g carbohydrate
52 g fat
8 g sat fat
255 mg cholesterol
1,570 mg sodium
25 g fiber

DAY 9

Breakfast

- 1 whole grain tortilla (8") spread with 2 tablespoons almond butter, rolled up
- 6 dried apricot halves
- Café au lait made with 8 ounces coffee and ½ cup fat-free milk

Lunch

- Seared Salmon BLT (page 89)
- 1 cup raw sugar snap peas
- ½ cup canned mandarin oranges

Dinner

- Butternut Squash Ravioli (page 136)

Snack

- Frozen Chocolate-Covered Bananas: Peel 1 banana and slice crosswise. Insert a Popsicle stick into the cut ends, lay on a baking sheet, and freeze for 1 to 2 hours, or until firm. Melt ¼ cup semisweet chocolate baking chips and coat the frozen banana halves, then roll in ½ cup crushed whole grain cereal. Return to the freezer until firm.

Nutrition for Total Day:
1,630 calories
64 g protein
182 g carbohydrate
77 g fat
15 g sat fat
110 mg cholesterol
1,350 mg sodium
25 g fiber

DAY 10

Breakfast

- 1 Berry Good Peanut Butter Scone (page 73)

Lunch

- Greek salad made with 2 cups romaine tossed with 1 tablespoon feta cheese, 10 kalamata olives, ½ cup sliced grape tomatoes, 1 cup peeled and chopped cucumber, and 2 tablespoons Greek salad dressing
- 1 whole wheat pita (6")

Dinner

- Chipotle Beef and Bean Chili (page 194)
- 6 whole grain crackers

Snack

- Apples with Honey-Yogurt Dip and Candied Walnuts (page 242)
- 1 cup sliced strawberries
- ½ cup fat-free milk

Nutrition for Total Day:
1,630 calories
64 g protein
219 g carbohydrate
72 g fat
12 g sat fat
70 mg cholesterol
2,290 mg sodium
26 g fiber

DAY 11	DAY 12

Breakfast

- O 1 cup whole grain cereal topped with 2 tablespoons pecans, ¼ cup raisins, and ½ cup fat-free milk

Lunch

- O Grilled Tomato and Cheese (page 84)
- O ½ cup fresh or canned juice-packed pineapple chunks

Dinner

- O 3 ounces baked tilapia
- O Creamy Sesame Greens (page 218)
- O ½ cup cooked whole wheat couscous

Snack

- O Lemon Bundt Cake (page 270)
- O 1 cup raspberries

Nutrition for Total Day:
1,630 calories
73 g protein
212 g carbohydrate
68 g fat
10 g sat fat
105 mg cholesterol
1,080 mg sodium
33 g fiber

Breakfast

- O 1 Banana Split Muffin (page 75)
- O 1 cup fat-free milk

Lunch

- O Quinoa Salad with Cherries and Pecans (page 99)

Dinner

- O 3 ounces precooked chicken breast
- O ⅔ cup cooked brown rice
- O Broccoli Rabe with Toasted Garlic (page 219)

Snack

- O 10 whole wheat crackers spread with 2 tablespoons peanut butter
- O 1 medium pear

Nutrition for Total Day:
1,560 calories
68 g protein
189 g carbohydrate
68 g fat
10 g sat fat
70 mg cholesterol
810 mg sodium
28 g fiber

DAY 13

Breakfast
o Smoothie made with 1 cup fat-free milk, ½ cup fat-free vanilla yogurt, ½ cup frozen blackberries, 2 teaspoons honey, and 1 tablespoon flaxseed oil

Lunch
o Pistachio Cheese Spread (page 243)

o 1 cup sliced red bell pepper

o 1 cup green or red grapes

Dinner
o Barbecue Turkey Burgers with Avocado Mash (page 123)

o 1 cup sliced zucchini, steamed

Snack
o 1 cup cooked shelled edamame

o 1 ounce baked multigrain chips

Nutrition for Total Day:
1,580 calories
85 g protein
197 g carbohydrate
59 g fat
9 g sat fat
75 mg cholesterol
1,240 mg sodium
29 g fiber

DAY 14

Breakfast
o Vegetable Frittata (page 67)

o 1 whole wheat English muffin spread with 2 teaspoons trans-free margarine

o ½ medium grapefruit

Lunch
o Chicken and Creamy Pepper Jelly Wrap (page 86)

o 1 cup baby carrots

o 1 cup blueberries

Dinner
o Cashew, Tofu, and Broccoli Stir-Fry (page 139)

Snack
o 1 cup fat-free milk

o ¼ cup semisweet chocolate baking chips mixed with ¼ cup dried cranberries

Nutrition for Total Day:
1,600 calories
58 g protein
220 g carbohydrate
60 g fat
14 g sat fat
255 mg cholesterol
1,840 mg sodium
28 g fiber

Endnotes

CHAPTER 1

1. C. Maffeis, A. Pietrobelli, A. Grezzani, S. Provera, and L. Tatò, "Waist Circumference and Cardiovascular Risk Factors in Prepubertal Children," *Obesity Research*, 9, no. 3 (2001): 179–87.

2. J. M. Sorof, D. Lai, J. Turner, T. Poffenbarger, and R. J. Portman, "Overweight, Ethnicity, and the Prevalence of Hypertension in School-Aged Children," *Pediatrics*, 113, no. 3 (2004): 475–82.

3. E. Lopez-Garcia, M. B. Schulze, J. B. Meigs, J. E. Manson, N. Rifai, M. J. Stampfer, W. C. Willet, and F. B. Hu, "Consumption of *Trans* Fatty Acids Is Related to Plasma Biomarkers of Inflammation and Endothelial Dysfunction," *Journal of Nutrition*, 135, no. 3 (2005): 562–66.

4. T. Psaltopoulou, A. Naska, P. Orfanos, D. Trichopoulos, T. Mountokalakis, and A. Trichopoulou, "Olive Oil, the Mediterranean Diet, and Arterial Blood Pressure: The Greek European Prospective Investigation into Cancer and Nutrition (EPIC) Study," *American Journal of Clinical Nutrition*, 80, no. 4 (2004): 1012–18.

5. L. A. Ferrara, A. S. Raimondi, L. d'Episcopo, L. Guida, A. D. Russo, and T. Marotta, "Olive Oil and Reduced Need for Antihypertensive Medication," *Archives of Internal Medicine*, 160, no. 6 (2000): 837–42.

6. M. D. Kontogianni, D. B. Panagiotakos, C. Chrysohoou, C. Pitsavos, A. Zampelas, and C. Stefanadis, "The Impact of Olive Oil Consumption Pattern on the Risk of Acute Coronary Syndromes: The Cardio2000 Case-Control Study," *Clinical Cardiology*, 30, no. 3 (125–29).

7. A. Garg, "High-Monounsaturated-Fat Diets for Patients with Diabetes Mellitus: A Meta-Analysis," *American Journal of Clinical Nutrition*, 67, no. 3 (1998): S577–S582.

8. K. C. Donaghue, M. M. Pena, A. K. F. Chan, B. L. Blades, J. King, L. H. Storlien, and M. Silink, "Beneficial Effects of Increasing Monounsaturated Fat Intake in Adolescents with Type 1 Diabetes," *Diabetes Research and Clinical Practice*, 48, no. 3 (2000): 193–99.

9. P. M. Kris-Etherton, T. A. Pearson, Y. Wan, R. L. Hargrove, K. Moriarty, V. Fishell, and T. D. Etherton, "High-Monounsaturated Fatty Acid Diets Lower Both Plasma Cholesterol and Triacylglycerol Concentrations," *American Journal of Clinical Nutrition*, 70, no. 6 (1999): 1009–15.

10. M. Sanchez-Bayle, A. Gonzalez-Requejo, M. J. Pelaez, M. T. Morales, J. Asensio-Anton, and E. Anton-Pacheco, "A Cross-Sectional Study of Dietary Habits and Lipid Profiles. The Rivas-Vaciamadrid Study," *European Journal of Pediatrics*, 167, no. 2 (2008): 149–54.

11. L. Hodson, C. M. Skeaff, and W-A. H. Chisholm, "The Effect of Replacing Dietary Saturated Fat with Polyunsaturated or Monounsaturated Fat on Plasma Lipids in Free-Living Young Adults," *European Journal of Clinical Nutrition*, 55, no. 10 (2001): 908–15.

12. G. Riccarfi, R. Giacco, and A. A. Rivellese, "Dietary Fat, Insulin Sensitivity and the Metabolic Syndrome," *Clinical Nutrition*, 23 (2004): 447–56.

13. D. Panagiotakos, C. Pitsavos, C. Chrysohoou, J. Skoumas, D. Tousoulis, M. Toutouza, P. Toutouzas, and C. Stefanadis, "Impact of Lifestyle Habits on the Prevalence of the Metabolic Syndrome among Greek Adults from the ATTICA Study," *American Heart Journal*, 147, no. 1 (2004): 106–12.

14. M. C. Morris, D. A. Evans, J. L. Bienias, C. C. Tangney, D. A. Bennett, N. Aggarwal, J. Schneider, and R. S. Wilson, "Dietary Fats and the Risk of Incident Alzheimer Disease," *Archives of Neurology*, 60, no. 2 (2003): 194–200.

15. J. A. Paniagua, A. Gallego dl la Sacristana, I. Romero, A. Vidal-Puig, J. M. Latre, E. Sanchez, P. Perez-Martinez, J. Lopez-Miranda, F. Perez-Jimenez, "Monounsaturated Fat-Rich Diet Prevents Central Body Fat Distribution and Decreases Postprandial Adiponectin Expression Induced by a Carbohydrate-Rich Diet in Insulin-Resistant Subjects," *Diabetes Care*, 3, no. 7 (2007): 1717–23.

16. K. J. Stewart, C. M. Seemans, L. D. McFarland, J. J. Weinhofer, and C. S. Brown, "Dietary Fat and Cholesterol Intake in Young Children Compared with Recommended Levels," *Journal of Cardiopulmonary Rehabilitation*, 19, no. 2 (1999): 112–17.

17. I. Shai, D. Schwarzfuchs, Y. Henkin, D. R. Shahar, S. Witkow, I. Greenberg, R. Golan, D. Fraser, A. Bolotin, H. Vardi, O. Tangi-Rozental, R. Zuk-Ramot, B. Sarusi, D. Brickner, Z. Schwartz, E. Sheiner, R. Marko, E. Katorza, J. Theiry, G. M. Fiedler, M. Blüher, M. Stumvoll, and M. J. Stampfer, "Weight Loss with a Low-Carbohydrate, Mediterranean, or Low-Fat Diet," *New England Journal of Medicine*, 359, no. 3 (July 17, 2008): 229–41.

18. K. McManus, L. Antinoro, and F. Sacks, "A Randomized Controlled Trial of a Moderate-Fat, Low-Energy Diet Compared with a Low-Fat, Low-Energy Diet for Weight Loss in Overweight Adults," *International Journal of Obesity*, 25, no. 10 (2001) 1503–11.

19. D. Romaguera, et al., "Adherence to the Mediterranean Diet Is Associated with Lower Abdominal Adiposity in European Men and Women," *Journal of Nutrition*, 129, no. 9 (2009): 1728–37.

CHAPTER 2

1. J. A. Fulkerson, M. Story, D. Newmark-Sztainer, and S. Rydell, "Family Meals: Perceptions of Benefits and Challenges among Parents of 8- to 10-Year-Old Children," *Journal of the American Dietetic Association*, 108, no. 4 (2008): 706–9.

2. M. W. Gillman, S. L. Rifas-Shiman, A. L. Frazier, H. R. H. Rockett, C. A. Camargo, A. E. Field, C. S. Berkey, and G. A. Colditz, "Family Dinner and Diet Quality among Older Children and Adolescents," *Archives of Family Medicine*, 9, no. 3 (2000): 235–40.

3. M. A. Eisenberg, R. E. Olson, D. Newmark-Sztainer, M. Story, and L. H. Bearinger, "Correlations between Family Meals and Psychosocial Well-Being among Adolescents," *Archives of Pediatric and Adolescent Medicine*, 158, no. 8 (2004): 792–96.

4. K. N. Boutelle, A. S. Birnbaum, L. A. Lytle, D. M. Murry, and M. Story, "Associations between Perceived Family Meal Environment and Parent Intake of Fruit, Vegetables, and Fat," *Journal of Nutrition Education and Behavior*, 35, no. 1 (2003): 24–29.

5. H. Patrick and T. Nicklas, "A Review of Family and Social Determinants of Children's Eating Patterns and Diet Quality," *Journal of the American College of Nutrition*, 24, no. 2 (2005): 83–92.

6. A. M. Andrade, G. W. Greene, and K. J. Melanson, "Eating Slowly Led to Decreases in Energy Intake within Meals in Healthy Women," *Journal of the American Dietetic Association*, 108, no. 7 (2008): 1186–91.

7. V. J. Rideout, U. G. Foehr, and D. F. Robert, "Generation M2: Media in the Lives of 8- to 18-Year Olds," Henry J. Kaiser Family Foundation, January 2010.

8. M. Bloxham, M. E. Holmes, J. Spaeth, and W. Moult, "Video Consumer Mapping Study. Council for Research Excellence," (2009). Reports, video, and presentation files available online at http://www.researchexcellence.com/vcmstudy.php.

9. United States Department of Agriculture, www.mypyramid.gov.

10. Center for Disease Control and Prevention, "Childhood Overweight and Obesity," http://www.cdc.gov/obesity/childhood/index.html.

11. G. C. Rampersaud, "Benefits of Breakfast for Children and Adolescents: Update and Recommendations for Practitioners," *American Journal of Lifestyle Medicine*, 3, no. 2 (2009): 86–103.

12. J. Fulkerson, D. Neumark-Sztainer, and M. Story, "Adolescent and Parent Views of Family Meals," *Journal of the American Dietetic Association*, 106, no. 4 (2006): 526–32.

13. P. M. Eng, I. Kawachi, G. Fitzmaurice, and E. B. Rimm, "Effects of Marital Transitions on Change in Dietary and Other Health Behaviors in US Male Health Professionals," *Journal of Epidemiology and Community Health*, 59, no. 1 (2005): 56–62.

14. E. A. Bergman, N. S. Buergel, T. F. Englund, and A. Femrite, "The Relationship between the Length of the Lunch Period and Nutrient Consumption in the Elementary School Lunch Setting," *Journal of Child Nutrition and Management*, 28, no.2 (2004).

15. B. Wansink, C. Payne, and C. Werle, "Consequences of Belonging to the 'Clean Plate Club,'" *Archives of Pediatrics and Adolescent Medicine*, 162, no. 10 (2008): 994–95.

16. J. Wardle, M. L. Herrera, L. Cooke, and E. L. Gibson, "Modifying Children's Food Preferences: The Effects of Exposure and Reward on Acceptance of an Unfamiliar Vegetable," *European Journal of Clinical Nutrition*, 57, no. 2 (2003): 341–48.

17. B. Wansink, M. Shimuzu, and C. Payne, "Nudging Healthy Food Consumption in a Preschool Setting" (2009), publication forthcoming.

18. K. E. Leahy, L. L. Birch, J. O. Fisher, and B. J. Rolls, "Reductions in Entrée Energy Density Increase Children's Vegetable Intake and Reduce Energy Intake," *Obesity*, 16, no. 7 (2008): 1559–65.

19. R. C. Whitaker, J. A. Wright, M. S. Pepe, K. D. Seidel, and W. H. Dietz, "Predicting Obesity in Young Adulthood from Childhood and Parental Obesity," *New England Journal of Medicine*, 337, no. 13 (1997): 869–73.

20. National Eating Disorders Association, "Fact Sheet on Eating Disorders," May 2008, www.nationaleatingdisorders.org.

CHAPTER 3

1. L. H. Eck Clemens, D. L. Slawson, and R. C. Klesges, "The Effect of Eating Out on Quality of Diet in Premenopausal Women," *Journal of the American Dietetic Association*, 99, no. 4 (1999): 442–44.

2. C. Zoumas-Morse, C. L. Rock, E. J. Sobo, and M. L. Neuhouser, "Children's Patterns of Macronutrient Intake and Association with Restaurant and Home Eating," *Journal of the American Dietetic Association*, 101, no. 8 (2001): 923–25.

3. O. M. Thompson, C. Ballew, K. Resnicow, A. Must, L. G. Bandini, H. Cyr, and W. H. Dietz, "Food Purchased Away from Home as a Predictor of Change in BMI z-score among Girls," *International Journal of Obesity*, 28 (2004): 282–89.

4. S. Paeratakul, D. P. Ferdinand, C. M. Champagne, D. H. Ryan, and G.A. Bray, "Fast-food Consumption among US Adults and Children: Dietary and Nutrient Intake Profile," *Journal of the American Dietetic Association*, 103, no. 10 (2003): 1332–38.

5. Food Marketing Institute, "2009 US Grocery Shopper Trends."

6. S. I. O'Donnell, S. L. Hoerr, J. A. Mendoza, and E. T. Goh, "Nutrient Quality of Fast-Food Kids' Meals," *American Journal of Clinical Nutrition*, 88, no. 5 (2008): 1388–95.

7. T. Liquori, P. D. Koch, I. R. Contento, and J. Castle, "The Cookshop Program: Outcome Evaluation of a Nutrition Education Program Linking Lunchroom Food Experiences with Classroom Cooking Experiences," *Journal of Nutrition Education*, 30, no. 5 (1998): 302–13.

8. N. I. Larson, M. Story, M .A. Eisenberg, and D. Neumark-Sztainer, "Food Preparation and Purchasing Roles among Adolescents: Associations with Sociodemographic Characteristics and Diet Quality," *Journal of the American Dietetic Association*, 106, no. 2 (2006): 211–18.

9. M. S. Nanney, S. Johnson, M. Elliott, and D. Haire-Joshu, "Frequency of Eating Homegrown Produce Is Associated with Higher Intake among Parents and Their Preschool-Aged Children in Rural Missouri," *Journal of the American Dietetic Association*, 107, no. 4 (2007): 577–84.

10. K. Alaimo, E. Packnett, R. A. Miles, and D. J. Kruger, "Fruit and Vegetable Intake among Urban Community Gardeners," *Journal of Nutrition Education and Behavior*, 40, no. 2 (2008): 94–101.

INDEX

Underscored page references indicate sidebars and tables. **Boldface** references indicate photographs.

Almonds
Almond, Oat, and Dried Cranberry-Cherry Granola, 62
Almond-Apple Crumble, 273
Broccoli Chicken Casserole, 188
Chicken and Almond Dumplings, 186, **187**
Chicken and Bok Choy with Almonds, 154
Haricot Verts, 220
as MUFA, 10
Sugar-Glazed Almond Trail Mix, 249
Alzheimer's disease, MUFAs preventing, 13
Apples
Almond-Apple Crumble, 273
Apples with Honey-Yogurt Dip and Candied Walnuts, 244
Fall Fruit Salad, 208
Orange, Apple, and Jicama Slaw with Shrimp, 101
Pan-Seared Chicken Breasts with Walnuts and Apples, 149
Apple shape, fat distribution in, 4
Apricot nectar
Apricot-Peach Smoothie, 60
Avocados
Avocado Ice Cream, 280
Avocado-Orange Salad, 100
Barbecue Turkey Burgers with Avocado Mash, 123
building meals with, 19
Chicken Cutlets Topped with Turkey Bacon and Avocado, 150, **151**
Chicken Tortilla Casserole, 189
Chilean Avocado, Bean, and Corn Salad, 202
Chili-Dusted Avocado Potatoes, 108, **109**
Citrus-Avocado Gelatin Mold, 257
Fast Tamale Casserole, 198
Grilled Shrimp and Zucchini Tostadas, 114
Mango-Avocado Salsa, 232, **233**
Mashed Avocado Cakes, 238
Mexican Corn Soup, 185

Mexican Eggs, 168
Mexican Pork Stew, 193
as MUFA, 10
in MUFA Serving Chart, 283
Mushroom, Onion, and Avocado Quesadillas, 137
Pan-Seared Shrimp Tacos, **142**, 143
Pork and Sweet Potato Skillet, 161
primer on, 53
Roasted Pepper–Corn Pasta Salad, **210**, 211
Salmon Salad with Avocado-Lime Dressing, 132
South-of-the-Border Baked Potato, 228
Spice-Rubbed Pork Tenderloin with Avocado, Cucumber, and Onion Salad, 126
Spinach-Avocado Caesar Salad, 216, **217**, 229
Super-Quick Breakfast Wraps, 78
Tropical Fruit Salad, 79, 256
Turkey, Avocado, and Cheddar Panini, 87

Bacon, turkey
Chicken Cutlets Topped with Turkey Bacon and Avocado, 150, **151**
Balsamic vinegar
Grilled Tilapia with Balsamic Vinaigrette, 118
Bananas
Bananas Imposter, 199, 278, **279**
Banana Split Muffins, 75
Banana-Walnut Cake, 272
Basic Banana Wrap, 78
Peanut Butter and Banana Malted Milk, 281
Tropical Fruit Salad, 79, 256
Barbecue sauce. *See also* Hoisin sauce
Barbecue Turkey Burgers with Avocado Mash, 123
Easy Barbecue Pita Pizzas, 51, **240**, 241

Shrimp and Broccoli with Peanut BBQ Sauce, 50, 144, 253
Bars
Oatmeal Cookie Bars, 264
Pecan Bars, 38, 265
Basil
Thai Basil-Coconut Chicken, 152
Beans
Chickpea Ragu with Polenta, 141
Chilean Avocado, Bean, and Corn Salad, 202
Chipotle Beef and Bean Chili, 194, **195**
Easy Creamy Bean Soup, 198
5-Bean Salad, 133, **204**, 205
Florentine Baked Beans, 176
Grilled Chicken with Italian Mashed Beans, 132
Super-Fast Chips and Dip, 252
Super-Quick Breakfast Wraps, 78
Beef
Beef Goulash Noodle Casserole, 196
Beefsteak Stuffed with Olives, 167
Caramelized Onion and Swiss Burgers, 51, 128, **129**
Chipotle Beef and Bean Chili, 194, **195**
Grilled Flank Steak with Chimichurri Sauce, 130
Lebanese Beef Patties, **162**, 163
Marinated Beef Tip Roast, 131
Oven-Baked Pot Roast, 197
Spaghetti and Meatballs, 164, **165**
Stovetop Meat Loaf with Mushroom Gravy, 33, 166
Beets
Roasted Beet Salad, 206, **207**
Belly fat
in children, 4–5
Flat Belly Diet for losing, 2, 37
health risks from, 4–5
metabolic syndrome and, 12, 12
MUFAs for losing, 13–14
stubbornness of, 2
subcutaneous, 4
visceral, 4, 13

Berries. *See also specific berries*
   Berry Good Peanut Butter Scones,
      73
Biscotti
   Pistachio Biscotti, 261
Blood sugar
   low, fatigue from, 14
   MUFAs for controlling, 10–11
   regular meals stabilizing, 17, 26
Blueberries
   Blueberry Pie, 133, 276
   Lemon-Blueberry Buttermilk
      Muffins, 74
Body mass index (BMI), 4
Bok choy
   Chicken and Bok Choy with
      Almonds, 154
   Grilled Turkey and Bok Choy with
      Chile-Garlic Sauce, **124**, 125
Bone health, calcium for, 28, 31
Brain development, nutrients for, 6, 18
Brain function, MUFAs improving, 13
Brazil nuts
   Chicken Picadillo, 159
Breads. *See also* Muffins; Pitas
   Cornbread, 199
   Dark Chocolate Zucchini Bread, 33,
      229, 269
   Tomato and Roasted Pepper
      Bruschetta, 236, **237**
Breakfasts
   Almond, Oat, and Dried
      Cranberry-Cherry Granola, 62
   Apricot-Peach Smoothie, 60
   Banana Split Muffins, 75
   Basic Banana Wrap, 78
   Berry Good Peanut Butter Scones,
      73
   Chocolate-Stuffed French Toast,
      70, 71
   Greek Shake, 78
   Honey-Walnut Oatmeal, 78
   Italian-Style Eggs, **64**, 65
   Lemon-Blueberry Buttermilk
      Muffins, 74
   Maple-Pecan Cinnamon Rolls,
      76, **77**
   Maple-Pecan Oatmeal, 61
   Pan-Fried Cheddar Polenta, 66
   Pesto Pinwheels, 68, **69**
   Pomegranate-Strawberry
      Smoothie, 58, **59**
   Scrambled Egg "Pizza," 63
   Super-Quick Breakfast Wraps, 78
   Vegetable Frittata, 67, 79
   Waffle Warm-Up, 78
   Walnut-Pear Pancake with Maple
      Syrup, 72
   for young schoolchildren, 28
Breastfeeding, calorie needs during, 18

Broccoli
   Broccoli Chicken Casserole, 188
   Broccoli Florets with Thai Cashew
      Dip, 239, 253
   Broccoli Pasta Salad, 213
   Cashew, Tofu, and Broccoli
      Stir-Fry, **138**, 139
   Italian Lentil-Broccoli Stew, 173
   Shrimp and Broccoli with Peanut
      BBQ Sauce, 50, 144, 253
Broccoli rabe
   Broccoli Rabe with Toasted Garlic,
      219
Brownies
   Fudgy Dark Chocolate–Raspberry
      Brownies, 262, **263**
Bruschetta
   Tomato and Roasted Pepper
      Bruschetta, 236, **237**
Burgers
   Barbecue Turkey Burgers with
      Avocado Mash, 123
   Caramelized Onion and Swiss
      Burgers, 51, 128, **129**
Buttermilk
   Lemon-Blueberry Buttermilk
      Muffins, 74
Butternut squash
   Butternut Squash Ravioli, 136

Cabbage

   Cucumber Coleslaw, 133
   Thai Peanut Slaw, 215
Cakes. *See also* Cupcakes
   Banana-Walnut Cake, 272
   Chocolate-Orange Snack Cakes, 268
   Lemon Bundt Cake, 270, **271**
   Strawberry Sponge Shortcake, 274,
      275
Calcium
   for children, 31
   for tweens and teens, 28
Calorie needs
   of children, 26, 27
   of men, 28–29
   during pregnancy and
      breastfeeding, 18
Calories. *See also* Calorie needs
   extra, from eating out, 42
   per meal, in Flat Belly Diet, 16–17
Cancer, vitamin E preventing, 31
Canola oil. *See also* Canola oil
      mayonnaise
   Bananas Imposter, 199, 278, **279**
   Beef Goulash Noodle Casserole, 196
   Blueberry Pie, 133, 276
   Carrot Cake Cupcakes with Orange
      Icing, 266, **267**

   Dark Chocolate Zucchini Bread, 33,
      229, 269
   5-Bean Salad, 133, **204**, 205
   Grilled Tomato and Cheese, 84, **85**
   Grilled Turkey and Bok Choy with
      Chile-Garlic Sauce, **124**, 125
   Italian-Style Eggs, **64**, 65
   Lemon-Blueberry Buttermilk
      Muffins, 74
   Pan-Fried Cheddar Polenta, 66
   Salt and Pepper Oven Fries, 224,
      225
   Strawberry Sponge Shortcake, 274,
      275
   Thai Basil-Coconut Chicken, 152
Canola oil mayonnaise
   Chicken and Creamy Pepper Jelly
      Wrap, 86
   Chicken Salad with Wheat
      Crackers, 91
   Fish Nuggets with Tartar Sauce,
      50, 177
   Grilled Shrimp Rolls, 51, 115
   Mexican Grilled Corn on the Cob,
      222, 223
   Salmon Surprise, 102
   Seared Salmon BLT, **88**, 89
   Tuna Noodle Casserole, 180
   Tuna Rotini Salad Toss, 92, **93**
   Turkey on Rye, 102
Carbohydrate, in restaurant meal, 44
Cardiovascular disease, 4, 5, 10, 11, 12
Carrots
   Carrot Cake Cupcakes with Orange
      Icing, 266, **267**
   Carrot Salad, 169
   Roasted Carrots and Hazelnuts,
      221, 229
Cashew butter
   Broccoli Florets with Thai Cashew
      Dip, 239, 253
Cashews. *See also* Cashew butter
   Cashew, Tofu, and Broccoli
      Stir-Fry, **138**, 139
   Cheese Plate, 252
   Chocolate-Covered Pretzels, **250**,
      251
   Indian Chicken in Cashew-Cilantro
      Sauce, 153, 169
Casseroles
   Beef Goulash Noodle Casserole, 196
   Broccoli Chicken Casserole, 188
   Chicken and Yellow Rice Casserole,
      184
   Chicken Tortilla Casserole, 189
   Crunchy Crust Mac and Cheese,
      178, 179, 229
   Fast Tamale Casserole, 198
   Rosemary Pork and Rice Bake, 192
   Tuna Noodle Casserole, 180

Vegetarian Lasagna with Tofu,
174, 175
Cereal
Marshmallow Cereal Bars, 246, 247
Cheeses
Caramelized Onion and Swiss
Burgers, 51, 128, 129
Cheese Plate, 252
Cheesy Baked Pasta, 198
Cheesy Chicken Quesadilla, 132
Crunchy Crust Mac and Cheese,
178, 179, 229
Grilled Tomato and Cheese, 84, 85
Pan-Fried Cheddar Polenta, 66
Pistachio Cheese Spread, 243
Turkey, Avocado, and Cheddar
Panini, 87
Cherries
Almond, Oat, and Dried Cranberry-
Cherry Granola, 62
Quinoa Salad with Cherries and
Pecans, 99
Chicken
Broccoli Chicken Casserole, 188
Cheesy Chicken Quesadilla, 132
Chicken and Almond Dumplings,
186, 187
Chicken and Bok Choy with
Almonds, 154
Chicken and Creamy Pepper Jelly
Wrap, 86
Chicken and Yellow Rice Casserole,
184
Chicken Cacciatore, 158
Chicken Cutlets Topped with
Turkey Bacon and Avocado,
150, 151
Chicken Picadillo, 159
Chicken Salad with Wheat
Crackers, 91
Chicken Tenders with Two Dips,
156, 157
Chicken Thighs with Green Beans,
160, 229
Chicken Tortilla Casserole, 189
Chinese BBQ Chicken Patties, 155
Curried Waldorf Salad, 98
Grilled Chicken Breasts with
Pan-Roasted Tomatoes and
Olives, 119
Grilled Chicken with Italian
Mashed Beans, 132
Indian Chicken in Cashew-Cilantro
Sauce, 153, 169
Mediterranean Chicken Kebabs with
Lemon-Tahini Sauce, 120, 121
Middle Eastern Chopped Salad, 96,
97, 103
Pan-Seared Chicken Breasts with
Walnuts and Apples, 149

poaching, 86
Tandoori Chicken Thighs, 122
Thai Basil-Coconut Chicken, 152
Walnut Chicken, 198
Chickpeas
Chickpea Ragu with Polenta, 141
Childhood obesity, 30
dietary fat and, 6
do's and don'ts about, 36
incidence of, 36
increases in, 5, 27
parental concern about, 3
Children. See also Childhood obesity
belly fat in, 4–5
calorie needs of, 26, 27
diets contraindicated for, 3, 27
exercise for, 15, 26
family meals benefiting, 22–23
fat intake recommendations for, 13
food shopping with, 49
garden grown by, 47
as kitchen helpers, 44–45, 45,
46–47
kitchen safety for, 48
limiting media time of, 25
making recipes appealing to,
48–51
meal frequency for, 26
meeting dietary needs of, 27–28, 29
milk fat recommended for, 6
modeling healthy eating for, 24
nutrients needed by, 30–31
obesity-related health problems
in, 5, 12
as picky eaters, 32–33
preventing emotional eating in,
34–35
preventing high cholesterol in, 8
restaurant meals eaten by, 42
Chile oil
Grilled Turkey and Bok Choy with
Chile-Garlic Sauce, 124, 125
Chili
Chipotle Beef and Bean Chili, 194,
195
Chili powder
Chili-Dusted Avocado Potatoes,
108, 109
Chimichurri sauce
Grilled Flank Steak with
Chimichurri Sauce, 130
Chipotle pepper
Chipotle Beef and Bean Chili, 194,
195
Chocolate, dark
building meals with, 19
Chocolate-Covered Pretzels, 250,
251
Chocolate-Orange Snack Cakes,
268

Chocolate-Stuffed French Toast,
70, 71
Dark Chocolate Swirled Meringues,
260
Dark Chocolate Zucchini Bread, 33,
229, 269
Emergency Fondue, 252
Fudgy Dark Chocolate–Raspberry
Brownies, 262, 263
Marshmallow Cereal Bars, 246,
247
vs. milk chocolate, 53
as MUFA, 10
in MUFA Serving Chart, 283
Oatmeal Cookie Bars, 264
primer on, 53–54
Cholesterol levels. See also HDL
cholesterol; LDL cholesterol
effect of dietary fats on, 8
effect of waist circumference on, 5
fiber lowering, 31
MUFAs improving, 11
type 2 diabetes and, 11
Chowder
Corn and Potato Chowder, 172
Cilantro
Indian Chicken in Cashew-Cilantro
Sauce, 153, 169
Cinnamon rolls
Maple-Pecan Cinnamon Rolls,
76, 77
Clams
Spaghetti with White Clam Sauce,
145
Coconut
Macadamia Coconut Clusters, 245
Coconut milk
Thai Basil-Coconut Chicken, 152
Cod
Fish Nuggets with Tartar Sauce,
50, 177
Cookies
Crunchy Peanut Butter Cookies, 38,
258, 259
Dark Chocolate Swirled Meringues,
260
Oatmeal Cookie Bars, 264
Pistachio Biscotti, 261
Cooking own meals
benefits of, 40, 42
family participation in, 43–47
Cooking techniques, 54–55
Cooking while dieting, challenges
of, 20
Corn
Chilean Avocado, Bean, and Corn
Salad, 202
Corn and Potato Chowder, 172
"Fried" Corn, 228
Mexican Corn Soup, 185

Corn (*cont.*)
  Mexican Grilled Corn on the Cob,
    222, 223
  Roasted Pepper–Corn Pasta Salad,
    210, 211
Cornmeal
  Cornbread, 199
Coronary artery disease, 5, 9
Coronary heart disease, 10
Couscous
  Middle Eastern Couscous, 168
Cranberries
  Almond, Oat, and Dried Cranberry-
    Cherry Granola, 62
Cravings, food, 17, 34
Crumble
  Almond-Apple Crumble, 273
Cucumbers
  Cucumber Coleslaw, 133
  Middle Eastern Chopped Salad, 96,
    97, 103
  Spice-Rubbed Pork Tenderloin with
    Avocado, Cucumber, and
    Onion Salad, 126
Cupcakes
  Carrot Cake Cupcakes with Orange
    Icing, 266, **267**
Curry powder
  Curried Waldorf Salad, 98

Dairy products, in Family Snack
    Pack Guide, 286

Dark chocolate. *See* Chocolate, dark
Desserts
  Almond-Apple Crumble, 273
  Avocado Ice Cream, 280
  Bananas Imposter, 199, 278, **279**
  Banana-Walnut Cake, 272
  Blueberry Pie, 133, 276
  Carrot Cake Cupcakes with Orange
    Icing, 266, **267**
  Chocolate-Orange Snack Cakes,
    268
  Citrus-Avocado Gelatin Mold, 257
  Crunchy Peanut Butter Cookies, 38,
    258, 259
  Dark Chocolate Swirled Meringues,
    260
  Dark Chocolate Zucchini Bread, 33,
    229, 269
  Fudgy Dark Chocolate–Raspberry
    Brownies, 262, **263**
  Lemon Bundt Cake, 270, **271**
  Mango Tart with Macadamia
    Crust, 169, 277
  Oatmeal Cookie Bars, 264
  Peanut Butter and Banana Malted
    Milk, 281

Pecan Bars, 38, 265
Pistachio Biscotti, 261
Strawberry Sponge Shortcake, 274,
  275
Tropical Fruit Salad, 79, 256
Diabetes, type 2
  from belly fat, 4
  blood sugar control in, 10–11
  in children, 5
  metabolic syndrome and, 5, 12
"Diet," redefining, 3
Dieting
  contraindicated for children, 3, 27
  cooking for others while, 20
Dill
  Pan-Roasted Sunflower Seeds with
    Dill, 234
Dips and spreads
  as appealing to children, 50
  Apples with Honey-Yogurt Dip and
    Candied Walnuts, 244
  Broccoli Florets with Thai Cashew
    Dip, 239, **253**
  Chicken Tenders with Two Dips,
    156, **157**
  Pistachio Cheese Spread, 243
  Super-Fast Chips and Dip, 252
Dumplings
  Chicken and Almond Dumplings,
    186, **187**

Eating disorders, signs of, 38
Eating frequency, on Flat Belly Diet,
  17, 26
Eating out
  vs. eating at home, 43
  extra calories from, 42
  Flat Belly Diet guidelines for, 44
Eating slowly, benefits of, 24
Edamame
  Pineapple-Edamame Salad, 102
  Steamed Edamame, 253
Eggplant
  Grilled Eggplant Pasta with Garlic
    Oil, 132
Eggs
  Italian-Style Eggs, **64**, 65
  Mexican Eggs, 168
  Pesto Pinwheels, 68, **69**
  Scrambled Egg "Pizza," 63
  Vegetable Frittata, 67, 79
Elderly people, nutritional needs of,
  27, 30
Emotional eating, preventing,
  34–35
Energy
  from exercise, 15
  from Flat Belly Diet, 14

English muffins
  English Muffin Pizzas, 242
Exercise, family activities for, 15, 26

Family. *See also* Family mealtime
  cooking with, 43–47
  Flat Belly Diet for, 3, 20, 22
    benefits of, 22–24
  naming dishes after, 46
  weight-loss support from, 37–38
Family mealtime
  avoiding arguments during, 35
  benefits of, 22–23
  finding time for, 23, 28
Family Snack Pack Guide, 285–87
Family-Style Buffet Menu, 229
Fast-food meals, 42, 43
Fat-free foods, problems with, 6
Fatigue, from low blood sugar, 14
Fats, dietary
  diets limiting, 6
  functions of, 6–7
  holding, in restaurant meals, 44
  monounsaturated fats (*see* MUFAs)
  in oils, 11
  polyunsaturated fats, 9, 12
  recommendations on, for children, 6
  saturated fats, 7–8, 13, 42
  trans fats, 7, 7, 8
Fiber, for children, 31
Fish. *See* Halibut; Salmon; Tilapia;
    Tuna
  Fish Nuggets with Tartar Sauce,
    50, 177
Flat Belly Diet
  benefits of, x, 2, 14–15, 22–24
  building meals in, 18–19
  eating out on, 44
  family-friendly plan for, 3, 20, 22
  meeting family needs with, 27–30
  MUFAs in (*see* MUFAs)
  principles of, for whole family,
    24–26
  rules of, 16–17, 37
  saving money with, 42
  weight loss from, 2, 37–39
Flat Belly Diet!, 16, 25
Flatbellydiet.com, 16, 39
Flat Belly Diet! Cookbook, 16
Flat Belly Diet! Diabetes, 2
Flat Belly Diet! for Men, 2, 29
Flat Belly Diet! Pocket Guide, 16
Flaxseed oil
  Greek Shake, 78
  Pomegranate-Strawberry
    Smoothie, 58, **59**
Fondue
  Emergency Fondue, 252

Food journal, 39
Food labels
    estimating nutrient values on, 54
    reading, with children, 49
    trans fats on, 7, 8
Food preparation techniques, 54–55
Food presentation, kid-friendly, 50
Food shopping, with children, 49
Food variety
    in Flat Belly Diet, 14–15
    for toddlers and preschoolers, 27
Four-Day Anti-Bloat Jumpstart, 16, 17
14-Day Meal Plan, 15, 18, 288–95
French toast
    Chocolate-Stuffed French Toast,
        70, 71
Frittata
    Vegetable Frittata, 67, 79
Fruit juice cubes, for smoothies, 58
Fruits. See also specific fruits
    Fall Fruit Salad, 208
    in Family Snack Pack Guide, 286
    Tropical Fruit Salad, 79, 256

Garden, benefits of growing, 47
Garlic
    Broccoli Rabe with Toasted Garlic,
        219
    Garlic Mashed Potatoes, 226
    Grilled Eggplant Pasta with Garlic
        Oil, 132
    Grilled Turkey and Bok Choy with
        Chile-Garlic Sauce, 124, 125
Gelatin
    Citrus-Avocado Gelatin Mold, 257
Grains. See also specific grains
    in Family Snack Pack Guide, 285
Granola
    Almond, Oat, and Dried Cranberry-
        Cherry Granola, 62
Gravy
    Stovetop Meat Loaf with
        Mushroom Gravy, 33, 166
Green beans
    Chicken Thighs with Green Beans,
        160, 229
    Green Bean and Pumpkin Seed
        Salad, 209
    Green Beans with Tapenade, 228
    Haricot Verts, 220
Greens. See also specific greens
    Creamy Sesame Greens, 218
Grilled dishes
    Barbecued Pork Tenderloin, 127, 133
    Barbecue Turkey Burgers with
        Avocado Mash, 123
    Caramelized Onion and Swiss
        Burgers, 51, 128, 129

Cheesy Chicken Quesadilla, 132
Chili-Dusted Avocado Potatoes,
    108, 109
Grilled Chicken Breasts with
    Pan-Roasted Tomatoes and
    Olives, 119
Grilled Chicken with Italian
    Mashed Beans, 132
Grilled Eggplant Pasta with Garlic
    Oil, 132
Grilled Flank Steak with
    Chimichurri Sauce, 130
Grilled Shrimp and Tapenade Pita,
    132
Grilled Shrimp and Zucchini
    Tostadas, 114
Grilled Shrimp Rolls, 51, 115
Grilled Tilapia with Balsamic
    Vinaigrette, 118
Grilled Tofu Cutlets, 111
Grilled Turkey and Bok Choy with
    Chile-Garlic Sauce, 124, 125
Grilled Zucchini Boats, 107
Italian Vegetable Spiedini, 106
Lemon Shrimp with Roasted
    Peppers, 112, 113
Marinated Beef Tip Roast, 131
Mediterranean Chicken Kebabs
    with Lemon-Tahini Sauce,
    120, 121
Salmon Salad with Avocado-Lime
    Dressing, 132
Salmon with Sizzling Sesame
    Scallions, 116, 117
Seared Portobello "Steaks," 110
Spice-Rubbed Pork Tenderloin with
    Avocado, Cucumber, and
    Onion Salad, 126
Tandoori Chicken Thighs, 122
Grilling, 54–55

Halibut
    Halibut with Chopped Olive Salad,
        146, 147
Ham
    Shrimp and Ham Jambalaya, 182,
        183, 199
Handheld foods, appeal of, 50–51
Haricot Verts, 220
Hass avocado. See Avocados
Hazelnuts
    Roasted Carrots and Hazelnuts,
        221, 229
HDL cholesterol, 5, 8, 11
Heart disease, 4, 8, 31
Hearty Picnic Menu, 103
High blood pressure, 5, 9–10, 12, 31
High-protein diets, problems with, 6

Hoisin sauce
    Chinese BBQ Chicken Patties, 155
Honey
    Apples with Honey-Yogurt Dip and
        Candied Walnuts, 244
    Honey-Walnut Oatmeal, 78
Hypertension. See High blood pressure

Ice cream
    Avocado Ice Cream, 280
    Caramel-Pecan Sundae, 252
    Peanut Butter and Banana Malted
        Milk, 281
Icing
    Carrot Cake Cupcakes with Orange
        Icing, 266, 267
Impromptu Party Menu, 253
Insulin resistance, 5, 10, 12

Jalapeño jelly
    Chicken and Creamy Pepper Jelly
        Wrap, 86
Jambalaya
    Shrimp and Ham Jambalaya, 182,
        183, 199
Jicama
    Orange, Apple, and Jicama Slaw
        with Shrimp, 101
Junk food, avoiding, 38–39

Kale
    Creamy Sesame Greens, 218
Katz, David, 2
Kebabs
    Italian Vegetable Spiedini, 106
    Mediterranean Chicken Kebabs with
        Lemon-Tahini Sauce, 120, 121
Kitchen safety, for children, 48
Kitchen scale, 90

Lasagna
    Vegetarian Lasagna with Tofu,
        174, 175
LDL cholesterol, 5, 8, 9, 10, 11
Legumes. See also specific legumes
    in MUFA Serving Chart, 283
Lemons
    Lemon-Blueberry Buttermilk
        Muffins, 74
    Lemon Bundt Cake, 270, 271
    Lemon Shrimp with Roasted
        Peppers, 112, 113

Corn (*cont.*)
  Mediterranean Chicken Kebabs
    with Lemon-Tahini Sauce,
    120, **121**
Lentils
  Italian Lentil-Broccoli Stew, 173
Limes
  Salmon Salad with Avocado-Lime
    Dressing, 132
Lunches
  Avocado-Orange Salad, 100
  Chicken and Creamy Pepper Jelly
    Wrap, 86
  Chicken Salad with Wheat
    Crackers, 91
  Curried Waldorf Salad, 98
  Grilled Tomato and Cheese, 84, **85**
  Middle Eastern Chopped Salad, 96,
    97, 103
  Nutty Noodles, 102
  Olive Spread Wrap, 102
  Orange, Apple, and Jicama Slaw
    with Shrimp, 101
  Peanut Butter–Strawberry Wrap,
    82, **83**
  Penne Pasta Salad, 95
  Pineapple-Edamame Salad, 102
  Quinoa Salad with Cherries and
    Pecans, 99
  Salmon Surprise, 102
  for schoolchildren, 28, 29
  Seared Salmon BLT, **88**, 89
  Sweet Potato Salad, 94
  Thai Butterfly Pasta Salad, 90
  Tuna Rotini Salad Toss, 92, **93**
  Turkey, Avocado, and Cheddar
    Panini, 87
  Turkey on Rye, 102

Macadamia nuts
  Macadamia Coconut Clusters,
    245
  Mango Tart with Macadamia
    Crust, 169, 277
Macaroni
  Crunchy Crust Mac and Cheese,
    178, 179, 229
Magnesium, for children, 30
"Make It a Team Effort" tips, 46
"Make It Faster" tips, 43
Mangoes
  Mango-Avocado Salsa, 232, **233**
  Mango Tart with Macadamia
    Crust, 169, 277
  Tropical Fruit Salad, 79, 256
Maple syrup
  Maple-Pecan Cinnamon Rolls,
    76, **77**

Maple-Pecan Oatmeal, 61
  Walnut-Pear Pancake with Maple
    Syrup, 72
Marshmallows
  Marshmallow Cereal Bars, 246,
    247
Meal frequency, on Flat Belly Diet,
    17, 26
Meal Plan, 14-Day, 15, 18, 288–95
Meal planning
  family involvement in, 46
  for weight loss, 39
Measuring foods, 37
  kitchen scale for, 90
Media time, limiting, 25
Mediterranean diet, 9, 14
Men, calorie needs of, 28–29
Menus
  Family-Style Buffet, 229
  Hearty Picnic, 103
  Impromptu Party, 253
  Perfect Summer Cookout, 133
  Watching the "Big Game," 199
  Weekend Brunch, 79, 169
Meringues
  Dark Chocolate Swirled Meringues,
    260
Metabolic syndrome, 5, 12, 12
Me-time, for women, 34
Milk
  fat in, for children, 6
  Peanut Butter and Banana Malted
    Milk, 281
  for tweens and teens, 28
Milk chocolate, 53
Money saving, from Flat Belly Diet,
    42
Monounsaturated fats. *See* MUFAs
MUFAs, **21.** *See also specific MUFAs*
  adding, to restaurant meal, 44
  building meals with, 18–19
  in Flat Belly Diet, 3
  health benefits from, 8, 9–13
  measuring, 37
  during pregnancy and
    breastfeeding, 18
  servings of, per meal, 16
  for vitamin absorption, 8
MUFA Serving Chart, 283
Muffins
  Banana Split Muffins, 75
  Lemon-Blueberry Buttermilk
    Muffins, 74
Mushrooms
  Mushroom, Onion, and Avocado
    Quesadillas, 137
  Seared Portobello "Steaks,"
    110
  Stovetop Meat Loaf with
    Mushroom Gravy, 33, 166

Nut allergies, 52
Nut butters. *See also specific nut
    butters*
  as alternative to peanut butter, 52
  primer on, 52–53
Nutrients, needed by children, 30–31
Nutrition Facts Panel
  for estimating nutrient values, 54
  trans fats on, 7, 8
Nuts. *See also specific nuts*
  building meals with, 18
  in MUFA Serving Chart, 283
  primer on, 52–53
  as snack, 16

Oats
  Almond, Oat, and Dried Cranberry-
    Cherry Granola, 62
  Honey-Walnut Oatmeal, 78
  Maple-Pecan Oatmeal, 61
  Oatmeal Cookie Bars, 264
Oils. *See also specific oils*
  building meals with, 18
  in MUFA Serving Chart, 283
  primer on, 51
  types of fats in, 11
Olive oil
  Bread Salad, 228
  Broccoli Rabe with Toasted Garlic,
    219
  Cheesy Baked Pasta, 198
  Cheesy Chicken Quesadilla, 132
  Chicken Tenders with Two Dips,
    156, **157**
  Crunchy Crust Mac and Cheese,
    178, 179, 229
  Cupboard Pasta, 168
  Easy Barbecue Pita Pizzas, 51, **240**,
    241
  Easy Creamy Bean Soup, 198
  Florentine Baked Beans, 176
  "Fried" Corn, 228
  Garlic Mashed Potatoes, 226
  Grilled Chicken with Italian
    Mashed Beans, 132
  Grilled Eggplant Pasta with Garlic
    Oil, 132
  Grilled Flank Steak with
    Chimichurri Sauce, 130
  Grilled Tilapia with Balsamic
    Vinaigrette, 118
  health benefits from, 9–10
  Italian Vegetable Spiedini, 106
  Lebanese Beef Patties, **162**, 163
  Marinated Beef Tip Roast, 131
  Middle Eastern Chopped Salad, 96,
    97, 103

Middle Eastern Couscous, 168
Oven-Baked Pot Roast, 197
Pasta Salad with Caramelized
    Onions and Zucchini, 212
Penne with Cherry Tomatoes, 140
Scrambled Egg "Pizza," 63
Shrimp and Ham Jambalaya, **182**,
    183, <u>199</u>
Southern-Style Baked Shrimp, 181,
    <u>199</u>
Spaghetti and Meatballs, 164,
    165
Spaghetti with White Clam Sauce,
    145
Super-Fast Chips and Dip, 252
Tomato and Roasted Pepper
    Bruschetta, 236, **237**
Olives. *See also* Tapenade
    Beefsteak Stuffed with Olives, 167
    Broccoli Pasta Salad, 213
    building meals with, 19
    Chicken and Yellow Rice Casserole,
        184
    Chicken Cacciatore, 158
    Grilled Chicken Breasts with
        Pan-Roasted Tomatoes and
        Olives, 119
    Grilled Zucchini Boats, 107
    Halibut with Chopped Olive Salad,
        146, **147**
    Italian Lentil-Broccoli Stew, 173
    in MUFA Serving Chart, <u>283</u>
    Olive Spread Wrap, 102
    primer on, 51–52
    Sicilian Tuna Salad, 214
    Spicy Spaghetti, 168
    Tomato-Olive Salad, 203
Omega-3 fatty acids, 9, <u>18</u>
Onions
    Caramelized Onion and Swiss
        Burgers, 51, 128, **129**
    Italian Vegetable Spiedini, 106
    Mushroom, Onion, and Avocado
        Quesadillas, 137
    Pasta Salad with Caramelized
        Onions and Zucchini, 212
    Spice-Rubbed Pork Tenderloin with
        Avocado, Cucumber, and
        Onion Salad, 126
    Vegetable Frittata, 67, <u>79</u>
Orange extract
    Chocolate-Orange Snack Cakes,
        268
Oranges
    Avocado-Orange Salad, 100
    Carrot Cake Cupcakes with Orange
        Icing, 266, **267**
    Citrus-Avocado Gelatin Mold, 257
    Orange, Apple, and Jicama Slaw
        with Shrimp, 101

Pancakes
    Walnut-Pear Pancake with Maple
        Syrup, 72
Panini
    Turkey, Avocado, and Cheddar
        Panini, 87
Pasta
    Beef Goulash Noodle Casserole, 196
    Broccoli Pasta Salad, 213
    Butternut Squash Ravioli, 136
    Cheesy Baked Pasta, 198
    Crunchy Crust Mac and Cheese,
        178, 179, <u>229</u>
    Cupboard Pasta, 168
    Grilled Eggplant Pasta with Garlic
        Oil, 132
    Italian Orzo Salad, 228
    Nutty Noodles, 102
    Pasta Salad with Caramelized
        Onions and Zucchini, 212
    Penne Pasta Salad, 95
    Penne with Cherry Tomatoes, 140
    Roasted Pepper–Corn Pasta Salad,
        210, 211
    Spaghetti and Meatballs, 164, **165**
    Spaghetti with White Clam Sauce,
        145
    Spicy Spaghetti, 168
    Thai Butterfly Pasta Salad, 90
    Tuna Noodle Casserole, 180
    Tuna Rotini Salad Toss, 92, **93**
    Vegetarian Lasagna with Tofu,
        174, 175
Peaches
    Apricot-Peach Smoothie, 60
Peanut allergy, <u>52</u>
Peanut butter
    alternatives to, <u>52</u>
    Barbecued Pork Tenderloin, 127,
        <u>133</u>
    Basic Banana Wrap, 78
    Berry Good Peanut Butter Scones,
        73
    Crunchy Peanut Butter Cookies, 38,
        258, 259
    Nutty Noodles, 102
    PB and Pineapple Snack Sandwich,
        252
    Peanut Butter and Banana Malted
        Milk, 281
    Peanut Butter–Strawberry Wrap,
        82, **83**
    Quick Peanut Stew, 198
    Shrimp and Broccoli with Peanut
        BBQ Sauce, 50, 144, <u>253</u>
    spreading, <u>82</u>
    Waffle Warm-Up, 78
Peanuts. *See also* Peanut butter
    Asian Snack Mix, 235, <u>253</u>

Chicken Thighs with Green Beans,
    160, <u>229</u>
Easy Peanut Brittle, 248
Thai Peanut Slaw, 215
Pears
    Fall Fruit Salad, 208
    Walnut-Pear Pancake with Maple
        Syrup, 72
Pear shapes, fat distribution in, 4
Pecans
    Caramel-Pecan Sundae, 252
    Maple-Pecan Cinnamon Rolls, 76, **77**
    Maple-Pecan Oatmeal, 61
    Pecan Bars, 38, 265
    Quinoa Salad with Cherries and
        Pecans, 99
Peppers
    Lemon Shrimp with Roasted
        Peppers, **112**, 113
    Middle Eastern Chopped Salad, 96,
        97, <u>103</u>
    Roasted Pepper–Corn Pasta Salad,
        210, 211
    Tomato and Roasted Pepper
        Bruschetta, 236, **237**
Perfect Summer Cookout Menu, <u>133</u>
Pesto sauce
    Lemon Shrimp with Roasted
        Peppers, **112**, 113
    Penne Pasta Salad, 95
    Pesto Pinwheels, 68, **69**
    Pesto Polenta, 168
    Vegetarian Lasagna with Tofu,
        174, 175
Picky eaters, 32–33, 48–49
Pie (dessert)
    Blueberry Pie, <u>133</u>, 276
Pie (savory)
    Turkey Pot Pies, **190**, 191
Pilaf
    Golden Rice Pilaf, <u>169</u>, 227
Pineapple
    PB and Pineapple Snack Sandwich,
        252
    Pineapple-Edamame Salad, 102
    Tropical Fruit Salad, <u>79</u>, 256
Pine nuts
    Chinese BBQ Chicken Patties, 155
    Italian Orzo Salad, 228
    Rosemary Pork and Rice Bake, 192
Pistachios
    Golden Rice Pilaf, <u>169</u>, 227
    Pistachio Biscotti, 261
    Pistachio Cheese Spread, 243
Pitas
    Bread Salad, 228
    Easy Barbecue Pita Pizzas, 51, **240**,
        241
    Grilled Shrimp and Tapenade Pita,
        132

Pizzas
    Easy Barbecue Pita Pizzas, 51, **240**, 241
    English Muffin Pizzas, 242
    Scrambled Egg "Pizza," 63
Poaching, 55
Polenta
    Chickpea Ragu with Polenta, 141
    Pan-Fried Cheddar Polenta, 66
    Pesto Polenta, 168
Polyunsaturated fats, 9, 12
Pomegranate juice
    Pomegranate-Strawberry Smoothie, 58, **59**
Popcorn
    Asian Snack Mix, 235, 253
Pork
    Barbecued Pork Tenderloin, 127, 133
    Mexican Pork Stew, 193
    Pork and Sweet Potato Skillet, 161
    Rosemary Pork and Rice Bake, 192
    Spice-Rubbed Pork Tenderloin with Avocado, Cucumber, and Onion Salad, 126
Potassium, for children, 31
Potatoes
    Chili-Dusted Avocado Potatoes, 108, **109**
    Corn and Potato Chowder, 172
    Garlic Mashed Potatoes, 226
    Oven Roasted Potatoes, 79
    Salt and Pepper Oven Fries, 224, **225**
    South-of-the-Border Baked Potato, 228
Pot pies
    Turkey Pot Pies, **190**, 191
Pregnancy, calorie needs during, 18
Pretzels
    Chocolate-Covered Pretzels, **250**, 251
Protein
    in Family Snack Pack Guide, 287
    in MUFAs, 42
    in restaurant meals, 44
    for seniors, 30
Pumpkin seeds
    Chipotle Beef and Bean Chili, 194, **195**
    Green Bean and Pumpkin Seed Salad, 209
    Orange, Apple, and Jicama Slaw with Shrimp, 101

Quesadillas
    Cheesy Chicken Quesadilla, 132
    Mushroom, Onion, and Avocado Quesadillas, 137

Quick-Fix Pantry Rescues
    breakfast, 78
    casseroles and stews, 198
    grilled dishes, 132
    lunch, 102
    on-the-go meals, 23
    salads and side dishes, 228
    for saving time, 43
    snacks, 252
    stovetop dishes, 168
    whole foods in, 25
Quinoa
    Quinoa Salad with Cherries and Pecans, 99

Raisins
    Fall Fruit Salad, 208
Raspberries
    Fudgy Dark Chocolate–Raspberry Brownies, 262, **263**
Ravioli
    Butternut Squash Ravioli, 136
Recipes. *See also specific recipes*
    as family-friendly, 15, 20, 22
    family members choosing, 46
    increasing family-friendly appeal of, 48–51
    shopping lists for, 39
Restaurant meals. *See* Eating out
Rice
    Chicken and Yellow Rice Casserole, 184
    Curried Waldorf Salad, 98
    Golden Rice Pilaf, 169, 227
    Rosemary Pork and Rice Bake, 192
Roasting, 54
Rosemary
    Rosemary Pork and Rice Bake, 192

Safety, kitchen, for children, 48
Safflower oil
    Lemon Bundt Cake, 270, **271**
    Turkey Pot Pies, **190**, 191
Salads
    Avocado-Orange Salad, 100
    Bread Salad, 228
    Broccoli Pasta Salad, 213
    Carrot Salad, 169
    Chicken Salad with Wheat Crackers, 91
    Chilean Avocado, Bean, and Corn Salad, 202
    Cucumber Coleslaw, 133
    Curried Waldorf Salad, 98
    Fall Fruit Salad, 208
    5-Bean Salad, 133, **204**, 205

Green Bean and Pumpkin Seed Salad, 209
    Halibut with Chopped Olive Salad, 146, **147**
    Italian Orzo Salad, 228
    Middle Eastern Chopped Salad, 96, **97**, 103
    Orange, Apple, and Jicama Slaw with Shrimp, 101
    Pasta Salad with Caramelized Onions and Zucchini, 212
    Penne Pasta Salad, 95
    Pineapple-Edamame Salad, 102
    Quinoa Salad with Cherries and Pecans, 99
    Roasted Beet Salad, 206, **207**
    Roasted Pepper–Corn Pasta Salad, **210**, 211
    Salmon Salad with Avocado-Lime Dressing, 132
    Sicilian Tuna Salad, 214
    Spice-Rubbed Pork Tenderloin with Avocado, Cucumber, and Onion Salad, 126
    Spinach-Avocado Caesar Salad, 216, **217**, 229
    Sweet Potato Salad, 94
    Thai Butterfly Pasta Salad, 90
    Thai Peanut Slaw, 215
    Tomato-Olive Salad, 203
    Tropical Fruit Salad, 79, 256
    Tuna Rotini Salad Toss, 92, **93**
Salmon
    Salmon Salad with Avocado-Lime Dressing, 132
    Salmon Surprise, 102
    Salmon with Sizzling Sesame Scallions, 116, **117**
    Seared Salmon BLT, **88**, 89
Salsa
    Mango-Avocado Salsa, 232, **233**
Sandwiches. *See also* Burgers; Wraps
    Grilled Shrimp Rolls, 51, 115
    Grilled Tomato and Cheese, 84, **85**
    PB and Pineapple Snack Sandwich, 252
    Seared Salmon BLT, **88**, 89
    Turkey, Avocado, and Cheddar Panini, 87
Sassy Water, 17
Satisfaction, from Flat Belly Diet, 14
Saturated fat, 7–8, 13, 42
Sauces
    Fish Nuggets with Tartar Sauce, 50, 177
    Grilled Flank Steak with Chimichurri Sauce, 130
    Grilled Turkey and Bok Choy with Chile-Garlic Sauce, **124**, 125

Indian Chicken in Cashew-Cilantro
    Sauce, 153, 169
Mediterranean Chicken Kebabs
    with Lemon-Tahini Sauce,
    120, **121**
Shrimp and Broccoli with Peanut
    BBQ Sauce, 50, 144, 253
Spaghetti with White Clam Sauce,
    145
Scale, kitchen, 90
Scallions
    Salmon with Sizzling Sesame
        Scallions, 116, **117**
Scones
    Berry Good Peanut Butter Scones,
        73
Seeds. *See also specific seeds*
    building meals with, 18
    in MUFA Serving Chart, 283
    primer on, 52–53
Seniors, nutritional needs of, 27, 30
Sesame seeds
    Salmon with Sizzling Sesame
        Scallions, 116, **117**
    Sesame-Crusted Tuna Steaks, 148
Shakes
    Greek Shake, 78
    Peanut Butter and Banana Malted
        Milk, 281
Shellfish. *See* Clams; Shrimp
Shopping for food, with children, 49
Shopping lists, for recipes, 39
Shrimp
    Grilled Shrimp and Tapenade Pita,
        132
    Grilled Shrimp and Zucchini
        Tostadas, 114
    Grilled Shrimp Rolls, 51, 115
    Lemon Shrimp with Roasted
        Peppers, **112**, 113
    Orange, Apple, and Jicama Slaw
        with Shrimp, 101
    Pan-Seared Shrimp Tacos, **142**, 143
    Shrimp and Broccoli with Peanut
        BBQ Sauce, 50, 144, 253
    Shrimp and Ham Jambalaya, **182**,
        183, 199
    Southern-Style Baked Shrimp, 181,
        199
Side dishes
    Broccoli Rabe with Toasted Garlic,
        219
    Creamy Sesame Greens, 218
    "Fried" Corn, 228
    Garlic Mashed Potatoes, 226
    Golden Rice Pilaf, 169, 227
    Green Beans with Tapenade, 228
    Haricots Verts, 220
    Mexican Grilled Corn on the Cob,
        222, 223

Roasted Carrots and Hazelnuts,
    221, 229
Salt and Pepper Oven Fries, 224,
    225
South-of-the-Border Baked Potato,
    228
Slaws
    Cucumber Coleslaw, 133
    Orange, Apple, and Jicama Slaw
        with Shrimp, 101
    Thai Peanut Slaw, 215
Smoothies
    Apricot-Peach Smoothie, 60
    fruit juice cubes for, 58
    Pomegranate-Strawberry
        Smoothie, 58, **59**
Snacks
    Apples with Honey-Yogurt Dip and
        Candied Walnuts, 244
    Asian Snack Mix, 235, 253
    Broccoli Florets with Thai Cashew
        Dip, 239, 253
    Caramel-Pecan Sundae, 252
    Cheese Plate, 252
    Chocolate-Covered Pretzels, **250**,
        251
    Easy Barbecue Pita Pizzas, 51, **240**,
        241
    Easy Peanut Brittle, 248
    Emergency Fondue, 252
    English Muffin Pizzas, 242
    Family Snack Pack Guide to,
        285–87
    Macadamia Coconut Clusters, 245
    Mango-Avocado Salsa, 232, **233**
    Marshmallow Cereal Bars, 246, **247**
    Mashed Avocado Cakes, 238
    nuts as, 16
    Pan-Roasted Sunflower Seeds with
        Dill, 234
    PB and Pineapple Snack Sandwich,
        252
    Pistachio Cheese Spread, 243
    Sugar-Glazed Almond Trail Mix, 249
    Super-Fast Chips and Dip, 252
    Tomato and Roasted Pepper
        Bruschetta, 236, **237**
Soups
    Chicken and Almond Dumplings,
        186, **187**
    Corn and Potato Chowder, 172
    Easy Creamy Bean Soup, 198
    Mexican Corn Soup, 185
Spices. *See also specific spices*
    Spice-Rubbed Pork Tenderloin with
        Avocado, Cucumber, and
        Onion Salad, 126
Spinach
    Spinach-Avocado Caesar Salad,
        216, **217**, 229

Spreads. *See* Dips and spreads
Squash. *See* Butternut squash; Yellow
    squash; Zucchini
Stews
    Chickpea Ragu with Polenta, 141
    Italian Lentil-Broccoli Stew, 173
    Mexican Pork Stew, 193
    Quick Peanut Stew, 198
Stir-fries
    Cashew, Tofu, and Broccoli Stir-
        Fry, **138**, 139
    Chicken and Bok Choy with
        Almonds, 154
Stir-frying, 55
Stovetop dishes
    Beefsteak Stuffed with Olives,
        167
    Butternut Squash Ravioli, 136
    Cashew, Tofu, and Broccoli Stir-
        Fry, **138**, 139
    Chicken and Bok Choy with
        Almonds, 154
    Chicken Cacciatore, 158
    Chicken Cutlets Topped with
        Turkey Bacon and Avocado,
        150, **151**
    Chicken Picadillo, 159
    Chicken Tenders with Two Dips,
        156, **157**
    Chicken Thighs with Green Beans,
        160, 229
    Chickpea Ragu with Polenta, 141
    Chinese BBQ Chicken Patties, 155
    Cupboard Pasta, 168
    Halibut with Chopped Olive Salad,
        146, **147**
    Indian Chicken in Cashew-Cilantro
        Sauce, 153, 169
    Lebanese Beef Patties, **162**, 163
    Mexican Eggs, 168
    Middle Eastern Couscous, 168
    Mushroom, Onion, and Avocado
        Quesadillas, 137
    Pan-Seared Chicken Breasts with
        Walnuts and Apples, 149
    Pan-Seared Shrimp Tacos, **142**,
        143
    Penne with Cherry Tomatoes, 140
    Pesto Polenta, 168
    Pork and Sweet Potato Skillet, 161
    Sesame-Crusted Tuna Steaks, 148
    Shrimp and Broccoli with Peanut
        BBQ Sauce, 50, 144, 253
    Spaghetti and Meatballs, 164, **165**
    Spaghetti with White Clam Sauce,
        145
    Spicy Spaghetti, 168
    Stovetop Meat Loaf with
        Mushroom Gravy, 33, 166
    Thai Basil-Coconut Chicken, 152

Strawberries
  Peanut Butter–Strawberry Wrap, 82, **83**
  Pomegranate-Strawberry Smoothie, 58, **59**
  Strawberry Sponge Shortcake, 274, **275**
Stroke, vitamin E preventing, 31
Sunflower seeds
  Pan-Roasted Sunflower Seeds with Dill, 234
  Sweet Potato Salad, 94
Sweet potatoes
  Pork and Sweet Potato Skillet, 161
  Sweet Potato Salad, 94
Syndrome X. *See* Metabolic syndrome

Tacos
  Pan-Seared Shrimp Tacos, **142**, 143
Tahini
  Creamy Sesame Greens, 218
  Mediterranean Chicken Kebabs with Lemon-Tahini Sauce, 120, **121**
  Seared Portobello "Steaks," 110
  Thai Butterfly Pasta Salad, 90
Tamale
  Fast Tamale Casserole, 198
Tapenade
  Caramelized Onion and Swiss Burgers, 51, 128, **129**
  Chickpea Ragu with Polenta, 141
  English Muffin Pizzas, 242
  Green Beans with Tapenade, 228
  Grilled Shrimp and Tapenade Pita, 132
  primer on, 51–52
  Vegetable Frittata, 67, 79
Tart
  Mango Tart with Macadamia Crust, 169, 277
Tilapia
  Grilled Tilapia with Balsamic Vinaigrette, 118
Tofu
  Cashew, Tofu, and Broccoli Stir-Fry, **138**, 139
  Grilled Tofu Cutlets, 111
  Vegetarian Lasagna with Tofu, **174**, 175
Tomatoes
  Grilled Chicken Breasts with Pan-Roasted Tomatoes and Olives, 119
  Grilled Tomato and Cheese, 84, **85**
  Italian Vegetable Spiedini, 106
  Middle Eastern Chopped Salad, 96, **97**, 103
  Penne with Cherry Tomatoes, 140
  Tomato and Roasted Pepper Bruschetta, 236, **237**
  Tomato-Olive Salad, 203
  Vegetable Frittata, 67, 79
Tortilla chips
  Chicken Tortilla Casserole, 189
  Super-Fast Chips and Dip, 252
Tostadas
  Grilled Shrimp and Zucchini Tostadas, 114
Trail mix
  Sugar-Glazed Almond Trail Mix, 249
Trans fats, 7, 7, 8
Triglycerides, 5, 10, 11, 12, 12
Tuna
  Sesame-Crusted Tuna Steaks, 148
  Sicilian Tuna Salad, 214
  Tuna Noodle Casserole, 180
  Tuna Rotini Salad Toss, 92, **93**
Turkey
  Barbecue Turkey Burgers with Avocado Mash, 123
  Grilled Turkey and Bok Choy with Chile-Garlic Sauce, **124**, 125
  Turkey, Avocado, and Cheddar Panini, 87
  Turkey on Rye, 102
  Turkey Pot Pies, **190**, 191

Vegetables. *See also specific vegetables*
  cooking methods for, 50
  in Family Snack Pack Guide, 287
  Italian Vegetable Spiedini, 106
  raw, 50
  Vegetable Frittata, 67, 79
Vitamin absorption, good fats for, 8
Vitamin D, for seniors, 30
Vitamin E, for children, 31

Waffles
  Waffle Warm-Up, 78
Walnut oil
  Apricot-Peach Smoothie, 60
  Fall Fruit Salad, 208
  Grilled Tofu Cutlets, 111
Walnuts
  Apples with Honey-Yogurt Dip and Candied Walnuts, 244
  Banana Split Muffins, 75
  Banana-Walnut Cake, 272
  Butternut Squash Ravioli, 136
  Corn and Potato Chowder, 172
  Curried Waldorf Salad, 98
  Honey-Walnut Oatmeal, 78
  Pan-Seared Chicken Breasts with Walnuts and Apples, 149
  Roasted Beet Salad, 206, **207**
  Stovetop Meat Loaf with Mushroom Gravy, 33, 166
  Tandoori Chicken Thighs, 122
  Walnut Chicken, 198
  Walnut-Pear Pancake with Maple Syrup, 72
Watching the "Big Game" Menu, 199
Water
  Sassy Water, 17
Weekend Brunch Menu, 79, 169
Weight loss
  from Flat Belly Diet, 2
  pointers for, 37–39
  meal plan for, 288
  MUFAs for, 13–14
Wheat crackers
  Chicken Salad with Wheat Crackers, 91
Whole foods, 25
Wraps
  Basic Banana Wrap, 78
  Chicken and Creamy Pepper Jelly Wrap, 86
  Olive Spread Wrap, 102
  Peanut Butter–Strawberry Wrap, 82, **83**
  Super-Quick Breakfast Wraps, 78

Yellow squash
  Italian Vegetable Spiedini, 106
Yogurt
  Apples with Honey-Yogurt Dip and Candied Walnuts, 244
  Avocado Ice Cream, 280
  Greek Shake, 78

Zucchini
  Dark Chocolate Zucchini Bread, 33, 229, 269
  Grilled Shrimp and Zucchini Tostadas, 114
  Grilled Zucchini Boats, 107
  Pasta Salad with Caramelized Onions and Zucchini, 212
  Vegetable Frittata, 67, 79

CONVERSION CHART

These equivalents have been slightly rounded to make measuring easier.

VOLUME MEASUREMENTS		
U.S.	IMPERIAL	METRIC
¼ tsp	–	1 ml
½ tsp	–	2 ml
1 tsp	–	5 ml
1 Tbsp	–	15 ml
2 Tbsp (1 oz)	1 fl oz	30 ml
¼ cup (2 oz)	2 fl oz	60 ml
⅓ cup (3 oz)	3 fl oz	80 ml
½ cup (4 oz)	4 fl oz	120 ml
⅔ cup (5 oz)	5 fl oz	160 ml
¾ cup (6 oz)	6 fl oz	180 ml
1 cup (8 oz)	8 fl oz	240 ml

WEIGHT MEASUREMENTS	
U.S.	METRIC
1 oz	30 g
2 oz	60 g
4 oz (¼ lb)	115 g
5 oz (⅓ lb)	145 g
6 oz	170 g
7 oz	200 g
8 oz (½ lb)	230 g
10 oz	285 g
12 oz (¾ lb)	340 g
14 oz	400 g
16 oz (1 lb)	455 g
2.2 lb	1 kg

LENGTH MEASUREMENTS	
U.S.	METRIC
¼"	0.6 cm
½"	1.25 cm
1"	2.5 cm
2"	5 cm
4"	11 cm
6"	15 cm
8"	20 cm
10"	25 cm
12" (1')	30 cm
2.2 lb 1kg	

PAN SIZES	
U.S.	METRIC
8" cake pan	20 × 4 cm sandwich or cake tin
9" cake pan	23 × 3.5 cm sandwich or cake tin
11" × 7" baking pan	28 × 18 cm baking tin
13" × 9" baking pan	32.5 × 23 cm baking tin
15" × 10" baking pan	38 × 25.5 cm baking tin
	(Swiss roll tin)
1½ qt baking dish	1.5 liter baking dish
2 qt baking dish	2 liter baking dish
2 qt rectangular baking dish	30 × 19 cm baking dish
9" pie plate	22 × 4 or 23 × 4 cm pie plate
7" or 8" springform pan	18 or 20 cm springform or
	loose-bottom cake tin
9" × 5" loaf pan	23 × 13 cm or 2 lb narrow
	loaf tin or pâté tin

TEMPERATURES		
FAHRENHEIT	CENTIGRADE	GAS
140°	60°	–
160°	70°	–
180°	80°	–
225°	105°	¼
250°	120°	½
275°	135°	1
300°	150°	2
325°	160°	3
350°	180°	4
375°	190°	5
400°	200°	6
425°	220°	7
450°	230°	8
475°	245°	9
500°	260°	–

The hottest diet in America!

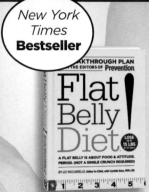
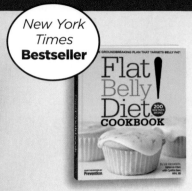
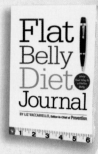
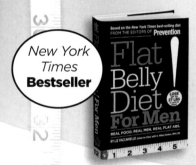
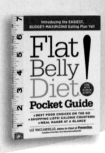
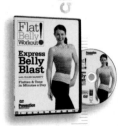
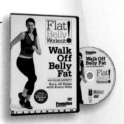